MAYO CLINIC

ON

ALZHEIMER'S DISEASE

and other dementias

MAYO CLINIC PRESS

MAYO CLINIC

Medical Editors
Jonathan Graff-Radford, M.D.
Angela M. Lunde, M.A.

Editorial Director
Paula M. Marlow Limbeck

Senior Editor
Karen R. Wallevand

Managing Editor
Stephanie K. Vaughan

Senior Product Manager
Daniel J. Harke

Art Director
Stewart J. Koski

Illustration, Photography and Production
Joanna R. King, Jamie Klemmensen,
Kent Mc Daniel, Gunnar T. Soroos

Editorial Research Librarians
Abbie Y. Brown, Edward (Eddy) S. Morrow Jr.,
Erika A. Riggin, Katherine (Katie) J. Warner

Copy Editors
Miranda M. Attlesey, Alison K. Baker,
Nancy J. Jacoby, Julie M. Maas

Indexer
Steve Rath

Contributors
Rachel A. Haring Bartony; Bradley F. Boeve, M.D.; Hugo Botha, M.B., Ch.B.; Guojun Bu, Ph.D.; Richard J. Caselli, M.D.; Tanis J. Ferman, Ph.D.; Neill R. Graff-Radford, M.D.; Sherrie M. Hanna, M.A., L.P.; Clifford R. Jack, M.D.; David T. Jones, M.D.; David S. Knopman, M.D.; Heather L. LaBruna; James F. Meschia, M.D.; Ronald C. Petersen, M.D., Ph.D.; Maisha T. Robinson, M.D.; Nikki H. Stricker, Ph.D., L.P.; Nilufer Taner, M.D., Ph.D.; Philip W. Tipton, M.D.; Ericka E. Tung, M.D., M.P.H.; Rene L. Utianski, Ph.D.; Prashanthi Vemuri, Ph.D.; Laura M. Waxman; Jenny Whitwell, Ph.D.; Bryan K. Woodruff, M.D.

Published by Mayo Clinic Press

Our heartfelt gratitude goes to all of the people living with dementia and their care partners who continue to help us understand the lived experience of Alzheimer's disease and related dementias. We extend a very special thank you to the team of people living with dementia and care partners who contributed input and guidance to this book's themes and content.

For bulk sales to employers, member groups and health-related companies, contact Mayo Clinic, 200 First St. SW, Rochester, MN 55905, call 800-430-9699, or send an email to *SpecialSalesMayoBooks@mayo.edu.*

Library of Congress Control Number: 2020934205

ISBN 978-1-893005-61-7

Printed in the United States of America

Contents

Letter from the editors

It's an exciting time in the field of Alzheimer's disease and other dementias. Significant progress has been made in the ability to diagnose dementia and detect Alzheimer's disease before symptoms develop. An early and accurate diagnosis offers a better understanding of how a person's illness will evolve.

Researchers have also discovered that dementia often has more than one cause, even though Alzheimer's disease is most common. This means that effective future treatment will be tailored to an individual.

Researchers are working diligently to develop therapies and, hopefully, prevent these diseases entirely. They understand the relationship between brain health and lifestyle behaviors, such as diet and exercise, much better than they have in the past. These are some of the reasons that there's hope in the world of dementia research.

As researchers work to develop new therapies, additional challenges must be addressed: reducing the stigma surrounding dementia and expanding care and support for those affected by dementia. These are urgent issues that require attention.

In *Mayo Clinic on Alzheimer's Disease and Other Dementias*, you'll gain an understanding of dementia based on what researchers and other medical experts know about it today. You'll also learn that dementia isn't just about loss and decline. For many, a good quality of life can — and does — continue.

Jonathan Graff-Radford, M.D.
Angela M. Lunde, M.A.
Medical Editors

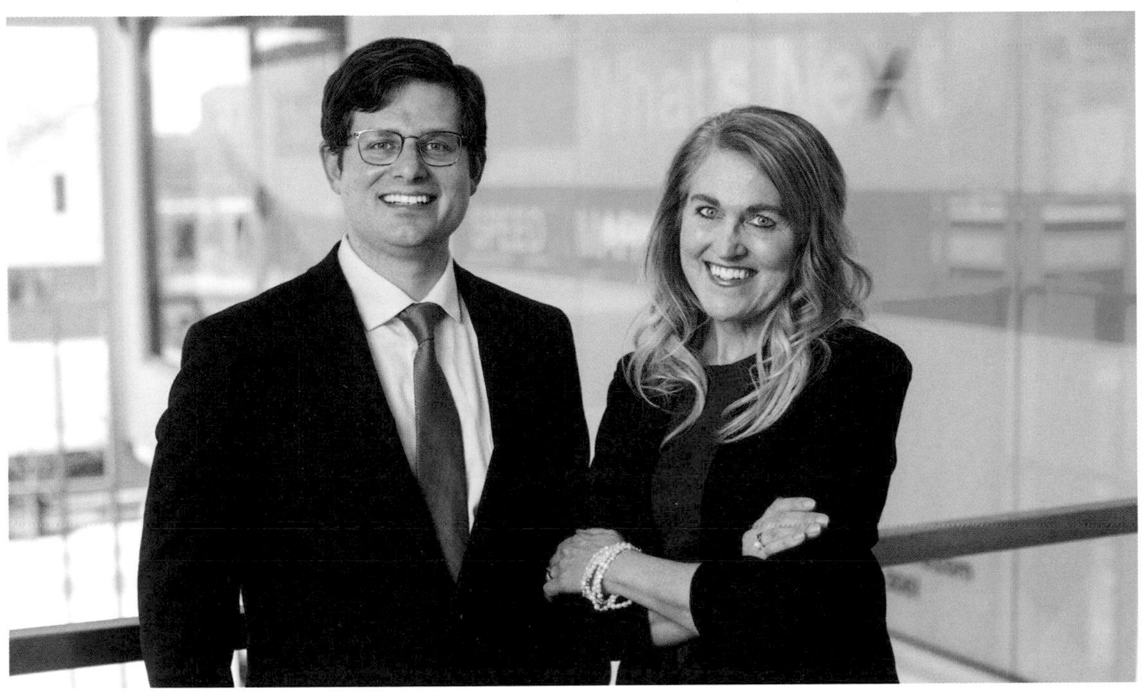

Jonathan Graff-Radford, M.D., is a behavioral neurologist at Mayo Clinic in Rochester, Minn., where he evaluates and treats patients with cognitive disorders, including dementia. An associate professor of neurology at Mayo Clinic College of Medicine and Science, Dr. Graff-Radford also serves as a co-investigator in the Mayo Clinic Alzheimer's Disease Research Center and the Mayo Clinic Study of Aging. Dr. Graff-Radford has published more than 100 articles and written chapters for books on cognition, Alzheimer's disease and related dementias. He was awarded the Paul B. Beeson Emerging Leaders Career Development Award in Aging for his research. During his training at Mayo Clinic, Dr. Graff-Radford received the Woltman Award for Excellence in Clinical Neurology and the Mayo Brothers Distinguished Fellowship Award.

Angela M. Lunde, M.A., has worked in dementia care for nearly 20 years. She is a co-investigator of the Outreach, Recruitment and Education Core in the Mayo Clinic Alzheimer's Disease Research Center, where she focuses on the emotional well-being and quality of life of those living with dementia and their care partners. Ms. Lunde is involved in state, national and international partnerships focused on reducing stigma, improving well-being, and supporting the inclusion and voice of people living with dementia. Awarded the recognition of associate in Mayo Clinic's Department of Neurology in 2012, Ms. Lunde has helped create innovative programs aimed at helping people affected by dementia live well. She has co-authored numerous articles, written several book chapters, and maintained an expert blog on dementia caregiving for more than a decade.

PREFACE

The lived experience

MIKE'S STORY: DEMENTIA AT AGE 52

The first warning signs started at work.

Tasks that would have taken me minutes to complete were taking longer and longer, and I was asking for help, often from people I had helped train. I got lost coming home from work. I always seemed ready for an argument if someone challenged me.

The turning point occurred when I couldn't recall an argument I had with my wife the night before.

She thought I was trying to make believe that it never happened, but when I told her I had no memory of the things I said, we cried and hugged because we knew something was seriously wrong.

At the age of 52, I was diagnosed with young-onset Alzheimer's. Three years later, the diagnosis was changed to Lewy body dementia. I am now 58 years old.

I can still learn new things, I can still do the things I enjoy doing, and most importantly, I still have a voice — and I plan on using that voice for as long as I can. One way I can do this is by dispelling some common myths about dementia.

Myth: People with dementia can no longer contribute in a meaningful way

The first thing I did when I retired from my career in telecommunications was to walk into my local senior center and ask if they had anyone helping them with computer and technology issues. They didn't, so I volunteered, and we started a group.

Myth: People with dementia can no longer learn new things

Since I retired, I've learned that I love to cook. For obvious reasons, I'm not allowed to use the stove when my wife isn't home, so we do it together. When needed, my wife helps me get through the recipe, but I'm involved in making the meal. The satisfaction I get from doing that makes me feel like I'm still contributing to my family.

I've also found a passion and talent for watercolor painting. I've always been able to draw pretty well, but painting always intimidated me for some reason. I took a painting class at the senior center. I fell in love with watercolor.

Myth: People with dementia are care *receivers* or *takers* and not care *givers*

This past March, my daughter told me that our granddaughter's favorite animal is a giraffe. Her birthday was coming up, so I painted her a giraffe for her eighth birthday.

I then quickly learned that you can't paint something for one grandchild and not paint something for the others. That led to paintings for each of our grandchildren.

This past April, I lost a very dear friend to dementia. I had never drawn a portrait of someone, let alone paint one. But I felt I needed to do this. I think it was therapy for me, but it was also a way to honor my friend Steve. That led me to paint six portraits of people who have passed away from a form of dementia, all for people I have known or their care partners. I've been posting these paintings online, which has also led to requests from friends.

Drawing and painting help relax me, especially when my anxiety is kicking in and I am very agitated. Painting helps me find fulfillment, helps me relax, and lets me contribute to others.

Myth: People with dementia are all the same

Anticipating what the future holds for me, I'm thinking about making a video of myself — a video that gives a clear picture of the real me. Who I am as a person, what my likes and dislikes are, what gives me passion, makes me tick.

My plan is that if I move into a care setting, everyone who cares for me needs to watch the video first to know the real me. This would also help them understand that if I'm agitated or upset, something must be bothering me, and it's their job to know me and to support my needs. I don't want people to settle for keeping me busy, for distracting me or entertaining me.

People who have been given this diagnosis can still contribute, learn and live a meaningful life. They also still have a voice even if they can't communicate in the ways they could before.

Please remember that dementia is a disease, not a personality trait.

FINDING HOPE IN DEMENTIA

Mike's story on the preceding pages offers one view into what it's like to live with dementia. When you've met one person living with dementia, it means just that — that you've met one person living with dementia. Everyone's experience with dementia is unique. If you're living with dementia, your experience will be different from Mike's in many ways, but in some ways, it may be similar.

The same can be said for the care partner experience. If you've met one care partner, you've gotten a glimpse into that care partner's life. Each care partner navigates this role in a different way, yet shares in the uncertainty of this unrequested role.

If you're living with dementia or providing support as a care partner, how do you move forward with this new reality? Can you feel hope again? Finding hope in the experience of a progressive disease may seem illogical and even insensitive to some.

However, Mike and care partners like Rosalie, whom you'll read about later in this book, would say that feeling hope alongside dementia is, indeed, possible.

In sharing their experiences, Mike and Rosalie demonstrate that when one hope fades, it's possible to infuse new hope into your life. Mike and Rosalie also offer the message that not all hope is the same; there's hope for things we can't control and hope for things we can.

Mike finds hope through what he can do — his new roles, hobbies and creative ways of adapting day to day. He finds hope through sharing his message that life goes on after a dementia diagnosis, and that people with dementia can still contribute in meaningful ways. Mike also has hope that as his disease progresses, those who care for and support him will get to know who he truly is — a whole person who feels emotions and who has likes, dislikes and a desire to engage meaningfully with life. He hopes for comfort, dignity, continued friendship and love.

Likewise, Rosalie and care partners like her will each define hope in their own way. Hope for care partners will likely change over time. For some, hope will be found in strengths that emerge in the caregiving role, including patience, resilience, and even humor and gratitude — qualities care partners may not know they had.

For people with dementia and care partners alike, hope is sometimes felt by supporting and mentoring others who are experiencing similar pain, or by advocating for human rights, laws or research funding.

Hope is a psychosocial and spiritual resource that offers up the possibility of joy alongside challenges. It becomes a source of inner strength.

A call to action

We each play a role in making sure that people living with dementia feel understood and respected, and are given opportunities to thrive. Worldwide, communities are taking action toward becoming more inclusive and dementia-friendly.

Whether or not your life is directly affected by dementia, you can help your community become:

- A place where people living with dementia, care partners and families feel supported and receive timely information and access to the services and resources available to them
- A place where those affected by dementia feel respected and understood, and where they're valued as contributing members of the community
- A place where every individual, business and organization receives education to increase awareness and understanding that translates into making a positive difference in the lives of the people with dementia they know and serve
- A place that offers people living with dementia and their families ways to stay engaged and connected through programs, clubs, experiences and the arts

This book is a resource that can help you learn everything you can about dementia. You may not read it from cover to cover in one sitting. Instead, you may read the portions of it that are relevant to you. As things change, you may find other sections more valuable or worth returning to.

Everyone plays an important role in learning about dementia, and this book is a good tool to do just that. However, the best learning and understanding comes from the real experts — people living with dementia and their care partners. May we stand by them, listen to them, and see them as the whole people they are, today and every day.

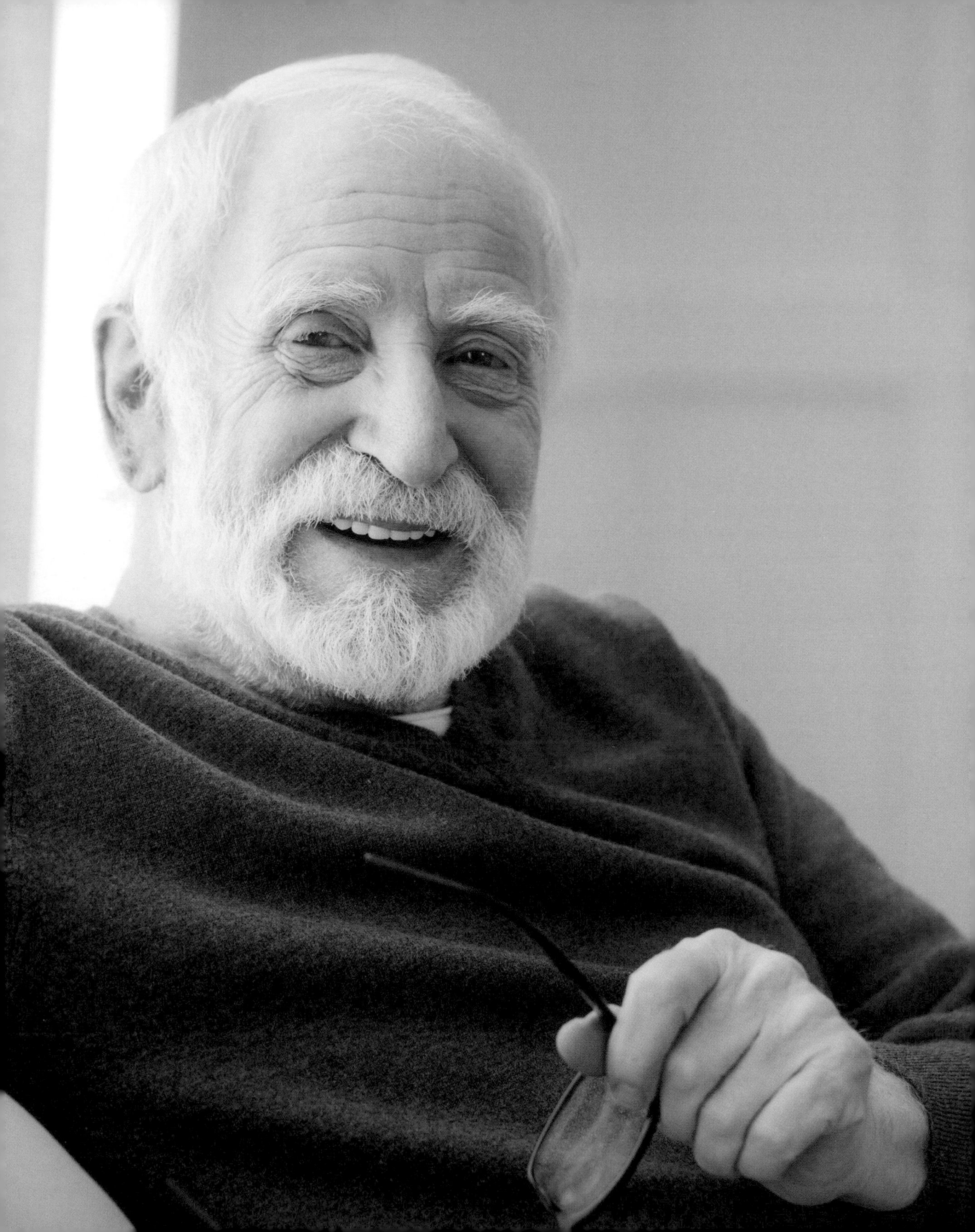

PART 1

Typical aging vs. dementia

People are living longer now than they ever have. In 2015, fewer than 1 in 10 people in the world was over the age of 65. By 2050, this number is expected to almost double. Since dementia is an age-related disease, the number of people living with dementia is expected to increase in the coming years. By some estimates, the number of people living with dementia could triple by 2050.

This makes the topic of healthy aging more critical than ever before.

Many of the strategies for living well as you age are ones you've likely heard many times. Getting regular physical activity, following a healthy diet, not smoking, managing stress and getting good-quality sleep are all ingredients for a long and healthy life.

But what about effective strategies for aging that are specific to brain health? Are there ways you can lower your risk of dementia? Can dementia be prevented entirely? If you have dementia, what can be done to treat it or slow its progression? Can you live well with dementia? If so, how?

These are important questions that scientists and researchers are seeking to answer, and in this book, you'll discover what they know currently.

In Part 1, you'll learn what's typical in aging — and what's not. You'll also get a brief introduction to the parts of the brain specific to memory and what dementia looks like. Part 1 closes with chapters that define dementia and outline steps that are commonly taken to tell if someone has dementia.

“WHILE IT’S POSSIBLE THAT ANY OLDER ADULT CAN DEVELOP A FORM OF DEMENTIA, DEMENTIA SHOULDN’T BE CONSIDERED A NORMAL PART OF AGING.”

CHAPTER 1

What's typical and what's not

No matter how healthy and injury-free you've kept yourself, the wear and tear that comes with age takes a toll on the body. You may start seeing changes as early as your 30s and 40s, when it's a little bit harder to bounce back from a cold or run as quickly as you used to.

Some of the physical changes of aging are easy to see, like graying or thinning hair. Your skin may wrinkle and sag as it becomes thinner, drier and less elastic. Age spots may appear, and your skin may bruise more easily.

Other physical changes may not be as easy to spot, at least at first. As you age, your eyes and mouth may start to feel drier. Vigorous exercise gets harder because your lungs can't take in as much air when you breathe. The walls of your bladder often become less elastic, making more-frequent bathroom trips necessary.

Some age-related changes are so subtle that you may not notice them until they're well established. Your digestive system naturally slows down, so you may have bouts of constipation more often. Your immune system doesn't work as well, so you may get sick more often. Kidney function declines, so it's easier to get dehydrated or retain fluid.

These are all typical changes that come with aging — changes that many people learn to adapt to in everyday life.

YOUR BRAIN AND TYPICAL AGING

As with other parts of your body, the brain undergoes changes with age. Weighing in at about 3 pounds, your brain is the most complex organ in your body — a master computer that controls actions you give thought to, like balancing your checkbook. It also manages actions you *don't* think about, like swallowing food or blinking.

When it's healthy, your brain keeps track of all your body's functions and actions. It stores your instincts and memories. It allows you to make decisions and be creative. It organizes and shapes emotions. And maybe most miraculously, the brain allows you to do all of these things at the same time.

Consider something as simple as reading. As you take in the meaning of each word, you're also likely holding a book or tablet upright, adjusting the distance from your eyes, and turning pages when you need to. You're studying what you read, recalling information you already know, and responding emotionally to the text.

At the same time, you're probably processing sounds and sensations from the environment around you. You might be doing other things at the same time, too, like keeping an eye on the clock or sipping from your coffee cup.

Your brain controls all of these actions. And while all of this is happening, your brain is managing vital functions that aren't directly related to what you're doing in the moment. It's making sure you're breathing, digesting food, and doing other things that are necessary for life.

The brain and memory

Your brain is made up of several structures that perform a variety of tasks. The structures in your brain work together to help you perform a cognitive function, like remembering something. These brain structures, working in concert with each other, may be located near or far away from each other in the brain.

The parts of the brain that work together to perform cognitive functions like thinking, learning and remembering are called a brain network. The parts of the brain linked most closely to memory are the cerebrum and the limbic system. Here's a little more on each.

Cerebrum The cerebrum is likely the one you're most familiar with. It's the largest part of the brain, and it rests on top of the brainstem. The cerebrum shapes who you are as a person.

A deep groove separates the cerebrum into left and right hemispheres. The hemispheres are connected by a thick band of fibers called the corpus callosum.

Each hemisphere has four lobes, as you'll see on the next page. Each lobe handles different functions. The temporal lobe, for example, is vital for memory. It sits at the side of your forehead, near your temple.

Limbic system The limbic system holds several small structures inside your brain. The limbic system processes the millions of messages bombarding your brain, both from within your body and from the outside environment. The limbic system is where you'll find the hippocampus (hip-o-KAM-pus). This is the central switchboard for your memory system.

The hippocampus sorts pieces of information, stores them in different parts of your brain and recalls them when you need them. It also moves information between your recent and remote memory. It helps you recall everything, from where you put your car keys this morning to the resort town you visited 20 summers ago.

In a healthy brain, all of the structures work together efficiently. They're protected by your skull and cushioned by layers of membrane. A network of blood vessels helps the brain survive and function.

Cognitive changes with typical aging

Many people begin to notice subtle changes in how well they remember, learn and make decisions. Their minds may not seem as nimble and sharp. These changes develop gradually and inconsistently in people in

STRUCTURES OF THE BRAIN

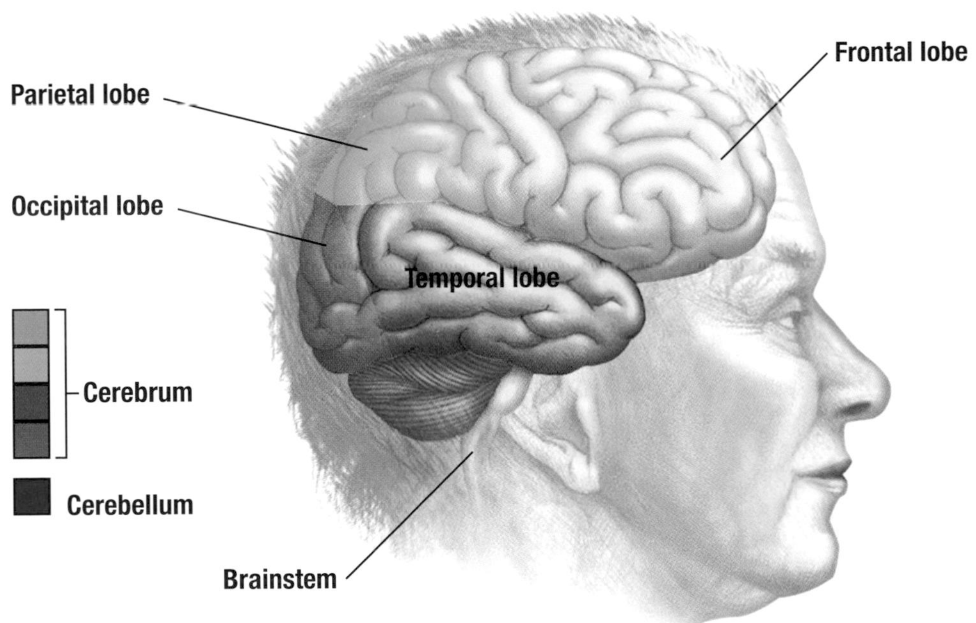

The cerebrum is divided into left and right hemispheres. Each hemisphere is divided into four sections (lobes). The lobes are separated from each other by surface grooves and connective tissue and by shape. The temporal lobe is vital for memory.

their 50s and 60s. Although you may find it unsettling to know that these changes can happen, the reality may be a little less foreboding than you think.

It's true that as you age, the number of neurons in your brain decreases. This means there will be less communication between your brain and the rest of your body. As this happens, you brain may shrink (atrophy). But with billions of neurons and trillions of connections between them, your brain's capacity far exceeds what you'll probably ever need in your lifetime. Even better, living neurons continue to make new connections, replacing at least some of the ones that are lost.

Nevertheless, neuron loss from aging will affect how well you think and learn to some extent. Here's more on the main changes in thinking that typically happen with age.

Processing speed How quickly you can process information and provide a response, like making a movement or giving an answer to a question, slows down with age. According to some estimates, an older adult's response time is about 1½ times slower than that of younger adults.

This means you may need more time to solve a complex problem than you did in your 30s, for example. Or you may need a little more time and a bit more instruction to master new skills. But when given enough time, older adults are able to come up with accurate, effective solutions that are equal to those of younger adults.

Memory Memory is a broad term that describes the ability to remember information.

With typical aging, older adults are generally good at retaining information and memories that they've previously acquired, like details about a family wedding or a child's graduation. It may just take longer to retrieve this information. The ability to perform well-learned procedures like riding a bike remains stable. This is an example of procedural memory, which you'll learn about on page 25.

Where older adults are likely to notice changes is in working memory. This is the ability to temporarily hold on to information, like hearing a new phone number and then remembering it long enough to dial it. Recent memory and the formation of new memories, however, are more vulnerable to aging.

Attention Attention is the ability to focus on something in order to process information. Simple or focused attention, like being able to watch and pay attention to a TV program, tends to be preserved in older age. But it's usually harder to do things that divide attention, like watching TV and talking on the phone at the same time. The brain can process only so much information at one time. With age, it's easier to lose focus. However, aging doesn't seem to affect the ability to focus on simple tasks as much.

Language Language skills describe how well you can understand and use language, whether it's written or spoken.

FUNCTIONAL AREAS OF THE BRAIN

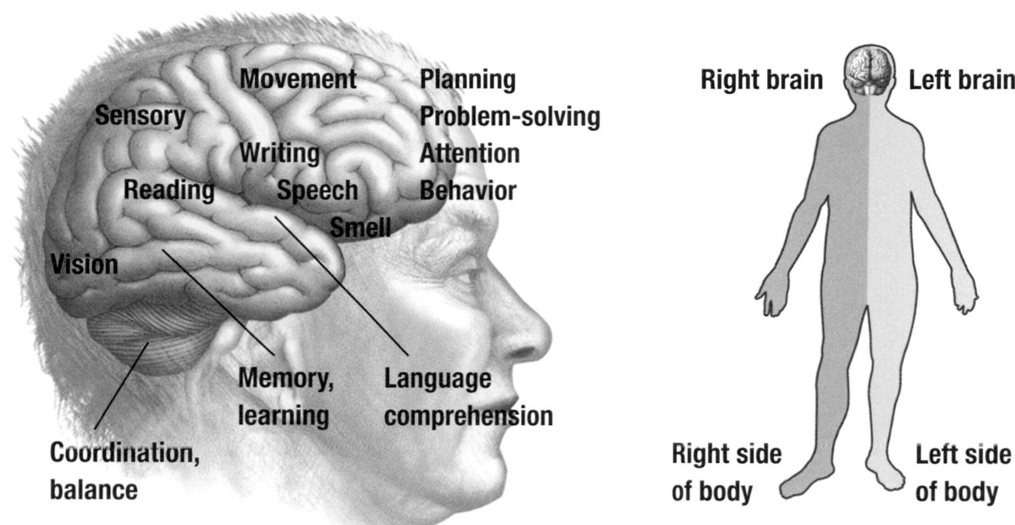

Functions like thinking, analyzing, remembering and speaking, as well as the processing of sensations, are associated with specific lobes of the brain. For example, vital structures of the brain for memory are located in the temporal lobe. Parts of the memory network are located in other lobes, too. Each side (hemisphere) of the cerebrum interacts with one half of the body, but the connections are crossed — the right hemisphere is connected to the left side of the body and the left hemisphere is connected to the right side.

With typical aging, older adults retain their vocabulary and their ability to understand written language. But understanding speech can get harder with age, especially in someone with hearing problems. It may take more time to find or retrieve a word, and spelling familiar words may become more difficult. But using a rich vocabulary and saying what you mean can actually improve with each passing year.

Executive function Executive function is a term that describes your mental agility. It includes the complex processes and abilities that make it possible for you to organize tasks, remember details, think abstractly, manage time and solve problems. These skills generally decline with age.

This doesn't mean that these skills aren't possible when you're older; they may just take you longer than they did when you were younger.

Emotional processing This is your ability to regulate your emotions so that you can respond appropriately, especially in negative situations. Research shows that older

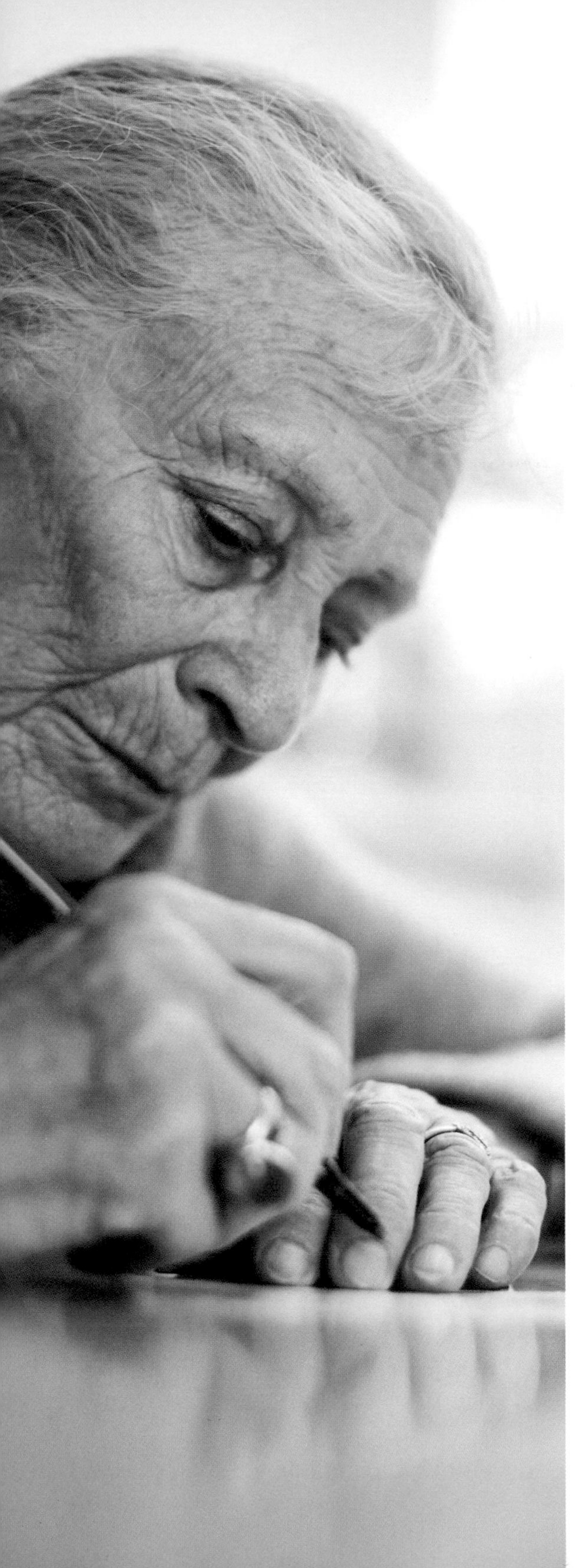

adults generally tend to react less to and recover more easily from negative situations. Older adults also focus on and remember more positive than negative information.

As you think about the cognitive changes that come with aging, the most important point to keep in mind is that while many thinking functions are affected by the process of aging, others are barely touched. Typical aging doesn't mean your cognitive skills will all decline. Many are preserved, and some may even improve over time.

Making memories

Occasional memory lapses are often a part of typical aging. They can trigger worry, anxiety and sometimes outright panic in older adults because memory loss is one of the earliest signs of dementia due to Alzheimer's disease.

Memory is how well you store, recall and reuse information. You may imagine your brain as a library filled with rooms of shelved books — or, in this case, memories just waiting to be checked out.

But this is only half true. Unlike a library's shelved books, your brain doesn't store an entire memory in a single place. Instead, the part of your brain called the hippocampus breaks memories down into pieces — like how an object looks, smells, sounds and feels. Then it stores these pieces in different parts of your brain.

For example, the melody of one of your favorite songs may be stored in your temporal lobes. These areas of your brain allow you to interpret sounds. What you know of the lyrics, on the other hand, may be stored in your frontal lobe. And then there may be emotions you associate with the song or information about the singer. This information may be stored in other parts of your brain.

Whenever you hear the melody on the radio, your brain goes to work, reassembling a single memory from many different loca-

NEURONS: YOUR BRAIN'S MESSENGERS

Nerve cells (neurons) are the basic units of your nervous system. In your brain alone, you have about 100 billion of them. Neurons collect and process messages by way of electric impulses and send information to other neurons. This is how your brain talks to other parts of your body.

Here's a little more about how neurons work. Thousands of neurons form pathways that let messages flow throughout the body. For one neuron to send a message, something must spur it into action. A neuron may relay an impulse to another neuron. Or something outside the body, like the pain of a paper cut or the smell of morning coffee, may cause a neuron to fire off an impulse. From there, the impulse travels like a wave and triggers the release of chemicals. All of this happens so that messages can travel from neuron to neuron and on to other parts of your body, like your brain.

Think of this as a version of the telephone game you may have played as a child. One child whispers a message into the ear of the child sitting beside him or her, who turns to whisper the message into the next child's ear, and so on, until an entire line of children has received the message — and can act on it together. In your brain and nervous system, this process happens at lightning speed and with far greater precision.

Dementia is caused by damage to or loss of nerve cells and their connections in the brain. You'll learn more about neurons as you continue to read this book.

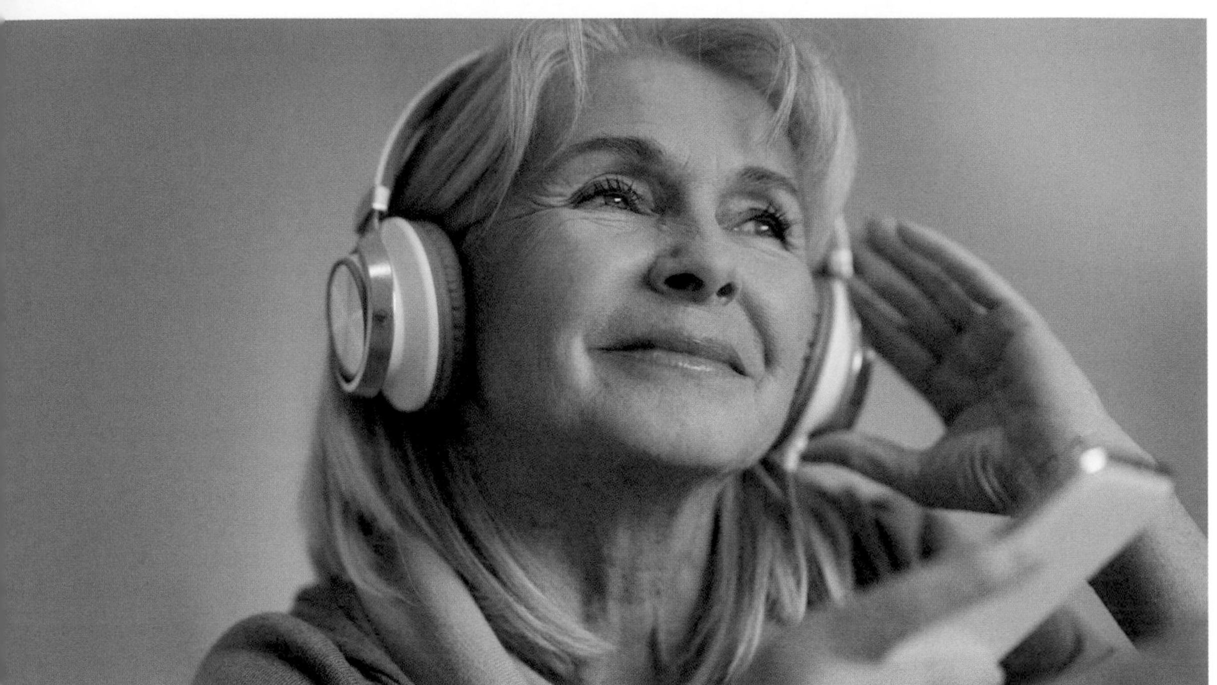

tions and — there you have it — you recognize the song and can sing along.

Different types of memory The memories stored in your brain are broken down into different categories. Later, you'll learn that different types of dementia target different types of memory. For now, learn about the main types of memory on the next page.

Your working memory lets you hold onto a small piece of information, like a phone number, for a short amount of time. Then the information is either discarded or moved into your long-term memory.

People who say they're having short-term memory problems are often actually describing trouble remembering information minutes to days after learning it — not problems with working memory.

While the transfer of information from your working memory to your longer term memory may sound simple, longer term memory itself is much more complex. Information in your working memory gets stored in your longer term memory. This happens through a process called consolidation. Learning a person's name is an example of how information in your working memory gets moved into your longer term memory. Your brain's longer term memory may store information anywhere from several minutes to a lifetime.

When you learn someone's name, that information forms a pathway in your brain.

Type of memory	How it works	How long information is stored
Episodic memory	This is a type of memory you have to consciously recall. Episodic memory is your memory of experiences and specific events. Your memories may be different from someone else's recollections of the same experiences. Specific details linked to episodic memory often include feelings, time and place. Experts believe that emotion plays a role in how these memories are formed. Examples of episodic memories may include the birth of a child, graduating from high school, your first date with your spouse or a vacation a few years back.	Minutes to years
Semantic memory	This is a type of memory you have to consciously recall. It involves what you know about the world around you. It's a structured record of facts, meanings of words, concepts and knowledge. These memories may have once had a personal context, but now they stand alone as simple knowledge. It includes things like an understanding of math, how objects function, definitions of words, knowledge about specific animals and recalling where a state is located. When older adults say they're having trouble remembering the words for objects and people's names, this is the part of the memory they're often describing.	Minutes to years
Procedural memory	This is the memory of how to do certain things. These memories are often formed early in life, for example, when you learned to tie your shoes and ride a bike, and later on, when you learned to drive a car. These tasks are done over and over and become so ingrained that they are almost automatic and don't require much, if any, conscious thought.	Minutes to years
Working memory	This is your memory for temporarily storing information, so it's readily accessible. Keeping a phone number in your head before dialing it, mentally following a route or rotating an object in your mind are examples.	Seconds to minutes; information is actively rehearsed or manipulated

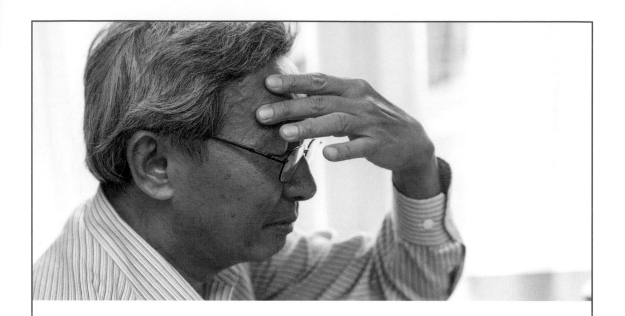

A NOTE ON THE TERM SHORT-TERM MEMORY

In common conversation, the term ***short-term memory*** can refer to both working memory and recent memory, so it sometimes leads to confusion. Often, people say they're having trouble with their short-term memory because they're forgetting information they've recently learned, also known as recent memory. Given this possible confusion, the term short-term memory is avoided in this book.

To become a longer term memory, the pathway must be strengthened. There are many ways this can happen: You may focus on the name when you first learn it, repeat the name afterward, or pair the name with something familiar. Any of these steps may help you remember. Say you just met a new neighbor and remembering names is a challenge for you. Her name is Sydney, so you associate her with Sydney, Australia. The next time you see her, if you don't recall her name, you may think *Australia* and that reminds you that her name is Sydney.

This association helps you recall her name quickly when you see her. In time, her name gets stored in your long-term memory, so you can recall it when you need to.

THE COGNITIVE SPECTRUM

It wasn't long ago that scientists thought there were clear boundaries between cognition that's considered normal versus cognition that's thought of as impaired.

Scientists thought people fell into one of two categories: either they had no disease-related changes in the brain, or they had changes in the brain that led to cognitive impairment.

Over the past 30 years, through the detailed study of normal aging and the development of cognitive impairment, scientists have learned more about how cognitive decline works. They can now identify small changes in mental performance that make it more likely that someone may eventually develop dementia.

Just as important, scientists have learned that changes in the brain can begin long before any signs and symptoms are evident — often, many years before. Put simply, brain health can't be described strictly in terms of "either-or:" It's in either a normal state or an abnormal state. These findings have caused specialists to reconsider their approach.

Experts know now that it may be more accurate to describe a person's cognitive status in terms of a wide, continuous range (spectrum). On one end of the spectrum is normal function, a state in which cognitive skills are intact. At the other end of the spectrum is dementia, a state in which disease has severely disrupted cognitive skills.

Between these extremes are many levels. In these levels, how a person thinks and learns may shift back and forth between normal

WHAT IS COGNITION?

The term *cognition* comes from a Latin word that means "the act of getting to know." It refers to all the processes of the brain that allow you to think and consciously act, to experience what's going on around you, and to feel emotions. These mental processes involve awareness, perception, judgment, reason, learning and memory.

Cognitive processes are in contrast to the many processes that your body undertakes without your thinking of them, such as heartbeat and respiration. You don't have to think in order for those functions to take place.

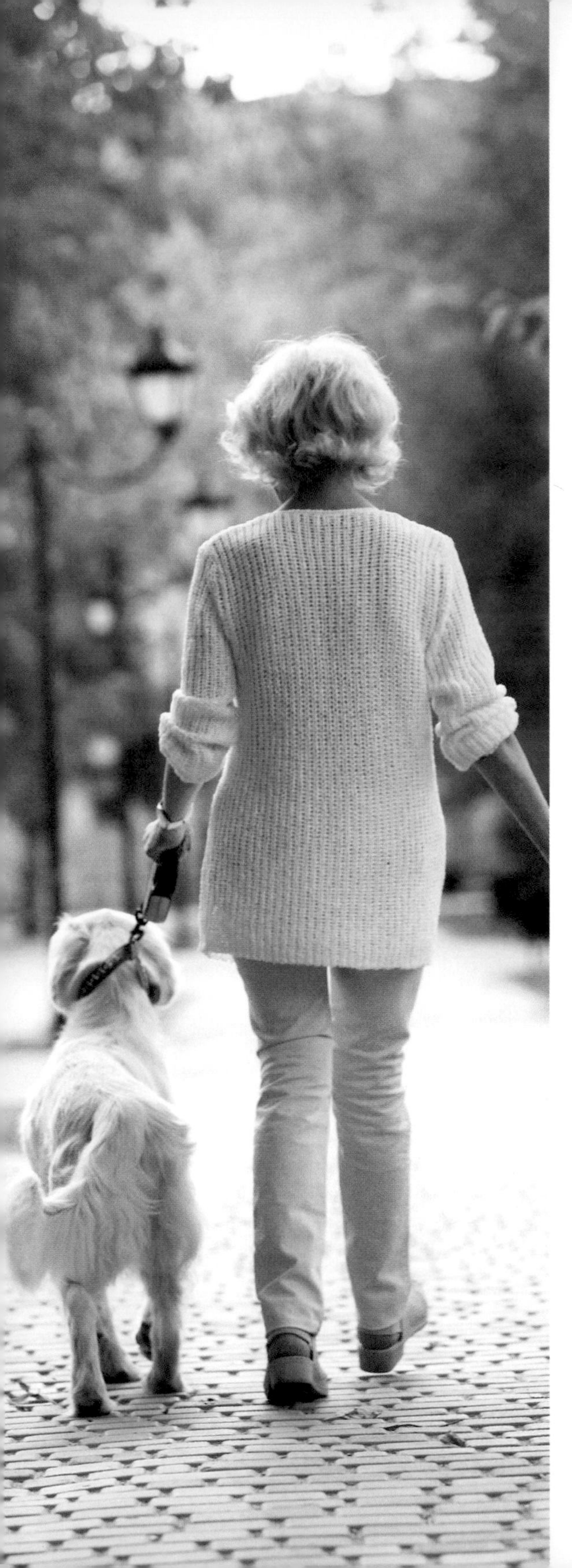

and poor. For example, some people have problems with memory loss, but their difficulties aren't enough to disrupt daily living. Their test results show some cognitive impairment, but they don't meet the criteria for dementia. These people may have mild cognitive impairment, a condition that's not as severe as dementia but of greater concern than the memory changes associated with typical aging. It's somewhere in the middle of the cognitive spectrum.

The line graph on the right illustrates the major role age plays in the cognitive spectrum. As people age, their risk of disorders that affect the brain increases. The disorders that can cause dementia are described in Chapter 3.

The top line on the graph shows typical aging. These are people who experience some degree of cognitive impairment as they get older. Many factors can reduce or disrupt cognition, like disease, injury and trauma, genes, substance abuse, and general wear and tear. In some cases, the cause of cognitive problems may be curable.

A metabolic problem caused by very low vitamin B-12 is an example.

How much cognition is impaired varies. Some people may get a little more forgetful but have no other symptoms. Other people may have trouble coming up with names or occasionally misplace their keys. Regardless of a drop-off in cognitive function, people who age "typically" are still able to function well in everyday life.

A small pool of people, most of whom have been blessed with both good health and good genes, represents what may be optimal aging. These are people who continue to enjoy good cognition as they grow old, including memory, reason, judgment, concentration, analytic skill, decision-making and language use.

The lower line on the graph represents abnormal aging, and with each passing year comes cognitive decline. The decline is often gradual, but it can be sharp.

Finally, the middle line represents a decline in thinking and memory that's more gradual than what's seen in abnormal aging.

AGING AND COGNITIVE CHANGE

This graph illustrates the different paths that cognition may take as people age. The vertical axis shows the cognitive spectrum, with good cognition (typical) at the top of the axis, poor or impaired cognition (abnormal) at the bottom, and a much more gradual decline in the middle. The horizontal axis shows years of age. Cognition levels range across the spectrum.

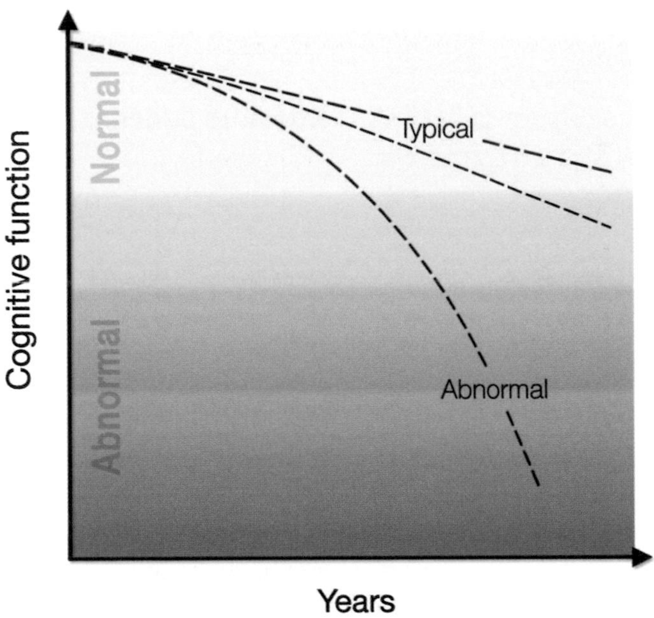

TYPES OF COGNITIVE AND FUNCTIONAL DECLINE

Dementia isn't a specific disease. It's a syndrome that can be caused by many different diseases. It's an umbrella term that refers to thinking (cognitive) symptoms that interfere with a person's ability to function from day to day. Dementia can affect behavior, decision-making, memory, language, visual or spatial skills, and attention. More than one of these areas is usually affected, but one area may be more impaired than another.

What causes dementia? Alzheimer's disease is the primary cause of dementia, but there are other causes of dementia, too, which you'll read about in this book. Each disorder has different characteristics that cause specific symptoms, but each individual's experience will vary.

Here are easy-to-understand explanations of the most common symptoms of dementia. These symptoms are most often associated with dementia due to Alzheimer's disease. See where different functional areas of the brain are located on page 21.

Memory loss and trouble recognizing familiar objects

Memory loss is the most common symptom that leads to a diagnosis of dementia. This common symptom of cognitive decline is marked by an inability to recall past events, either partially or in full. Problems with recent memory are often the earliest and most noticeable signs of this decline. The hippocampus, as you learned earlier, is the memory system of the brain.

Another effect of damage to the brain is the inability to recognize familiar objects. The technical term for this is agnosia. Agnosia often occurs later in the disease than other symptoms of dementia, but in rare instances can be an early symptom. Agnosia means not being able to recognize or identify objects despite being able to see, hear and feel them. Or maybe someone can't identify the shape of a fork at the dinner table. As dementia progresses, agnosia can make it difficult for people to recognize their children or spouses and partners. They may even deny that they have an illness at all. The term for this is anosognosia.

Attention deficit

This is when it's hard to concentrate on words being spoken or on tasks that need to be accomplished. It may cause someone to feel scatterbrained and highly distracted.

Difficulties understanding spatial relationships

Feeling easily disoriented and having a hard time moving about are examples of visuospatial decline. This type of decline in a person can cause problems with judging the height of a step or the distance around an obstacle in his or her path.

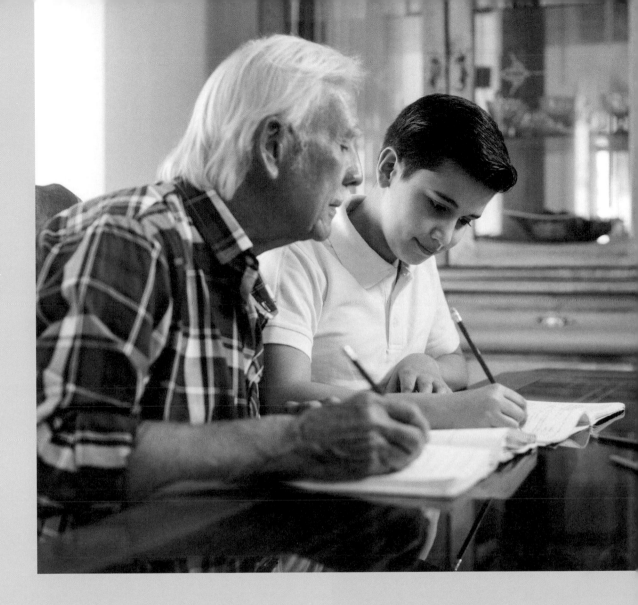

Difficulties managing time and effort

These difficulties may make it hard to organize, prioritize and think abstractly. The term for making decisions and carrying them out is executive functioning. Tasks like managing finances, outlining a report, organizing a family vacation or hosting a dinner party may be too difficult.

Difficulties with language use

Language difficulties may include having a hard time coming up with the names of familiar people, places and objects. In the later stages, speech often doesn't make sense, is repetitive, and is peppered with nonspecific words like *thing* and *it*. It may be hard to understand spoken and written language.

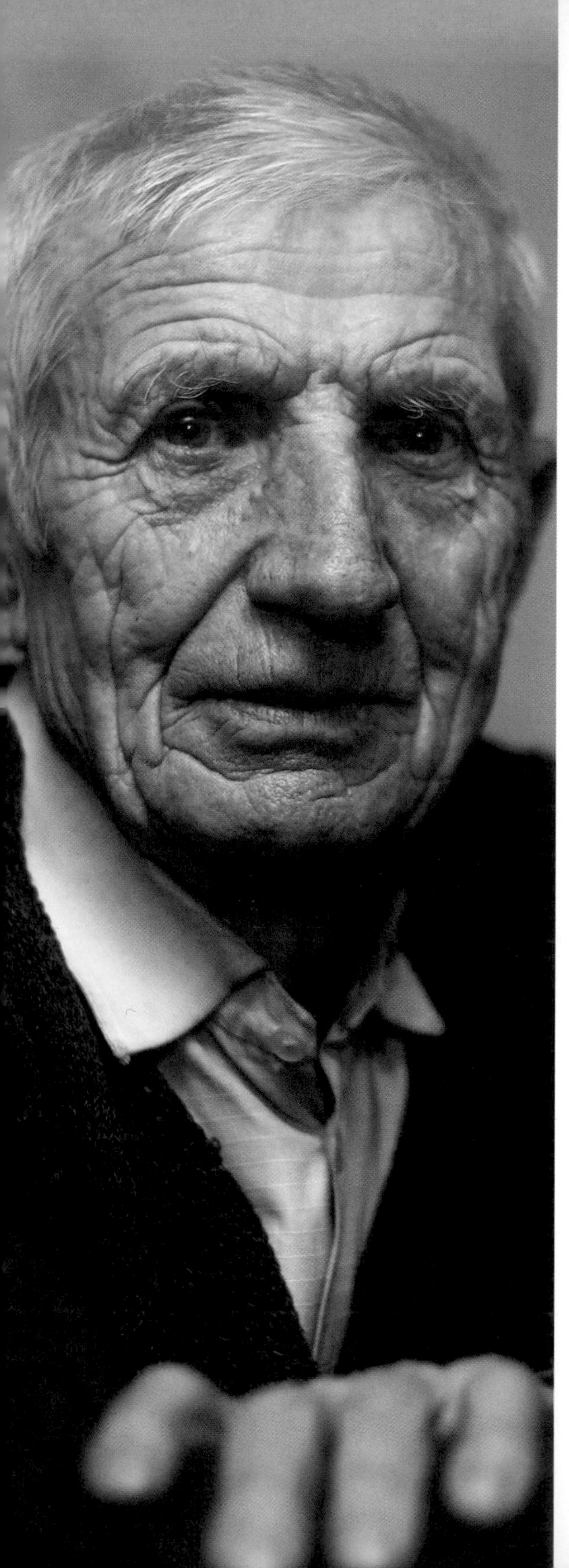

The symptoms of cognitive impairment often develop in people in their 70s or 80s. Many diseases can cause cognitive impairment later in life, but Alzheimer's disease is the most common.

As you'll learn later, researchers now know that the changes that happen in Alzheimer's disease and other types of brain diseases begin many years before the first symptom.

AGING THAT'S NOT TYPICAL

At 75 years old, Frank is proud to say that he's lived in a house for the past 40 years that he built with his own two hands. Though his wife died years ago, he feels like he is doing OK on his own and doesn't ask for a lot of help from family and friends.

For years, Frank liked to tinker in his workshop, fixing cars, lawn mowers, appliances — basically anything with a motor in need of repair. Almost every day, he dropped by a neighborhood diner to drink coffee and talk with other regulars. On weekends, he enjoyed visits from his grandchildren.

Months ago, people began noticing changes in Frank's behavior. Now, he's constantly misplacing keys, tools, glasses, food items and anything else he carries in his hands. Several times, he's started out for the diner, only to become confused about where he was going and try to turn back — but unfortunately, remembering how to get back home also was a struggle for him.

WHAT IS 'TYPICAL'?

When it comes to cognitive functions — thought, perception, memory, problem-solving, decision-making — what age-related changes are typical and what may be cause for concern? You may be surprised to learn that research into the answer to this question is lacking. In part, this is because the answer isn't as straightforward as you may think.

For example, take a woman in her early 90s whose mind is as sharp as a tack. She still lives at home, takes few medications, walks her dog every day and meets regularly with friends. People like this exist. Does "typical" apply to this woman? In terms of the actual number of people who age this way, this may not be typical. Instead, experts refer to this as successful aging or optimal aging — the kind that most people would want to experience.

Typical aging can have many variations. More often than not, aging includes illnesses and conditions like heart disease, decreased bone density, and hearing or vision loss. Many people also think of slight forgetfulness as a common part of aging. The changes that come with aging may be inconvenient and frustrating, but they don't stop you from living an active, independent life.

The challenge in defining what's "typical" lies in telling the difference between elements of typical aging from abnormal changes that may signal dementia and Alzheimer's disease. By being able to spot a disorder in its earliest stages, scientists hope to capture Alzheimer's when it may be most treatable.

At the same time, researchers are looking into the concept of optimal aging and what can be done to promote lifelong health. Both tracks of research may provide valuable insight into how to prevent cognitive decline and treat dementia.

The most important point to remember is that dementia is *not* part of typical aging.

He can't seem to finish projects anymore. And according to one grandchild, Frank says he's recently talked with his wife.

Family members are concerned about these changes, which seem to affect Frank's cognition — his ability to reason, decide and remember. They also notice that Frank seems more depressed, anxious and short-tempered than he used to be. They worry that whatever is causing Frank's problems will only get worse.

What abnormal aging looks like

How well people retain their cognitive skills as they get older varies widely.

While some people begin to struggle with memory lapses in their 50s, other people retain good memory well into their 90s — and their reasoning and judgment stay sharp to boot. The changes that occur don't seem to disrupt everyday life, and cognition remains intact. It's all part of typical aging.

But not all changes that occur later in life are typical. Some people, particularly after age 65, experience a sustained decline in many parts of cognition. They start having trouble processing information, especially when it's new. Memory problems and periods of confusion are frequent. They struggle to think abstractly, concentrate, express ideas clearly and work with numbers. Some may undergo personality changes, have trouble controlling emotions, and become paranoid or withdrawn.

Although these signs and symptoms are often associated with getting older, they aren't part of typical aging. They're signs and symptoms of *abnormal* aging.

Some of Frank's changes are abnormal, and it's unlikely they're solely a result of getting older. Not every older adult experiences the kind or amount of cognitive impairment Frank seems to have.

There's a strong chance that disease-related changes in Frank's brain are causing his symptoms. These changes may have started many years before anyone noticed a difference in his personality and behavior. As the disease progresses, the symptoms may worsen and Frank's cognition will continue to decline.

Right now, Frank seems unaware that a problem exists. He's not concerned because he doesn't see his own failing memory and troubling behavior. But the symptoms are affecting how well he can carry out the tasks of daily living.

Family members are beginning to wonder whether Frank may have a serious medical problem. And they're questioning whether it's still a good idea for Frank to be living alone.

The best action that the family could take would be to schedule a visit for Frank with his doctor or with someone who specializes in cognitive disorders that happen later in life, like a neurologist, geriatrician or geriatric psychiatrist.

COGNITIVE HEALTH: BY THE NUMBERS

Cognitive health isn't an either-or scenario. It isn't as if you're either in good cognitive health or you aren't. Instead, as you learned in this chapter, cognitive health is a spectrum. Dementia is part of that spectrum, and it can have many different causes.

A population-based study that followed adults around age 77 for four years showed that about 1 in 5 will develop mild cognitive impairment or dementia.

Most of the time, more than one disease causes a person's dementia. For example, people with Alzheimer's disease also often have vascular cognitive impairment, Lewy body disease, and sometimes both. A mix of causes happens more often as people age.

SOME REASSURANCE

As you continue to read this book, it's important to understand that minor memory lapses happen to almost everyone as they age. The lapses don't mean that dementia is just around the corner. While it's possible that any older adult can develop a form of dementia, dementia shouldn't be considered a typical part of aging.

Sometimes, when older adults feel lonely, worried or bored, they show signs and symptoms associated with dementia. For example, coping with emotional trauma or the death of a spouse can cause extreme changes in personality and behavior. Only an experienced doctor who can carefully interpret someone's signs and symptoms and family history can say whether or not they're being caused by dementia.

"MANY EXPERTS SEE MILD COGNITIVE IMPAIRMENT AS AN OPPORTUNITY TO ACT EARLY AND HELP DELAY DEMENTIA OR PREVENT IT ALTOGETHER WITH THE RIGHT TREATMENT."

CHAPTER 2

Mild cognitive impairment

Alzheimer's disease and other dementias don't usually come on quickly or out of the blue. It's not as if one month everything's fine and the next month you're struggling with memory loss and mood swings.

Instead, the onset tends to take place little by little. Mild symptoms turn more severe over time. As you learned in Chapter 1, this takes place along a spectrum.

The word *spectrum* means "a range or a continuous whole." In this case, it refers to a person's history of cognitive change and how it relates to aging and disease. It's a collection of signs and symptoms from their onset to a point where they produce the extreme changes seen in dementia.

For many years, scientists focused on the severe end of this spectrum. This is largely because at that stage, people tend to need immediate and extensive care. But researchers are now paying more attention to the milder end of the spectrum, when symptoms are more severe than typical aging but aren't severe enough to be dementia.

The common term for this stage is mild cognitive impairment. Mild cognitive impairment can be caused by Alzheimer's disease or another similar disorder.

WHAT IS MILD COGNITIVE IMPAIRMENT?

Mild cognitive impairment is when someone develops trouble with cognitive skills. It's clearly different from the person's previous cognitive level, but not severe enough to interfere with daily functioning.

In people with mild cognitive impairment, many aspects of cognition may be fairly normal. There may be new patterns of forgetfulness that are noticeable. However, people with mild cognitive impairment are generally still able to live on their own, handle their own finances, perform household tasks and drive a car just as they did before these changes began.

Someone with mild cognitive impairment is most likely to see a doctor when forgetfulness becomes a concern. When memory is tested, the person doesn't do as well as expected for someone around the same age and education level. However, the impairment isn't severe enough to show that the person has dementia due to Alzheimer's disease or another cause of dementia.

Not everyone with mild cognitive impairment will develop dementia. People with mild cognitive impairment have a higher risk of eventually getting dementia, but some people stay at this stage. Others may even return to a normal cognitive status.

In other words, having mild cognitive impairment doesn't mean you're guaranteed to develop dementia. Each year, about 1 in 10 people with mild cognitive impairment develops dementia.

As research reveals more about how cognitive decline progresses, knowing more about mild cognitive impairment will offer clues about how dementia develops. This understanding may offer more options for treating conditions that cause dementia.

Subcategories

Mild cognitive impairment is broken down into two broad categories: amnestic and nonamnestic. Each has different signs and symptoms, but both types seem to affect men more often than they do women.

Here's more about each type.

Amnestic MCI The term for this type of mild cognitive impairment comes from the word *amnesia*. As you may have guessed, its main symptom is memory loss. Other functions like attention and language use may be affected, too, but usually only slightly. People with this type of mild cognitive impairment are likely able to live on their own and function relatively fully within the community. However, some may tend to avoid socializing because they may fear feelings of embarrassment if they forget details of a conversation.

This type of mild cognitive impairment is broken down into two more categories. One is for cases when only memory loss is present. The other is for people who have memory loss as well as problems in other areas. They may struggle with forgetfulness but also have trouble focusing or coming up with names, for example.

Amnestic MCI is the most common form of mild cognitive impairment. It's also the type that researchers study most. Generally, it's thought to be an early stage of Alzheimer's disease. This makes amnestic MCI a risk factor for Alzheimer's disease dementia.

Nonamnestic MCI With this type of mild cognitive impairment, someone has trouble in a cognitive area *other than* memory. Examples include trouble with reasoning, judgment, language and communication skills. Another example involves difficulty with visuospatial skills, like moving about or judging the height of a step or the distance around an obstacle. As with amnestic MCI, one or many cognitive skills may be affected.

Researchers think that a mild yet constant problem with skills like decision-making and prioritizing may mean that someone is in the early stages of a non-Alzheimer's type of dementia, like frontotemporal degeneration (see Chapter 9). It could also be a sign of an atypical form of Alzheimer's disease where memory is relatively spared (see Chapter 7).

Researchers also think that mild language issues may be linked to different types of dementia. In addition, mild problems with reasoning, judging and solving problems (executive skills) are often seen early on in Lewy body dementia (see Chapter 10).

Causes

As with dementia, mild cognitive impairment isn't the name of a disease. It's a syndrome — a set of symptoms — with many underlying causes. Mild cognitive impairment can have more than one cause. Causes are grouped into several categories, which you'll learn about starting on the next page.

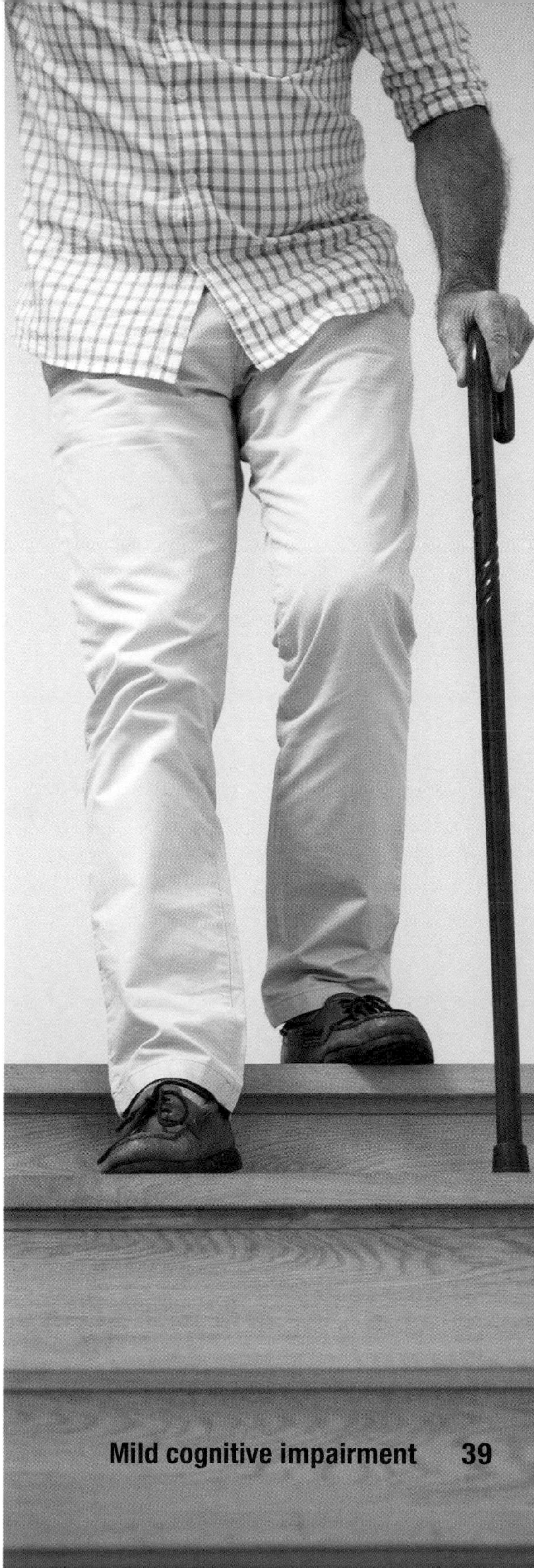

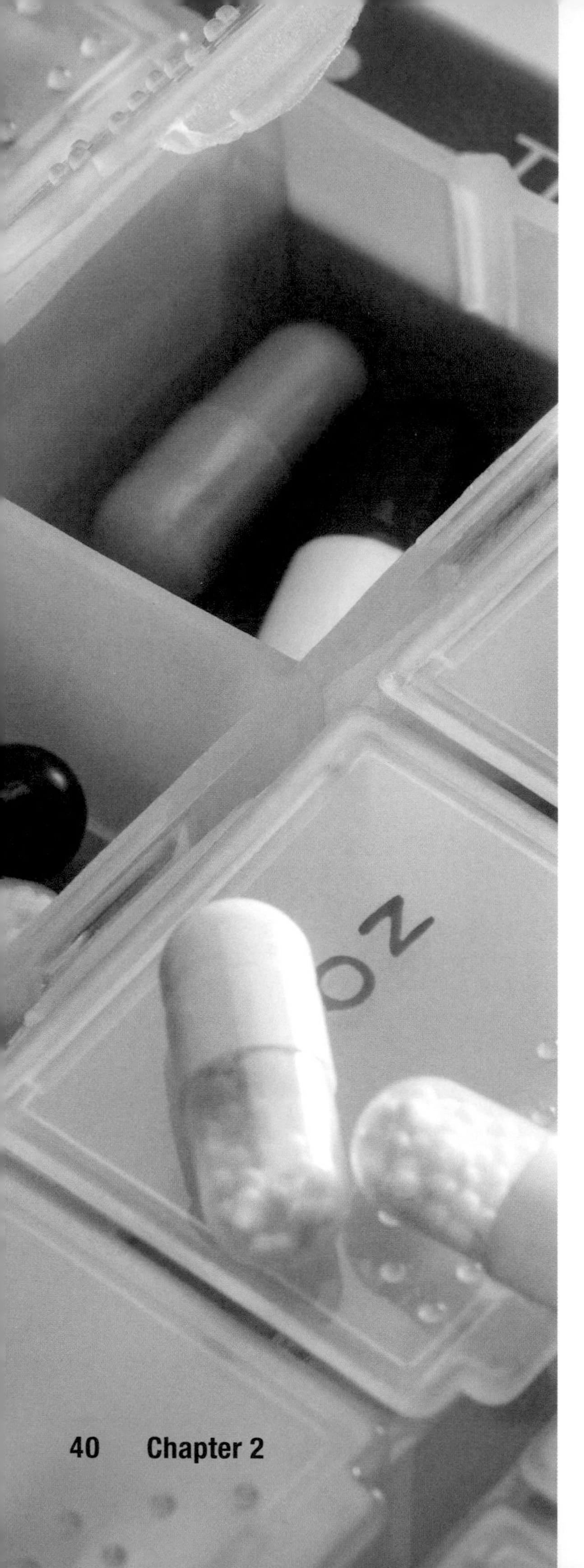

Neurodegenerative A disorder that destroys nerve cells (neurons) in the brain and gets worse over time. Alzheimer's disease, Lewy body dementia and frontotemporal degeneration are examples.

Vascular A disorder that affects blood vessels of the brain. Blood supply is limited, causing cell damage and death. This is known as vascular dementia.

Psychiatric Conditions that affect memory, concentration and mood. Depression is an example.

Medications Certain drugs can cause side effects that affect brain function. There are many examples; in general, anytime someone experiences changes in cognition after starting a new medication, the drug's effects may be to blame. Examples include pain-relieving opioids and any drug that alters brain function, like drugs used to treat anxiety (benzodiazepines).

Sleep disturbances Not getting enough good-quality sleep can affect how well someone thinks and learns. This can be due to insomnia, sleep apnea or other problems.

Metabolic disturbances Metabolism includes all the processes the body needs to maintain life. A disruption to these processes can cause mild cognitive issues. Thyroid problems and not getting enough vitamin B-12 are examples.

Some of these causes can be reversed. If you notice mild changes in cognitive function, a visit with your doctor may help show if these changes can be treated.

Making a diagnosis

No one test can determine if someone has mild cognitive impairment. Instead, doctors use a set of criteria to make a diagnosis.

The criteria doctors use to diagnose mild cognitive impairment include:

- Evidence of a cognitive decline when compared to previous tests and exams. This often involves memory loss but may also include trouble with focus, decision-making, language, and visuospatial, motor or social skills. It's best for these issues to be confirmed by family or friends, or through testing.
- Being able to still complete the activities of daily living. These include household tasks, taking medications, work responsibilities and social functions.
- Symptoms that aren't the result of delirium or another mental health disorder, like depression.
- Symptoms that aren't severe enough to be dementia because the person can still perform the activities of daily living.

It can be hard to diagnose mild cognitive impairment. Memory issues vary from person to person based on the impact they have. Often, people with memory issues don't realize that they have them. It can be valuable for someone who knows the person well to be able to describe incidents that involve memory loss.

Usually, people bring up forgetfulness after they notice a new pattern, like asking the same question over and over or having trouble keeping track of dates and names that once were easy to remember. Forgetting an appointment here and there is fairly normal, but regular slips in routine may be signs of a serious underlying condition.

A doctor will ask several questions and check a person's mental status to look for signs of cognitive decline. A doctor may suspect that a person has mild cognitive impairment if it seems like there's more change than is typical for someone at a certain age and similar education level, but not enough change to signal dementia.

Certain tests can help show if a person's memory and other cognitive functions are impaired. The results of these tests are compared to other people in the same age group. A series of tests over time is best, as they capture the signs of decline.

Even with this criteria, a diagnosis of mild cognitive impairment partly depends on a doctor's judgment, within the context of each person's case. In general, an experienced doctor will combine personal interviews, medical history and test results to identify and measure cognitive change when making a diagnosis.

Determining a cause

Once a doctor has diagnosed someone with mild cognitive impairment, the next step is to figure out what's causing it. A number of imaging tests may be used to determine what's causing mild cognitive impairment.

For example, magnetic resonance imaging (MRI) can show if a tumor or the effects of a head injury are causing symptoms. An MRI can also be used to look for damage to the brain's blood vessels, which may be caused by a stroke.

Imaging tests can also find shrinkage in the brain (atrophy) that may tell a doctor if mild cognitive impairment is being caused by a disease that destroys neurons in the brain (neurodegenerative disease).

These tests can also help a doctor look at a person's hippocampus, a part of the brain important for memory. Studies suggest that people with mild cognitive impairment who progress to dementia often have a smaller hippocampus.

Researchers are studying other forms of imaging that may also help evaluate mild cognitive impairment. These tests may also help predict whether mild cognitive impairment is likely to develop into dementia.

For example, functional imaging — imaging that looks at brain activity rather than physical structure — shows that certain changes in brain activity may take place with mild cognitive impairment. In turn, these changes may serve as markers that show if someone has a higher risk of progressing from mild cognitive impairment to Alzheimer's dementia.

Molecular imaging tests may be another valuable tool. For example, positron emission tomography (PET) scans use tracers that stick to beta-amyloid in the living brain. These PET scans can help doctors see if someone has amyloid plaques in the brain. It's important to note that in general, functional and molecular imaging are used mostly for research and aren't routine parts of an exam.

When treatments to prevent Alzheimer's dementia are discovered and readily available, tests for mild cognitive impairment will be even more important than they are today. That's because these tests will be able to show if someone with mild cognitive impairment is likely to develop Alzheimer's dementia. This group of people will benefit most from early treatment.

OUTLOOK

Mild cognitive impairment is common in older people, and the risk of developing it increases with age. People with less education also seem to be at a higher risk. As researchers learn more about what causes people with mild cognitive impairment to have dementia at some point, they're also learning about the people with mild cognitive impairment who *don't* go on to develop dementia.

A review of 17 studies, for example, showed that people with mild cognitive impairment who are more likely to return to normal cognition have several things in common.

OTHER TESTS USED TO STUDY MILD COGNITIVE IMPAIRMENT

Several studies suggest that using a spinal tap to measure the levels of specific forms of beta-amyloid and the tau protein in the fluid around the brain and spinal cord may help show if someone with mild cognitive impairment is undergoing changes in the brain that will turn into a disorder like dementia due to Alzheimer's disease.

PET scans may also be helpful. First, some background: Beta-amyloid is a protein that clumps together and hardens into plaques that cause nerve cells in the brain to die. This process is what leads to Alzheimer's disease, a common cause of dementia. You'll learn more about beta-amyloid in Chapter 5.

Using a radiotracer that binds to beta-amyloid, like the Pittsburgh Compound B (PiB), PET scans can show a buildup of beta-amyloid in the living brain over time. As the color bar below indicates, cooler colors like blue and green show lower levels of beta-amyloid, while warmer colors like yellow and orange show higher levels.

The left image is of a brain that's cognitively normal. It has normal levels of beta-amyloid, as you'll notice with the blue and green colors. The image in the middle is a brain with mild cognitive impairment. It shows a buildup of beta-amyloid. The image on the right shows a brain of someone who's been diagnosed with Alzheimer's disease dementia. It shows areas with abnormally high levels of beta-amyloid.

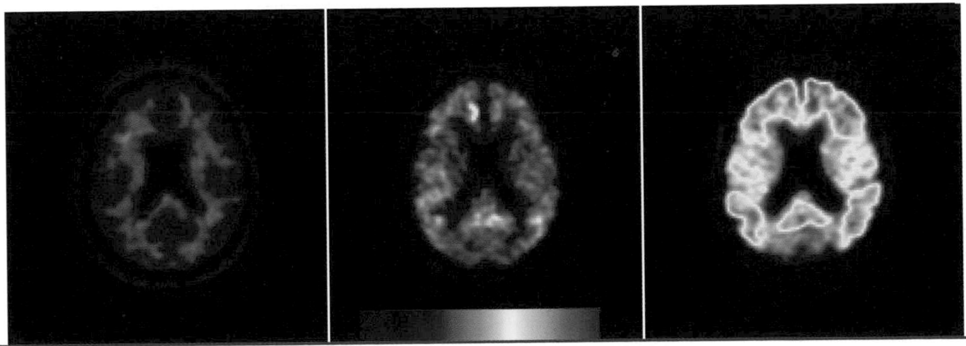

SPOTTING ALZHEIMER'S DISEASE EARLIER

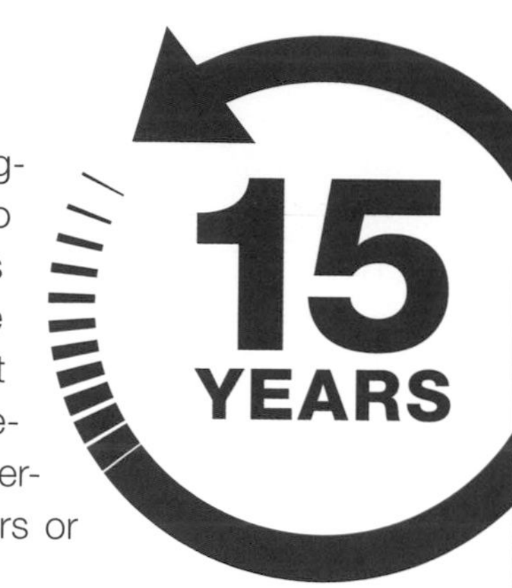

Most research suggests that by the time a person is diagnosed with dementia due to Alzheimer's disease, it's too late to stop the disorder or reverse the damage it's caused. That's what makes research on mild cognitive impairment so important; it may lead to strategies that help delay a shift to Alzheimer's disease dementia or prevent it entirely. In fact, researchers are beginning to understand that Alzheimer's disease begins in the brain years or even decades before symptoms are noticed.

The key idea is to use biomarkers to spot disease before it has a chance to take hold, similar to the idea of treating heart disease before a heart attack ever happens. Researchers are studying changes in the brain that happen early on to help predict if dementia is in someone's future, rather than waiting until symptoms start to develop. The hope is that these markers in the brain will be used as part of a preventive strategy in the future.

The researchers found that people with mild cognitive impairment who are more likely to return to normal cognition are younger, have more education, don't have high blood pressure, haven't had a stroke and don't have the APOE e4 allele, a gene variant linked to Alzheimer's disease. (You'll learn more about this gene variant in Chapter 5.)

Researchers have also learned that treating high blood pressure and other risk factors for heart disease can reduce the risk of mild cognitive impairment and dementia.

Each year, about 1 in 10 people with mild cognitive impairment develops dementia. For example, for every 100 people with mild cognitive impairment, 10 will develop dementia a year later. That means if you have mild cognitive impairment, it's more likely that you'll develop dementia — but it's not guaranteed.

Some people with mild cognitive impairment improve over time or stay at the same cognitive level. In fact, between 5% and 10% percent return to normal in terms of their thinking abilities.

It's also important to know that people with mild cognitive impairment can still take part in the activities of daily living. This means that they can generally:

- Perform complex tasks, like paying bills and managing medications, although sometimes help is needed
- Live independently

Many experts see mild cognitive impairment as an opportunity to act early and help delay dementia or prevent it altogether with the right treatment.

When does MCI shift to dementia?

Researchers are working to figure out what causes someone to move from mild cognitive impairment to dementia. Genetics is one factor. The e4 variant of the apolipoprotein E (APOE) gene is one example. Diseases that affect blood flow in the brain, like high blood pressure and diabetes, are another factor that can increase the risk of progressing from mild cognitive impairment to dementia.

It's likely that a combination of risk factors will predict dementia better than any one single factor. By learning the elements that point to early signs of a process that may lead to dementia, doctors hope to be able to say who will be most likely to benefit from taking part in clinical trials geared toward slowing or stopping the progression to dementia. They also hope to be able to predict who will benefit most from monitoring, which could allow for an early diagnosis.

INSIDE THE MCI BRAIN

Scientists are studying disease-related changes that happen with mild cognitive impairment and their effects on the brain. Knowing more in this area offers a step toward understanding the earliest stages of dementia and maybe providing new treatment options.

So far, researchers have learned that the brain of a person with mild cognitive impairment doesn't always show the heavy load of amyloid plaques and neurofibrillary tangles seen in the Alzheimer's brain. However, some changes are underway. These changes especially affect parts of the brain vital to memory and learning.

Current evidence also shows that mild cognitive impairment often, but not always, develops from a lesser degree of the same types of brain changes seen in Alzheimer's disease or other forms of dementia.

Research findings also suggest that at the mild cognitive impairment stage, Alzheimer's disease and other similar disorders are at an earlier stage of the disease. This opens up the possibility of treating the disorder early and preventing it from getting worse.

TREATMENT

Researchers have tested different compounds to see how much they can affect the brain of someone who is in the process of moving from mild cognitive impairment to dementia due to Alzheimer's disease.

As a starting point, researchers looked at drugs and other substances that have already shown some effect on dementia due to Alzheimer's disease. Cholinesterase inhibitors were a primary target. These drugs boost levels of a brain chemical called acetylcholine. This chemical usually decreases as Alzheimer's develops, so the idea behind using this drug is to stabilize cognitive function in the early stages of the disease. However, experts don't recommend these drugs for routine treatment of mild cognitive impairment. (Learn more about these medications and how they work in Chapter 8.)

Other drugs and supplements also have been studied for use with mild cognitive impairment, but none has shown promise. Examples include memantine, vitamin E, rofecoxib, piracetam, donepezil, galantamine, rivastigmine, homocysteine-lowering B-vitamins and a flavonoid-containing drink.

SLOWING THE DECLINE

Outside of medications, these steps may help slow cognitive decline.

Treating depression

Depression is common in people with mild cognitive impairment. Treating depression can help improve memory.

Treating sleep apnea

This condition causes breathing to start and stop repeatedly during sleep, making good-quality rest difficult, if not impossible. Getting treatment for sleep apnea can restore sleep and make it easier to concentrate during the day.

Controlling high blood pressure

Blood vessel damage can cause damage to the brain. Doctors think that controlling high blood pressure and other diseases that can affect the blood vessels may help prevent dementia.

Following a healthy lifestyle

Evidence suggests that a healthy diet and regular physical activity may help reduce the risk of cognitive decline and dementia.

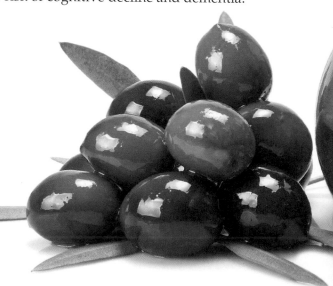

Exercise, for example, has been shown to improve some thinking-related functions. In turn, it may delay the onset of dementia in people with mild cognitive impairment. In terms of diet, researchers have found that following an eating pattern similar to the Mediterranean diet may offer more benefits for thinking-related functions than a low-fat diet does.

Unfortunately, no research has confirmed what will delay or keep mild cognitive impairment from progressing to dementia. But researchers are hopeful that a better understanding of the disease process and better tools for identifying those at risk will lead to research studies that will offer more answers. In turn, this research may lead to more-effective treatments, especially ones focused on prevention. You'll learn more about preventive strategies later in this book.

MAKING PROGRESS

Most scientists are confident that treatment to prevent Alzheimer's will be developed in the next few decades. It stands to reason that being able to identify those at high risk of the disease, like people with mild cognitive impairment or those at an even earlier, pre-mild cognitive impairment stage, will help experts get treatment to those who can benefit most from it.

The challenge facing scientists who study mild cognitive impairment is twofold: One direction lies in narrowing down how to diagnose the condition and identify the people with mild cognitive impairment who will go on to develop dementia. The other direction lies in identifying and developing treatments that keep mild cognitive impairment from progressing into dementia.

“DEMENTIA IS A SYNDROME LINKED TO PROBLEMS WITH REMEMBERING, LEARNING NEW THINGS, FOCUSING AND MAKING DECISIONS THAT AFFECT EVERYDAY LIFE.”

CHAPTER 3

What is dementia?

In Chapter 1, you read about Frank. At 75 years old, Frank has always enjoyed working on anything with a motor that's in need of repair. He's lived in the same house for 40 years, a house he built himself. But lately, Frank is constantly misplacing things. And he has set out for the diner he frequents regularly and then gotten confused about where he's going. When he tries to turn back, he's confused about how to get home. Frank also mentions talking to his wife, even though she died years ago.

If Frank's symptoms make it so that he can't perform daily functions, like managing his finances, cooking or managing his medications, then a doctor may diagnose Frank with dementia. If his doctor thinks that the cause of Frank's dementia is Alzheimer's disease, Frank would be diagnosed with dementia due to Alzheimer's disease.

DEMENTIA 101

Around 50 million people around the world have dementia. Each year, nearly 10 million new cases are reported. The World Health Organization defines dementia as a syndrome that causes memory, thinking, behavior and the ability to perform everyday activities to worsen over time. Dementia is *not* a normal part of aging.

A key word in this definition is *syndrome*. Many people think of dementia as a disease. But in fact, it's a syndrome. Here's the difference: A syndrome is a collection of signs and symptoms *caused by* disease. Signs and symptoms vary based on what's causing the syndrome.

A variety of diseases and conditions can cause dementia; you'll learn about them in detail in this chapter. Regardless of its cause, dementia means that certain cognitive functions have become severely impaired. These are the most common signs and symptoms of dementia:

- Memory loss, usually noticed by a spouse or someone else
- Having trouble using or finding words
- Trouble with visual and spatial skills; for example, getting lost while driving
- Difficulty reasoning or solving problems
- Problems with planning and organizing
- Lack of coordination and motor function
- Personality changes
- Inappropriate behavior
- Paranoia
- Agitation
- Seeing or hearing things that aren't real

Memory loss is a common symptom of dementia. In fact, it's a hallmark of dementia due to Alzheimer's disease. But memory loss on its own doesn't mean you have dementia.

Having dementia means having significant problems with cognitive functions, one of which may be memory. These issues have to be severe enough to interfere with day-to-day function. For example, dementia could be signaled by memory loss plus feeling easily disoriented and having a hard time coming up with words. It's the *combination* of signs and symptoms and how severe they are that shows if someone has dementia.

Scientists hope to one day be able to spot different patterns of cognitive change in their earliest stages and from there, pinpoint what causes dementia. Many experts think the best time to treat dementia is when it's just beginning, before the condition is well established in the brain.

Scientists also hope to find links between a person's signs and symptoms and how fast or how far someone may shift from normal function to dementia. For example, why does memory stabilize for some people after mild to moderate memory loss while others decline quickly? The brain is so complex that answers to questions like this are hard to come by.

Dementia is a major cause of disability among older people. As the disease progresses, people living with dementia may need help with or depend on others for personal care, like eating, bathing, dressing and using the bathroom. They may not be able to live on their own. They may become unable to use and understand language, written or spoken. Some of these capacities may be retained longer than others.

Dementia affects people physically, psychologically, socially and economically. Dementia impacts a person's career, family and the society around them.

COMMON CAUSES OF DEMENTIA

Cognition refers to brain processes that allow you to think, reason and interact with the world around you. Dementia happens when these processes become seriously impaired. Most times, impairment is caused

WHAT'S A SYNDROME?

A syndrome is a collection of signs and symptoms that occur in a consistent pattern. This pattern often points to a specific condition as the cause. For example, many women regularly have headaches, breast tenderness, irritability and fatigue before their menstrual cycles. These signs and symptoms point to premenstrual syndrome (PMS).

If an older adult has memory issues that are getting worse over time and the person is having trouble with attention and getting lost, a doctor may suspect that the signs and symptoms are caused by dementia and that the dementia is due to Alzheimer's disease. A different set of symptoms may signal a different condition as the cause of dementia.

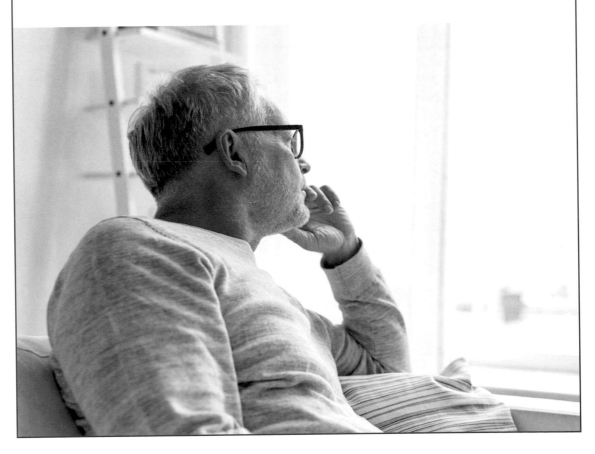

DEMENTIA: AN UMBRELLA TERM

Dementia is a syndrome linked to problems with remembering, learning new things, focusing and making decisions that affect everyday life. It's an umbrella term that includes thinking (cognitive) problems that interfere with someone's normal day-to-day functioning.

Dementia can affect behavior, decision-making, memory, language, visual or spatial perception, and attention, among other areas of daily living. More than one of these areas is usually affected, but one area may be more affected than another.

The four main causes of dementia are listed below. Each one has different characteristics and causes specific symptoms. With that said, the experience of dementia will be unique for each person. Not everyone will experience all of the symptoms of the disorder.

Because dementia describes a range of symptoms and many disorders, it's possible to have symptoms of more than one disorder at the same time.

Here's a brief breakdown of the four main causes of dementia and how they compare, in terms of the number of people they affect. You'll learn more about each of these disorders starting on the next page.

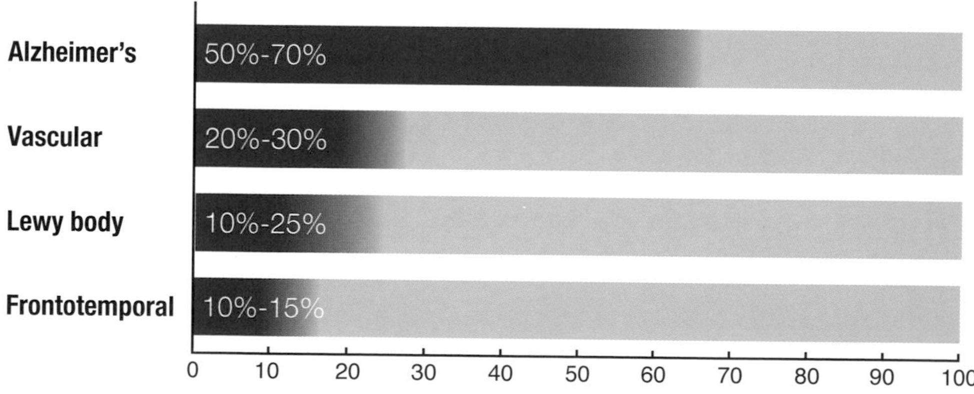

ALZHEIMER'S DISEASE VS. DEMENTIA

Although the terms ***Alzheimer's disease*** and ***dementia*** are often used to mean the same thing, they actually mean two different things. Dementia is a syndrome, not a specific disease. It's an overall term — sometimes referred to as an umbrella term — that describes a range of symptoms. These symptoms impact a person's ability to perform everyday activities.

Alzheimer's disease is one cause of dementia, but it's not the only one, as you'll learn in this chapter.

by disorders that affect the brain (neurodegenerative), the blood vessels (vascular) or both.

While treatment can help ease the symptoms of dementia, it often can't cure its causes. But sometimes, dementia may arise from conditions that *can* be treated, like medication side effects or infection. Here's a little more on the most common causes of dementia.

Neurodegenerative disorders

These disorders cause a breakdown in the brain that leads to dementia. Here's some information about each disorder. You'll learn more in later chapters.

Alzheimer's disease dementia Alzheimer's disease is the most common cause of dementia. In Alzheimer's disease, brain cells break down due to the buildup of amyloid plaques and neurofibrillary tangles. The result is a steady decline in memory and mental function.

The rate at which symptoms worsen varies from person to person. Memory loss is one of the first symptoms. Learn more about Alzheimer's disease dementia in Part 2.

Lewy body dementia Lewy body dementia is the second most common type of neurodegenerative dementia after Alzheimer's disease. It's an umbrella term that includes dementia with Lewy bodies and Parkinson's disease dementia.

As its name suggests, Lewy body dementia happens when protein deposits called Lewy bodies develop in nerve cells in the parts of the brain involved in thinking, memory and movement. Some people with Lewy body dementia see things that aren't real (visual hallucinations), act out their dreams while sleeping, and experience fluctuations in alertness and attention. Other effects may include Parkinson's disease-like signs and symptoms like rigid muscles, slow movement and tremors.

Unlike Alzheimer's disease, in which memory loss is one of the first symptoms, memory isn't usually affected until later on in Lewy body dementia. Learn more about Lewy body dementia in Chapter 10.

Frontotemporal degeneration Frontotemporal degeneration is an umbrella term for a diverse group of uncommon disorders that mostly affect the frontal and temporal lobes of the brain. This group of disorders also includes a mild cognitive impairment stage and a frontotemporal dementia stage.

Some people with frontotemporal degeneration undergo changes in personality and social skills and can be impulsive or emotionally indifferent. In others, the ability to use language is affected. Learn more about frontotemporal degeneration in Chapter 9.

Vascular disorders

Your vascular system involves the heart and a network of blood vessels that make blood flow throughout your body, from your head to your feet and everywhere in between. This book focuses on disorders that affect the blood vessels in the brain.

Conditions like high cholesterol, high blood pressure, diabetes and smoking can lead to a buildup of substances that can restrict blood flow (atherosclerosis). This can increase your risk of heart disease, a heart attack or stroke. In turn, these conditions can lead to forms of dementia known as vascular cognitive impairment.

One of the most common forms of vascular cognitive impairment results from a series of small strokes to the brain. These strokes damage brain tissue after the blood supply is blocked, creating areas of dead tissue. This dead tissue looks like spots in the brain's white matter.

Vascular cognitive impairment may come on suddenly if strokes are severe and affect critical parts of the brain. It may get worse, little by little, each time the person has another stroke.

Symptoms of vascular cognitive impairment may include problems thinking or paying attention, walking unsteadily, confusion, or depression. Depending on where the dead tissue is located in the brain, symptoms may be limited to just one side of the body or to a couple of functions.

Damage to brain tissue from strokes can't be reversed. However, the chance of future strokes can be reduced by controlling high blood pressure and other conditions that affect the blood vessels. This can help prevent further damage. Learn more about vascular cognitive impairment, including ways to prevent it, in Chapter 11.

OTHER CAUSES OF DEMENTIA

Dementia is sometimes caused by conditions that aren't linked to your brain or blood vessels. And sometimes these causes can be treated and even reversed; normal-pressure hydrocephalus is an example.

Normal-pressure hydrocephalus, Huntington's disease and Creutzfeldt-Jakob disease are conditions that can cause dementia-like symptoms. You may have heard of these conditions without knowing that they can cause dementia-like symptoms.

These conditions illustrate why it's important to talk to your doctor if you're having any significant problems with memory and focus. Here's more on each one.

Normal-pressure hydrocephalus

Hydrocephalus is a condition that happens when the fluid that surrounds and cushions the brain doesn't reabsorb into the bloodstream as it should. Instead, the fluid builds up and puts pressure on the brain.

Normal-pressure hydrocephalus is a variation of this condition. As with hydrocephalus, a buildup of fluid puts pressure on the brain, but not as much. This type of hydrocephalus is mostly seen in older adults. It may be the result of an injury or illness, but in most cases, the cause is unknown. Sometimes, this type of hydrocephalus can be treated.

Signs and symptoms Walking slowly with short, shuffling steps is usually the first sign of normal-pressure hydrocephalus. A person may walk with feet spread wide and may have trouble turning and starting to move. Balance problems and falls also are common.

After developing problems walking, people with normal-pressure hydrocephalus may feel more-frequent urges to urinate, leading

NORMAL-PRESSURE HYDROCEPHALUS

With normal-pressure hydrocephalus, fluid in the brain builds up. This excess fluid disrupts brain function, causing changes in how someone walks. It also often causes problems with thinking abilities.

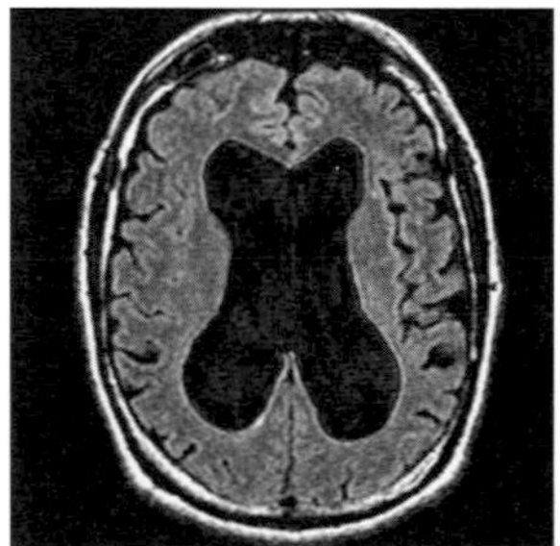

"WITH AN EARLY DIAGNOSIS IN PLACE, TREATMENT CAN START QUICKLY FOR PEOPLE WHO MAY BENEFIT FROM IT."

to loss of bladder control (incontinence). People with normal-pressure hydrocephalus may think and process information more slowly. They may not pay attention as well, and they may be forgetful.

But symptoms may not be as severe as they are with the dementia disorders described in other parts of this book. Unlike Alzheimer's disease, for example, people with normal-pressure hydrocephalus usually can answer questions correctly, but it may take a bit longer to reply.

Signs and symptoms of normal-pressure hydrocephalus are sometimes similar to other types of dementia, which can sometimes lead to a misdiagnosis. Certain tests are done to tell the difference. With an early diagnosis in place, treatment can start quickly for people who may benefit from it.

How it's treated A long, flexible tube called a shunt is typically used to drain excess fluid from the brain to treat normal-pressure hydrocephalus. The tube tunnels under the scalp and skin along the neck and chest down to the belly, where the fluid drains into a container. Draining the fluid may help relieve symptoms and bring the fluid level in the brain back to normal.

Although treatment can help many people with this condition, the procedure carries risks. And while some research shows that using a shunt to treat normal-pressure hydrocephalus improves symptoms in most people long term, how well a shunt works varies from person to person. Some symptoms disappear right away, while others take more time to resolve.

A doctor may test you to see how well you respond to the fluid drainage before placing a permanent shunt. For example, your doctor may want to test how well you walk to see if it's improved.

Huntington's disease

Huntington's disease is an inherited disease that usually develops in middle age. It causes uncontrolled movements, emotional disturbances and mental decline. In younger adults, symptoms are often more severe and may get worse quickly. In rare cases, children can develop this condition.

Signs and symptoms Huntington's disease usually develops slowly. How severe it is depends on how much damage has been done in the brain. Emotional changes like irritability, anger and paranoia are early signs and symptoms. Depression also is common. Huntington's disease can cause problems with making decisions, learning new things, answering questions and remembering facts. Early movement disorders include mild balance problems, facial twitches and grimaces, and clumsiness.

As the disease gets worse, the body's movements may become sudden and jerky. A person with the disease may walk with a wide, prancing gait. Speech may be halting or slurred. Dementia is another symptom.

People with this disease usually die between 10 and 30 years after symptoms first appear. Death is often caused by an infection related to pneumonia or injuries and complications from a fall. Typically, the earlier symptoms appear, the more quickly the disease progresses.

Screening and diagnosis A single abnormal gene causes Huntington's disease. Normally, this gene controls the production of a protein called huntingtin (note the difference in spelling between the protein and the disease). It's possible that the mutated gene produces a toxic form of huntingtin that destroys nerve cells in the brain.

To tell if Huntington's disease is causing symptoms, a doctor performs a physical exam and looks at a person's medical history and family medical history. A doctor may ask about recent changes with emotions or intellect. Imaging tests of the brain and blood tests also may be done.

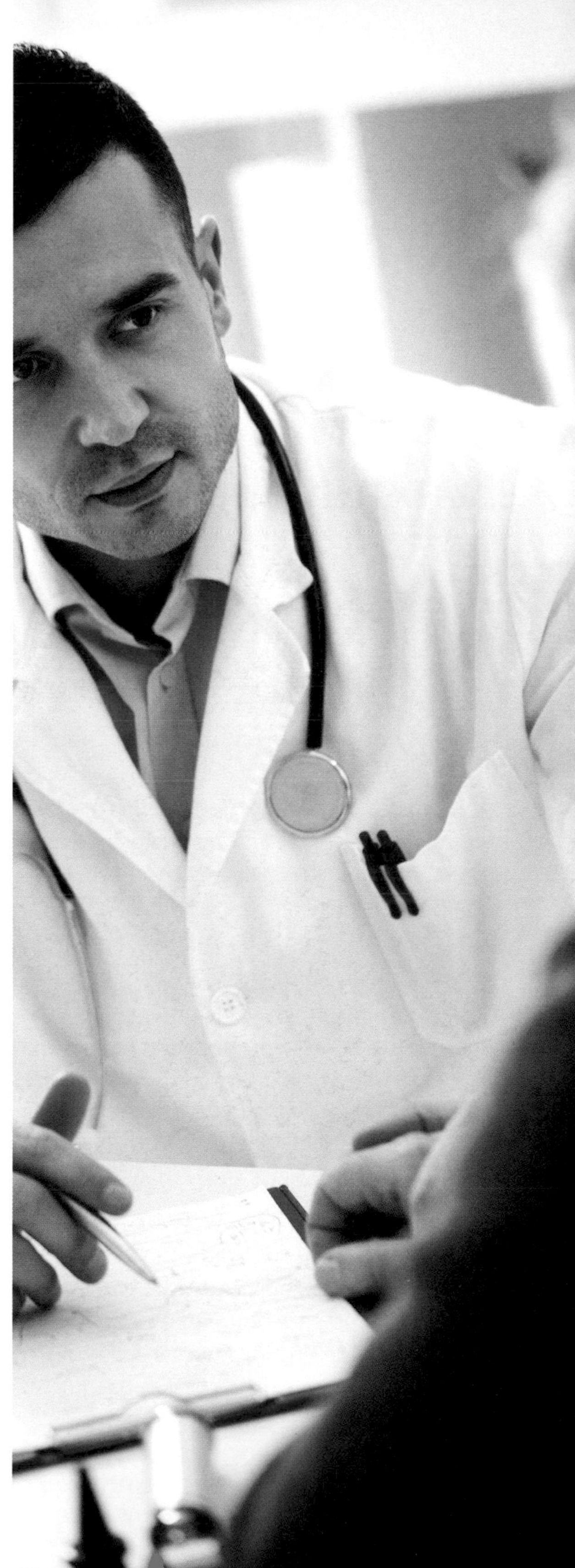

A blood test can also show if someone carries the gene that causes this disease. Some people with a family history of the disease choose to take the test even before symptoms develop.

Deciding whether to be tested early is a personal decision. If you're not sure if you should have the test, a genetic counselor can help you weigh the pros and cons and understand the implications of the test result.

How it's treated No treatment can stop or reverse the development of Huntington's disease. However, several approaches can help with signs and symptoms.

Tetrabenazine (Xenazine) is approved by the Food and Drug Administration to control jerking and writhing movements. Among its side effects, this drug may worsen or cause depression and other mental health conditions. It can also cause drowsiness, nausea and restlessness.

Antipsychotic drugs like haloperidol (Haldol) and chlorpromazine can help with uncontrolled movements and may help with violent outbursts, agitation and mood disorders. However, they may cause muscles to become stiff and rigid.

Drugs aimed to help with mood include ones typically used to treat seizures, like valproate, carbamazepine (Carbatrol, Epitol, Tegretol) and lamotrigine (Lamictal).

Antidepressants are sometimes used to help with obsessive-compulsive habits that are common with Huntington's disease, but they can cause nausea, diarrhea, drowsiness and low blood pressure.

Talk therapy, physical therapy and speech therapy may help, especially in the early stages. These therapies can improve quality of life and may help reduce the risk of side effects from taking medications.

Following a balanced diet and maintaining a normal body weight are also important for people with Huntington's disease. That's because people with this disorder may burn as much as 5,000 calories a day — much higher than the average person. Extra vitamins and supplements may be used if a doctor thinks they would be helpful.

Help with meals may also be needed. For example, cutting food into small pieces or pureéing it may make eating easier. Allowing plenty of time for eating is also helpful.

Creutzfeldt-Jakob disease

Creutzfeldt-Jakob disease affects about 1 out of every 1 million people every year. It's thought to occur when misshapen proteins attack brain cells and kill them in a way that's far more rapid than what occurs in Alzheimer's disease. The disorder leads to dementia and, ultimately, death.

Creutzfeldt-Jakob disease typically occurs around the age of 60. Once a person becomes sick with this disease, it worsens quickly. A person with this disease usually

TREATABLE CAUSES OF COGNITIVE IMPAIRMENT

As with normal-pressure hydrocephalus, other conditions that can cause cognitive impairment can be treated or reversed. Here are several examples.

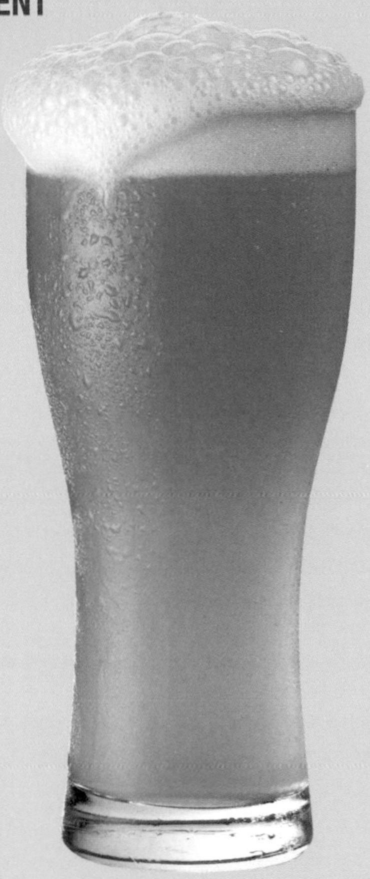

Infection Meningitis, for example, can cause confusion, impaired judgment and memory loss. If it's caught early, however, meningitis can be cured.

Reaction to medication Side effects from some drugs can cause short-term problems with memory and focus.

Metabolic or endocrine imbalances Diseases of the thyroid, kidney, pancreas and liver can upset the chemical balance of your blood, causing dementia.

Brain tumor Some tumors can cause dementia symptoms. A tumor that presses against the parts of the brain that controls hormone levels is an example.

Subdural hematoma This is when blood collects between the brain's surface and its thin outer covering.

Substance abuse Misuse of some prescription drugs may cause dementia symptoms. Street drugs, especially in high doses, can have a similar effect.

Chronic alcoholism The complications of chronic alcoholism, like liver disease and not getting enough nutrients, especially thiamin, can lead to dementia.

Nutritional deficiencies Not getting enough nutrients, like B vitamins, may cause dementia-like symptoms.

Poisoning Exposure to toxic solvents or fumes without protective equipment can damage brain cells. In time, this can lead to dementia.

Autoimmune system issues Sometimes, memory and thinking problems can be a sign of a problem with the immune system. In these cases, treatment with steroids can improve symptoms.

dies from complications within months. At this time, no treatment can stop the disease or keep it from getting worse.

Creutzfeldt-Jakob disease captured the public eye in the 1990s when a form of it developed among people in Great Britain who had eaten beef from cows that had mad cow disease, also known as bovine spongiform encephalopathy.

Signs and symptoms Symptoms of dementia that worsen quickly is the main feature of Creutzfeldt-Jakob disease. At first, a person with this disease may have problems with muscle coordination, personality changes, sleeplessness and blurred vision. Signs and symptoms get dramatically worse, leading to severe mental impairment. Muscles may jerk, it may be hard to move or speak, and blindness may occur.

Many people with this disease eventually fall into a coma. From there, heart or lung failure or an infection like pneumonia leads to death. Death usually occurs within a year after signs and symptoms first appear.

The type of this disease that's linked to mad cow disease affects people at a younger age and usually starts with symptoms like depression, anxiety, apathy, and seeing or hearing things that aren't real. Cognitive impairment comes later. This form of the disease lasts a little longer (12 to 14 months).

What causes it The proteins that cause Creutzfeldt-Jakob disease are called prions. Prion proteins are normally harmless, but when they're misshapen, they can cause disease. These proteins perform as they're supposed to when they're folded into a specific 3D shape. Proteins that don't fold properly are sent away to a recycling center of sorts in the body. However, as people age, the recycling process may not work as well. As a result, proteins that don't fold properly may start to build up in the brain.

Proteins that don't fold properly and build up in the brain may force other proteins to misfold, too. Then, the infected cells die. In turn, large clusters of cells die, leaving the brain riddled with holes. The disease may not show up for years after changes in the proteins have occurred.

How the disease develops People can get Creutzfeldt-Jakob disease in one of three ways. It may develop for no apparent reason; this happens in more than 85% of all cases. It may run in families. In the United States, this happens in 5% to 10% of cases.

This disease may also occur from exposure to the proteins that cause it, during a skin transplant or from an injection of growth hormone. The risk of this happening is low, however. Since 1985, for example, all human growth hormone in the U.S. has been genetically reengineered, eliminating the risk of Creutzfeldt-Jakob disease for people receiving growth hormone treatment.

There's also a very slight risk that instruments used in some types of brain surgery can transmit this disease. That's because the misshapen proteins that cause this disease

> **"IN SOME CASES, SOMEONE CAN HAVE SIGNS AND SYMPTOMS OF DEMENTIA BUT NOT HAVE DEMENTIA AT ALL."**

aren't affected by standard methods used to sterilize medical instruments.

Studies suggest that contaminated blood and related products may transmit the disease in animals, but this hasn't been seen in humans.

How it's diagnosed Doctors can be fairly sure someone has Creutzfeldt-Jakob disease based on a medical exam, personal history, brain exam, and a test of the fluid around the brain and spinal cord (cerebrospinal fluid). But first, other causes of the symptoms often need to be ruled out.

MRI scans and brain wave tests may be used to look for signs of the disease. A spinal tap may be used to check for certain proteins in the spinal fluid. A specific test for Creutzfeldt-Jakob disease called real-time quaking-induced conversion (RT-QuIC) may be used to detect the proteins that cause it in a person's cerebrospinal fluid.

The only way to know for sure if someone has the disease is to examine brain tissue after death.

How it's treated Although many drugs have been tested, there's no effective way to treat either type of Creutzfeldt-Jakob disease. Doctors focus on relieving pain and other symptoms and making people with the disease as comfortable as possible.

CAUSES OF DEMENTIA-LIKE SYMPTOMS

In some cases, someone can have signs and symptoms of dementia but not have dementia at all. For example, mild memory loss may simply be a natural slowing down of mental processing.

Two conditions in particular, depression and delirium, may look like dementia, but they're not. Plus, they're both treatable. Here's more on each condition.

Depression

People often use the term *depression* to describe a temporary low mood that comes from a bad day or bad feeling.

But as a medical term, *depression* denotes a serious illness that affects thoughts, emotions, feelings, behaviors and physical health.

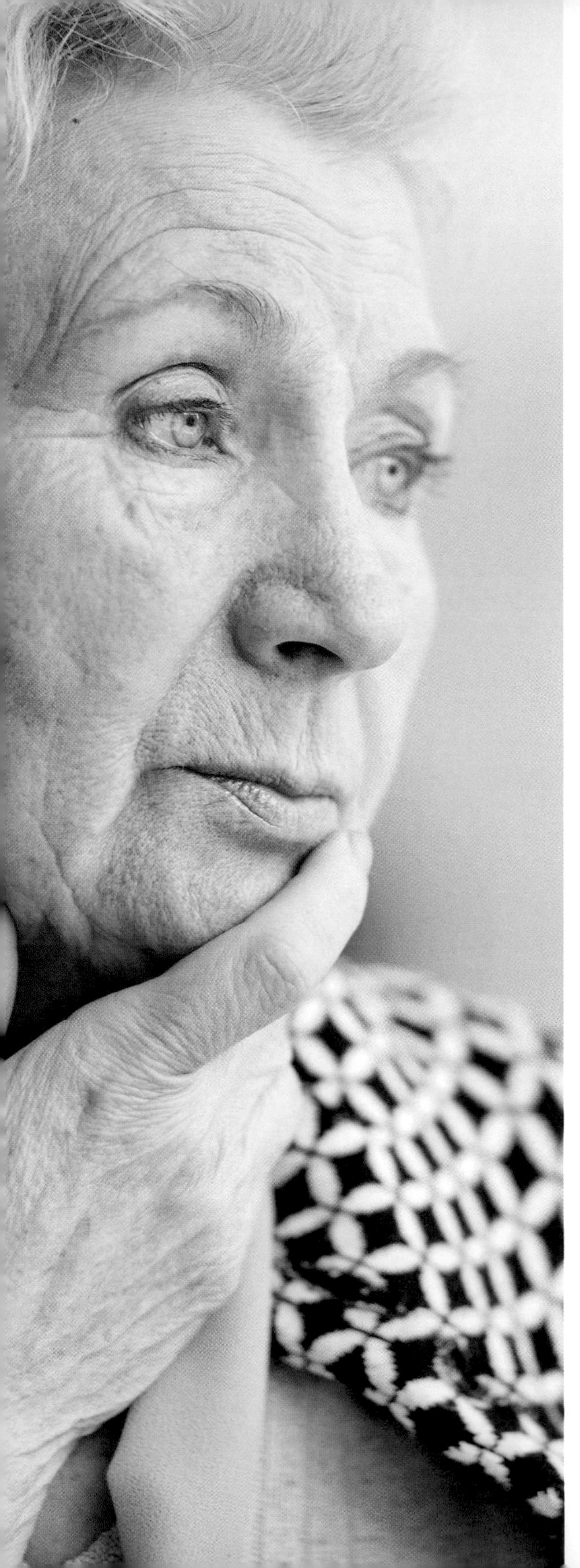

People used to think depression was "all in your head" and that if you really tried, you could pull out of the mood. Doctors now know that depression isn't something you can treat on your own. It's a medical disorder with a biological or chemical basis.

Sometimes a stressful event, like the death of a spouse, triggers depression. Other times, depression seems to happen on its own with no cause you can pinpoint. Either way, depression is much more than grieving or a bout of the blues.

Similar to people with dementia, people with depression may be confused, forgetful and slow to respond. That's because depression affects how someone feels, thinks, eats, sleeps and acts.

Two hallmark symptoms of depression are an ongoing sense of sadness and despair and loss of interest in activities that once brought pleasure. People with depression often have trouble concentrating, which makes it look like they have dementia.

It's important to see your doctor if you're concerned about changes that may signal depression. Symptoms may not get better on their own — and depression may get worse if it isn't treated. Even if symptoms aren't associated with depression, it's important to identify the reasons for distress.

Depression is also common with dementia. In fact, more than a third of people with Alzheimer's disease also have depression. Brief periods of discouragement and apathy may be expected when someone is dealing with a diagnosis of Alzheimer's. But it's important not to let prolonged sadness go untreated. When it's added to dementia, the negative impact of depression on emotions and intellect can be even more extreme.

Delirium

Delirium is a state of mental confusion and clouded consciousness. People with delirium go through a range of extreme emotions.

Delirium may cause trouble with focus or attention. Memory, especially of recent events, may be poor. Speech may be rambling or not make sense. People with delirium may get disoriented, restless, irritable or combative. They may see or hear things that aren't real (hallucinate), or they may not be able to sleep well.

Though the signs and symptoms of delirium may be mistaken for those of dementia, there are important differences. For example, signs and symptoms of delirium usually appear over a short period of time, from a few hours to a few days. And symptoms may get better or worse over that time.

Another difference is that delirium is often caused by a treatable condition. In these cases, emergency medical treatment is critical. A serious infection or exposure to a toxin, for example, may be causing the delirium.

Delirium may affect older adults who have lung or heart disease, long-term infections, poor nutrition, or hormone disorders. It may also stem from the way one drug acts with another, or from alcohol or drug abuse or emotional stress.

In addition, someone with dementia can develop delirium, often due to another medical condition like a urinary tract infection.

Whether depression or delirium occurs on its own or along with dementia, both are treatable conditions. That makes it critical to talk to a doctor if you're seeing signs and symptoms of cognitive impairment in yourself or a loved one.

RISK FACTORS FOR DEMENTIA

Now that you know a little more about dementia and its possible causes, what factors can put you at risk? You can't avoid some, like age and family history. But others are within your control.

As you review these risk factors, keep in mind that if several apply to you, it doesn't mean that dementia is in your future. Calculating risk is an inexact science. It estimates what your chances are of getting a disease over a certain period of time — and by no means is your risk result definitive.

Age

The risk of getting dementia nearly doubles every five years after you reach age 65. The risk reaches nearly one-third after age 85.

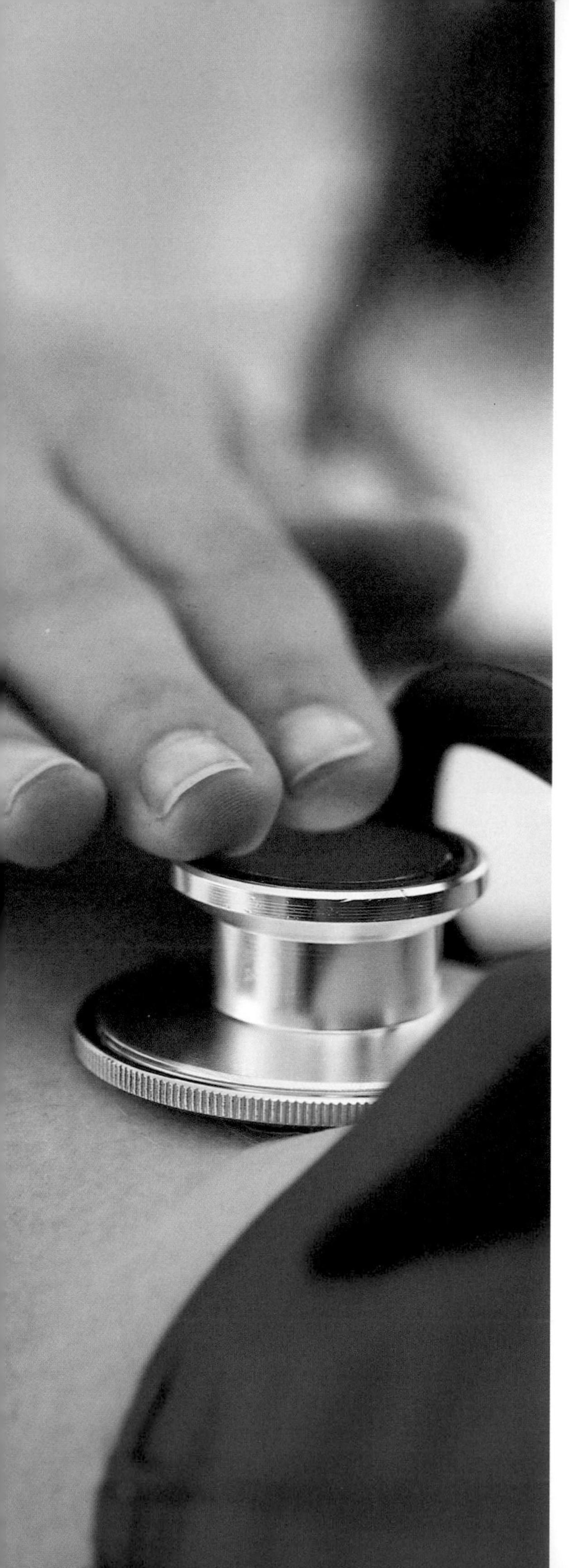

Family history and genetics

As a rule, people with a family history of Alzheimer's are thought to have a higher risk than those without that family history. Researchers have found genes and gene changes that increase the risk of dementia. But some people with this particular genetic makeup never develop Alzheimer's. The bottom line: It's still not possible to predict the risk of dementia strictly based on genetic evidence.

Heart problems

There seems to be a link between the health of the brain and of the heart. Risk of stroke and vascular dementia increases with the buildup of fats, cholesterol and other substances in and on the arteries of your heart. High levels of low-density lipoprotein (LDL, or "bad") cholesterol and high blood pressure can also increase your risk.

Diabetes

Diabetes can damage blood vessels in the brain, increasing the risk of vascular dementia. In addition, ongoing research is uncovering possible links between diabetes and Alzheimer's disease.

Smoking

Although the link between smoking and dementia is somewhat controversial, some studies suggest that people who smoke have a higher risk of dementia. One reason for this may be that smokers have a higher risk of heart disease that, in turn, makes dementia more likely.

Blood pressure

High blood pressure can make dementia more likely for a number of reasons. High blood pressure in midlife has been shown to increase the risk of dementia.

Hearing loss

Research shows that hearing loss is linked to a higher risk of dementia. In fact, hearing loss can almost double the risk.

Hearing loss may make someone feel more alone socially, leading to lifestyle habits — like smoking, drinking alcohol and gaining weight — that may make dementia more likely. Hearing loss may also cause changes in the part of the brain responsible for hearing, which may lead to dementia. Certain parts of the brain may be more likely to shrink with hearing loss.

Physical inactivity

Physical activity protects against dementia. Put simply, getting more exercise makes it less likely that you'll develop dementia. Not getting enough physical activity has been shown to increase the risk of dementia.

Poor dental health

Preliminary research suggests that people who have severe dental disease that leads to tooth loss also have a higher risk of dementia. However, it's too soon to make claims about the link between dental disease and dementia and if one causes the other. This is an active area of research.

Lack of education

Many studies suggest that a low level of education early in life may be linked to developing dementia later in life. Some research shows that a quarter to one-third of dementia cases could possibly be delayed or prevented by improving a person's educational level.

REDUCING YOUR RISK

Although there are no exact conclusions, more and more evidence suggests that some lifestyle factors may actually protect the brain and help reduce the risk of dementia. Physical activity, social engagement, and continuing to learn and challenge your brain are all examples. Learn more in Chapter 19.

“NO SINGLE TEST CAN SHOW WHETHER OR NOT SYMPTOMS ARE BEING CAUSED BY DEMENTIA. IT TAKES A PROCESS, WHICH USUALLY STARTS WITH A DOCTOR.”

CHAPTER 4

Getting an accurate dementia diagnosis

In Chapter 3, you got a brief introduction to dementia, including what it is and what causes it. In short, dementia is defined as cognitive impairment that affects a person's ability to independently perform the functions of daily life.

You also learned that having dementia-like symptoms doesn't always mean you have a neurodegenerative disease like Alzheimer's. You could have other reasons for cognitive issues, like an infection, a reaction to a medication you're taking or depression. You also learned that several factors can increase your risk of developing dementia at some point.

With this background in mind, it's time to learn how a doctor can tell if you have dementia — or if something else is causing your symptoms. In this chapter, you'll get the step-by-step process that helps a doctor determine what's causing someone's symptoms. A doctor has to see a pattern of loss of skills and function and see what a person can do and what struggles a person is having. You'll also learn what tests help confirm the cause of dementia.

It's important to remember that dementia is a clinical diagnosis. Several tests can help determine the cause of a person's symptoms, show whether or not someone has dementia, and pinpoint the best way to move forward with treatment, whether dementia is present or not. Because no single test can diagnose dementia or determine its cause, several tests are often needed.

To determine if someone has dementia, a doctor will start by answering the following questions: *(continued on page 69)*

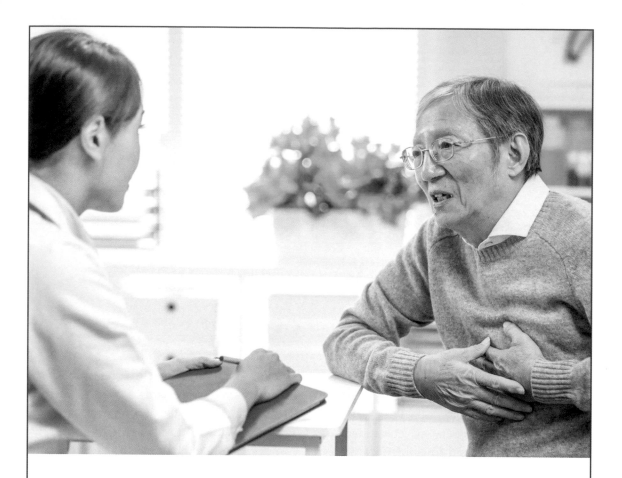

EXPERTS WHO HELP DIAGNOSE DEMENTIA

While a primary care doctor often starts the process of diagnosing or ruling out dementia, other specialists and medical experts are sometimes also involved. They include:

- A neurologist, who specializes in the brain and nervous system
- A psychiatrist or another licensed mental health specialist
- A psychologist or neuropsychologist, who specializes in assessing memory and mental functions
- A geriatrician, who specializes in the care of older adults

(continued from page 67)

- Does the individual have cognitive impairment?
- If the person has cognitive decline, could it be mild cognitive impairment, or is it severe enough to be dementia?
- If a condition that looks like dementia is actually something else, is it something that can be improved or reversed?
- If the person has dementia, what's causing it? Examples include Alzheimer's disease and Lewy body disease.

Here are the steps a doctor will take to answer these questions.

COMMON TESTS AND EVALUATIONS

No single test can show whether or not symptoms are being caused by dementia. It takes a process, which usually starts with a doctor.

During a basic dementia evaluation, a doctor will interview you and someone who knows you well — like a family member or close friend — about your symptoms. A doctor will also take your medical history, conduct a physical exam that includes certain cognitive tests and do basic lab tests. You'll also likely have an imaging test, like a computerized tomography (CT) scan of the head or a magnetic resonance imaging (MRI) scan of the brain.

The doctor will then put all of this information together to make a diagnosis. If this evaluation shows that dementia is causing the symptoms, the next step is to find out what's causing the dementia. Here's a closer look at each step of the process.

History of issues with thinking or behaviors

To gather a medical history, a doctor usually starts by interviewing the person with cognitive signs and symptoms.

From there, the doctor will often interview someone the person spends a lot of time with. A spouse, partner, family member or friend can shed additional light on possible examples of the symptoms and how they've affected day-to-day functioning.

These interviews help the doctor come up with a timeline of events, spot signs and symptoms that could be linked to dementia, and find out the effects these signs and symptoms are having. The doctor will want to record personality and mood changes and learn how the person with the symptoms performs tasks now compared with the past. Household chores, mental abilities and interacting with others are a few areas a doctor may focus on.

The doctor may ask these questions:

- What's your daily routine like?
- What were the first symptoms? When did you notice them?
- Have the symptoms gotten worse or stayed mostly the same? If they've gotten worse, how quickly have they worsened?

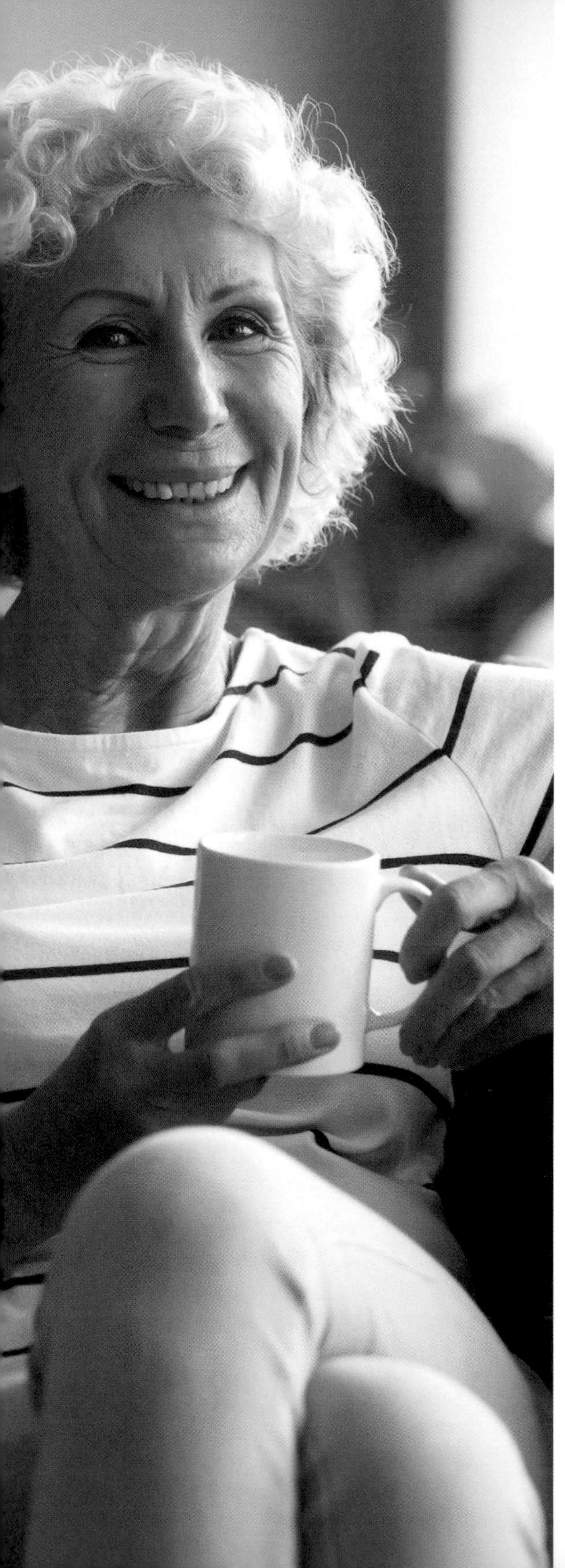

- Are the symptoms severe enough to cause problems with daily activities? Examples include needing help with activities like eating, personal hygiene or dressing. Other examples may include difficulty with more-complex tasks, like writing checks, paying bills, balancing a checkbook, shopping alone for groceries, playing a game of skill, like chess, working on a hobby, following a recipe, taking medication, traveling out of the neighborhood or driving.

The doctor will also ask about:
- Past or ongoing medical and psychiatric concerns
- Any over-the-counter or prescription drugs being taken
- A family history of dementia and other diseases
- The family's social and cultural background

Physical exam

Testing physical health is another important step. A number of factors, like heart disease, thyroid disease, or vision or hearing problems, may affect how well someone can think and learn. A general physical exam helps show if anything physical is contributing to the signs and symptoms of dementia.

As part of a physical exam, you'll have a neurological exam. This looks at how well the brain, spinal cord, and the system of nerves that sends information from your brain and spinal cord to the rest of your

PREPARING FOR AN APPOINTMENT

A past medical history is important when a doctor is evaluating possible signs of dementia. Before an appointment, it's helpful to take these steps:

- Be prepared to talk about the main reason for the appointment.
- Prepare and bring with you a list of symptoms that are unusual or concerning. Include details about when the problems began, how often they happen, and how they affect daily activities, like work, household responsibilities, personal care, decision-making, and remembering appointments or other information.
- Bring a list of current and past medical problems. Include when they were diagnosed and how they were treated.
- Be prepared to share a family history of medical issues that may be related to what you want to discuss. For example, maybe your older sister was diagnosed with Alzheimer's at age 65. Include the issue, who it affected, the person's age when the issue was diagnosed, and the person's relationship to you.
- Prepare and bring a list of medications you're currently taking. Include how much and how often you take any prescription and over-the-counter drugs, as well as herbal and dietary supplements.

body (peripheral nervous system) works. A doctor may test strength, balance, reflexes and how different sensations feel. These tests also help show how strong your muscles are and how well your nerves are working. A neurological exam may spot signs of Parkinson's disease, evidence that you've had a stroke, and other medical issues that can be associated with impaired thinking and physical ability.

As part of the neurological exam, you may have a mental status evaluation. These brief tests help show which thinking and learning functions may be impaired. For example, you may be asked to recite three to five words immediately and then after a five-minute delay.

After a doctor takes a person's medical history and performs a physical exam, lab tests and imaging tests are often done. A person's history, a physical exam, screening and lab tests, and certain imaging tests like an MRI or a CT scan of the head make up a basic dementia evaluation.

OTHER QUESTIONS A DOCTOR MAY ASK

In addition to the general questions usually asked during a basic exam, a doctor may ask several other questions. These are questions that help show trouble in certain areas that are linked to specific types of dementia.

Here are several examples of questions a doctor might ask.

To evaluate memory problems, a doctor may ask if you're:	• Having trouble remembering appointments and medications • Forgetting details of recent conversations • Repeating questions or statements
To evaluate language skills, a doctor may ask if you're having trouble:	• Recalling people's names consistently • Finding the words you want to use • Writing or spelling words
To test visuospatial skills, which help you judge the height of a step or find your way around familiar places, a doctor may ask if you:	• Are having trouble reading • Get lost while driving • Have trouble with depth perception
To test executive function, which involves organizing tasks, thinking abstractly and solving problems, a doctor may ask if you have trouble with:	• Multitasking • Following directions that involve several steps • Organizing bills and finances

A doctor may look for neuropsychiatric symptoms by asking questions like these:	• Have you been experiencing depression or anxiety? • Have you seen objects, animals or people that were not actually there (visual hallucinations)? • Has there been any change in behavior or any socially inappropriate behavior? • Has there been less interest (apathy) in things or activities that used to be important? • Have there been any new food preferences, like sweets?
To evaluate motor symptoms, a doctor may want to see if you:	• Have tremors • Speak more softly than you used to • Walk with a stooped posture or a shuffling gait • Have experienced any changes in your handwriting • Have trouble buttoning buttons • Have had issues with falling • Twitch repeatedly in any muscles • Have trouble swallowing
To look for sleep issues that may be related to dementia, a doctor may ask a person's bed partner questions like:	• Have you ever seen the person appear to act out his or her dreams while sleeping, including punching or flailing arms in the air, screaming, or shouting? • Does the person snore or stop breathing during sleep?
A doctor may also ask about other symptoms, including:	• Lightheadedness upon standing • Constipation • Not being able to hold urine or stool (incontinence) • Loss of sense of smell

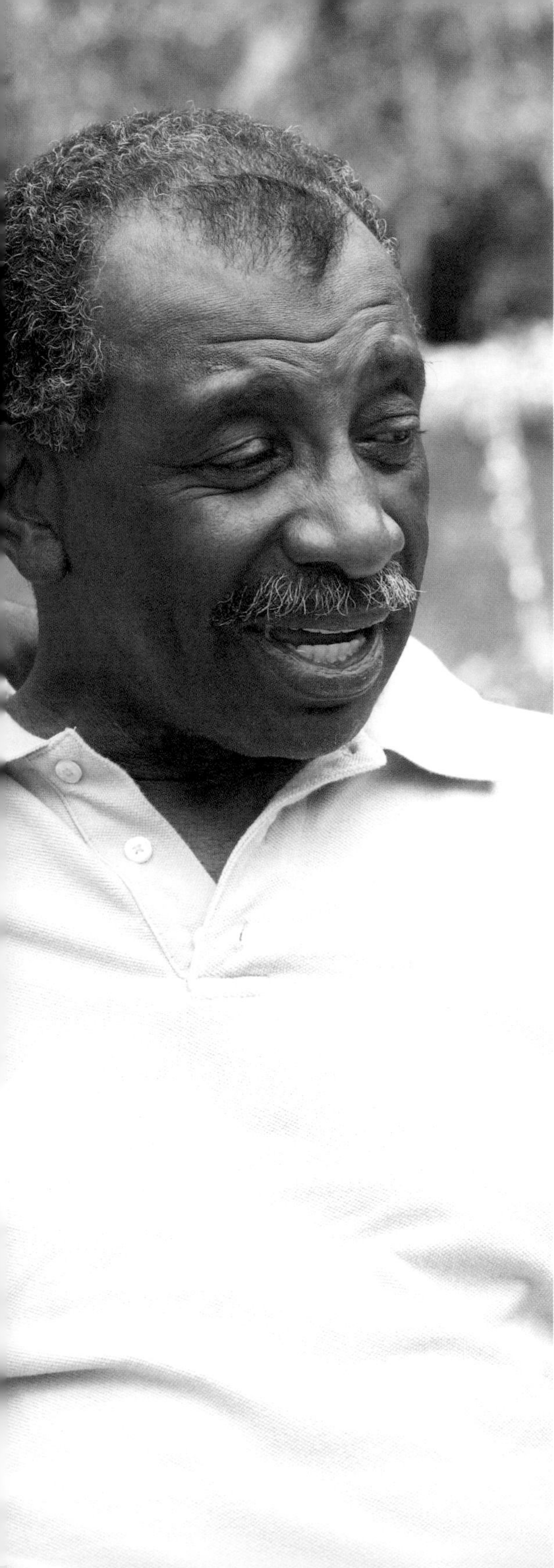

In most cases, the information from this basic evaluation will tell a doctor if dementia is present and what's likely causing it. However, sometimes other tests are needed. You'll learn about these tests next.

WHEN OTHER TESTS ARE NEEDED

If a basic evaluation doesn't yield all the answers a doctor is looking for, other tests may be done. Additional tests aren't often needed and not everyone will get them, but they can help a doctor decide if a person's cognitive issues are part of typical aging or not. If the symptoms seem to be caused by dementia, these tests help show which type of dementia may be causing the symptoms.

Neuropsychological tests

These tests show what cognitive changes a person may be having and how much these changes are affecting the person. They assess the following skills:

- ***Memory and learning.*** This tests how well someone learns and retains new information.
- ***Visuospatial skills.*** This identifies how well someone can navigate when driving, dress, recognize faces or objects, find objects in plain view, and copy designs.
- ***Executive skills.*** This tests how well someone can reason, judge and solve problems.
- ***Thinking speed.*** This tests how quickly someone can process information.

(continued on page 78)

COMMON NEUROPSYCHOLOGICAL TESTS

Here are some of the most common neuropsychological tests doctors use. While these tests may sound simple in some cases, they're designed to be challenging.

What is tested	What the doctor may ask
Recent memory	Learn a list of words and repeat them, and then recall them after a delay of several minutes; after that, identify the words from a longer list of words
Remote memory	Relate facts from personal history, like where the person lived as a child, worked or went to school, or information learned in school
Language skills	• Name common objects in the room, like a desk, light switch or curtain • Follow commands, like repeating a simple phrase or pointing at different items
Motor skills	• Manipulate small pegs • Tap the fingers so that tapping speed can be measured • Grip something so that grip strength can be measured
Executive skills	• Point out the similarities and differences in related words • Solve problems
Visuospatial skills	• Copy figures with blocks • Match figures that look alike • Draw a clock or a complex figure

DRUGS USED FOR SOME CONDITIONS CAN AFFECT MEMORY

If you're concerned about memory lapses, ask your doctor about side effects from the drugs you're taking. Some, including these examples, can affect how well you remember things.

Note that just because you're using one of these medications doesn't mean you'll have memory problems. Also note that medications that aren't on this list may also cause forgetfulness.

Conditions	Drug generic name (brand name)
Anxiety	• Alprazolam (Xanax) • Clonazepam (Klonopin) • Diazepam (Valium)
Depression	• Amitriptyline • Clomipramine • Desipramine (Norpramin) • Doxepin • Imipramine (Tofranil) • Nortriptyline (Pamelor) • Protriptyline (Vivactil)
Allergies	• Brompheniramine (Veltane) • Carbinoxamine • Chlorpheniramine • Clemastine • Cyproheptadine • Diphenhydramine (Benadryl, Aleve PM) • Hydroxyzine • Meclizine
Schizophrenia, bipolar disorder and other mental health conditions	• Clozapine (Clozaril) • Olanzapine (Zyprexa) • Promethazine
Cramps or spasms of the stomach, intestines, bladder; ulcers; and preventing nausea, vomiting and motion sickness	• Atropine products (such as Lomotil) • Dicyclomine (Bentyl) • Homatropine • Hyoscyamine products (Levsin, Levbid) • Propantheline • Scopolamine (Transderm Scop)

Heartburn	• Cimetidine (Tagamet HB) • Famotidine (Pepcid AC)
Heart rhythm problems or heart failure	• Sotalol • Digoxin (Lanoxin)
Muscle pain and spasms	• Carisoprodol • Cyclobenzaprine (Amrix) • Orphenadrine • Tizanidine (Zanaflex)
Pain (opioids)	• Meperidine (Demerol) • Fentanyl (Duragesic) • Oxycodone (Oxycontin, Roxicodone, others) • Tramadol (Ultram, ConZip, others)
Parkinson's disease	• Benztropine (Cogentin) • Trihexyphenidyl
Sleep	• Flurazepam • Temazepam (Restoril) • Triazolam (Halcion) • Zaleplon (Sonata) • Zolpidem (Ambien) • Diphenhydramine (Benadryl, Aleve PM, others) • Doxylamine succinate (Unisom SleepTabs)
Urinary incontinence	• Darifenacin (Enablex) • Fesoterodine (Toviaz) • Oxybutynin (Ditropan XL) • Flavoxate • Solifenacin (Vesicare) • Tolterodine (Detrol, Detrol LA)

(continued from page 74)

- ***Attention.*** This shows how well someone pays attention over time, even with distractions or while doing more than one thing.
- ***Language use.*** This indicates how well someone writes, and understands when being spoken to. And it shows how often someone has trouble thinking of common words while speaking or makes errors in word use or spelling.

Your current level of cognition (memory, language, reasoning, visuospatial ability, judgment and attention) may be tested and compared with normal values or previous levels to show if brain function has changed.

The results of these tests help assess how well someone is likely to handle a variety of common but complex tasks, like following recipes and managing finances. They can also provide information that may help families make decisions regarding safety at home, living alone, and what other assistance and support may be needed.

A doctor can also use these tests to spot the difference between dementia and another condition, like depression, to see if they're occurring at the same time. This can be helpful in the early stages of dementia.

Imaging tests

As you've learned, brain imaging tests are part of an evaluation for dementia. They're used to get a better picture of what's going on inside the brain. Brain imaging offers additional information that may help a doctor figure out what's causing symptoms. Some imaging tests are routine. Some are used when the diagnosis is uncertain. And others are used mostly for research.

Brain imaging tests are generally described as structural, functional or molecular. While the type of imaging needed depends on what information will help a doctor most, structural imaging tests are used most often to help determine the cause of dementia.

Structural imaging shows the size, shape and location of the structures in your brain. It can detect strokes, tumors, prior traumatic brain injury, hydrocephalus or other structural issues in the brain. It can also show brain shrinkage (atrophy). Computerized tomography (CT) and magnetic resonance imaging (MRI) are examples; they're the structural imaging tests doctors use for an overall assessment of dementia.

When it's available, MRI is the structural imaging test most doctors prefer for cognitive concerns. The pattern of changes seen on MRI can provide clues as to what's causing symptoms of dementia.

For example, in Alzheimer's disease dementia, MRI may show shrinking (atrophy) in the hippocampus, a part of the brain that's involved in memory. MRI is also more likely to help determine if blood vessel (cerebrovascular) disease, like a stroke, is contributing to the dementia.

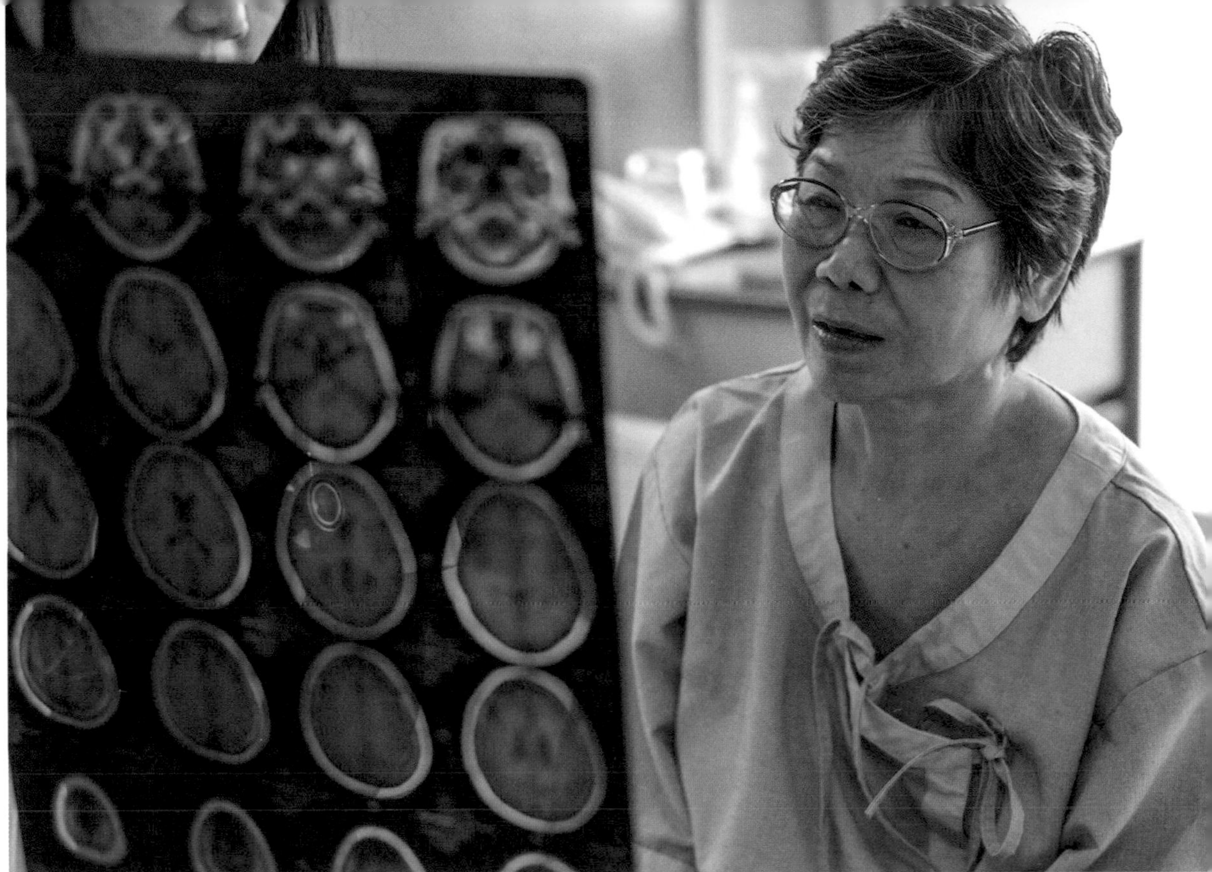

Here's more on MRI and CT scans.

Computerized tomography (CT) A CT scan takes a series of images from different angles. The angles are combined to show a picture of the brain, including bones, blood vessels and soft tissues.

When you have a CT scan, you lie on a table inside a doughnut-shaped machine. A scanner inside the machine rotates around you, emitting a series of X-ray beams. A computer collects and processes these scans, combining them into a single, detailed image. A CT scan offers more-detailed pictures than an X-ray does.

Magnetic resonance imaging (MRI) For this medical imaging technique, you lie on a table inside a long, tubelike machine that produces a magnetic field. The magnetic field aligns atoms in your body, and radio waves cause these atoms to emit faint signals. These signals create images of the brain, similar to slices in a loaf of bread. An MRI offers a more detailed picture than a CT scan does.

Functional and molecular imaging

Other imaging tests are occasionally used as part of a dementia exam. They're sometimes used when a diagnosis isn't clear after a routine exam. These tests are described as functional imaging or molecular imaging.

Functional imaging shows brain activity rather than brain structure. It detects changes in the chemical makeup of brain tissue, like how energy is processed or blood flows in the brain. These images help link functions, like listening to a conversation or recalling a memory, to different parts of the brain.

Based on the changes seen in functional images, a doctor may be able to spot a pattern of abnormal brain activity that's seen in

CT SCAN VS. MRI SCAN

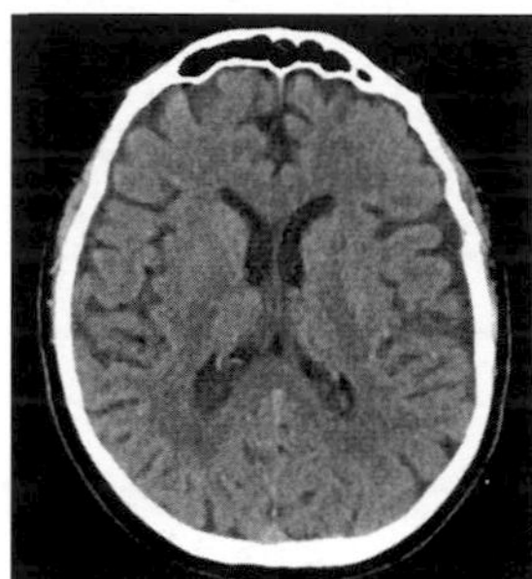

Structural imaging shows the size and shape of structures inside the brain. This image is a computerized tomography (CT) scan of a healthy brain.

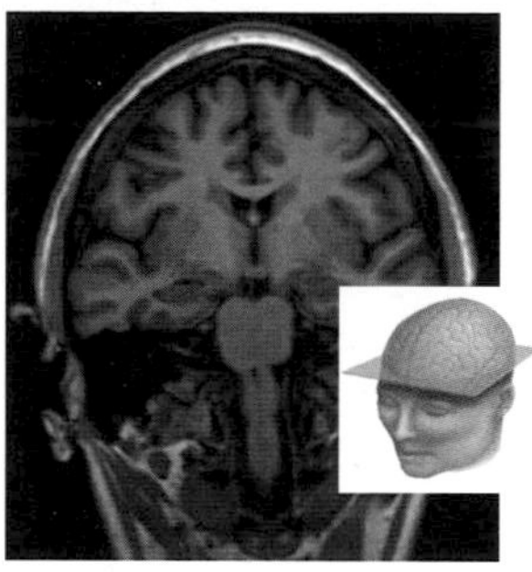

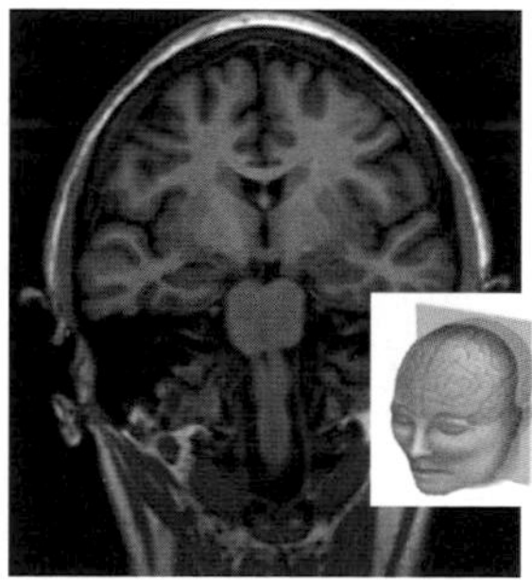

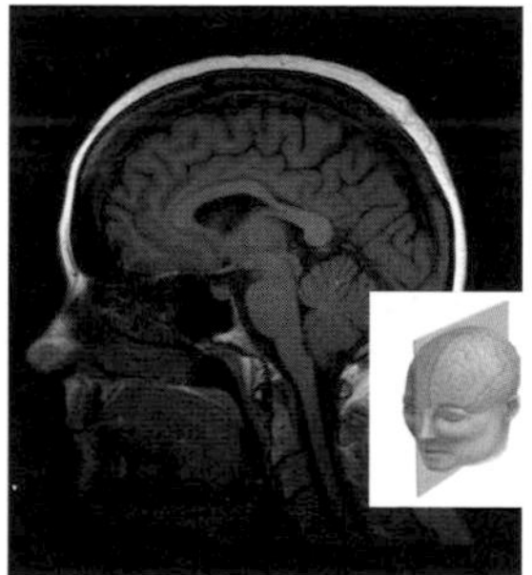

These are magnetic resonance imaging (MRI) scans, which offer a little more detail than CT scans do. Different views of the brain are helpful because each one provides different details about the brain.

Alzheimer's disease or a related dementia. Examples of functional imaging tests include a fluorodeoxyglucose PET-CT scan and single-photon emission computerized tomography (SPECT).

Molecular imaging creates pictures that show and measure brain disease. It uses radioactive tracers (radiotracers) with positron emission technology (PET) or MRI technology. Molecular imaging lets researchers see processes in the brain down to the molecule. When tracers are released into the brain, they trigger chemical changes that are picked up in images.

Molecular imaging tests are currently used mostly for research. They offer information that other tests can't; for example, they can spot clumps of beta-amyloid (plaques) in the living brain. These plaques are a hallmark of Alzheimer's disease.

Functional and molecular neuroimaging tests used mostly by researchers include functional magnetic resonance imaging (fMRI) and tau PET. Functional magnetic resonance imaging (fMRI) uses the magnetic properties of blood to record activity in different areas of the brain and detect changes in this activity over short periods of time.

FUNCTIONAL MRI (FMRI)

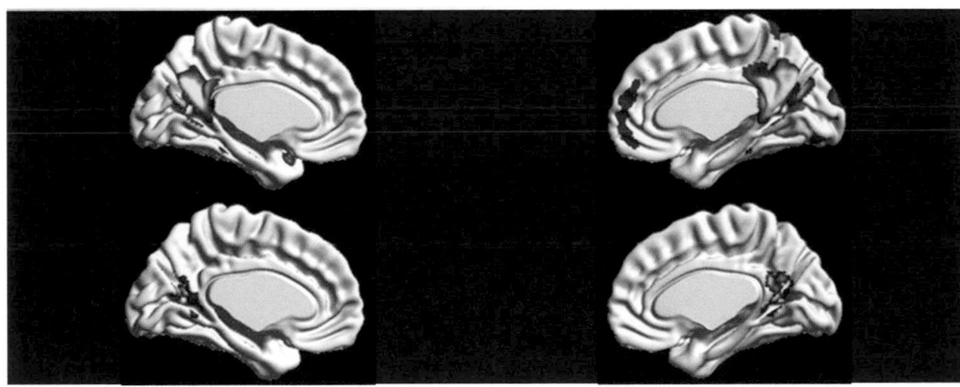

In these functional MRI (fMRI) images, the two on top highlight the areas of the brain that seem to be affected by Alzheimer's disease. In the top images, activity in these areas is normal. The bottom two images show how Alzheimer's disease leads to less activity in the same areas of the brain.

PET scans and single-photon emission computerized tomography (SPECT) are examples of fMRI.

Positron emission tomography (PET) A positron emission tomography (PET) scan is seen both as a functional imaging test and a molecular imaging test. It provides information about the metabolic or molecular activity in the brain. A small amount of a radioactive drug called a tracer is injected into the body. See how a PET scan shows if someone is experiencing dementia in the images below.

In a fluorodeoxyglucose (FDG) PET scan, the tracer collects in areas that have higher levels of brain activity. These are often areas of disease. Diseased areas of the brain are less active, so they take up less of the tracer. In turn, less metabolism can be seen in the PET scan.

POSITRON EMISSION TOMOGRAPHY (PET) SCAN

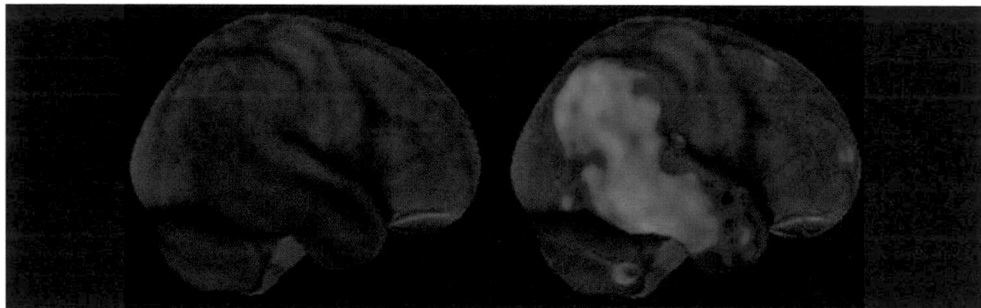

A PET scan uses a radioactive drug called a tracer to spot areas of disease. These images are of a type of PET scan called a fluorodeoxyglucose (FDG) PET scan. This type of PET scan shows areas of the brain where there's decreased glucose metabolism, meaning that fewer nutrients are broken down. Showing the areas of the brain where nutrients are broken down poorly can help show if someone is experiencing Alzheimer's disease dementia or another type of dementia. In these images, cool colors show areas of normal activity, making a normal brain look almost black. Warm colors (green, yellow and red) show areas of abnormally low activity. The left image is from a person with normal brain metabolism. The right image shows the brain of a person with Alzheimer's dementia. Green and yellow colors show decreased brain metabolism.

Tau PET scan Tau is a protein that's considered a hallmark of Alzheimer's. PET scans that detect tau (see page 84) aren't used in doctors' offices yet, but they're commonly used by researchers in clinical trials.

Just as there are tau and amyloid PET scans today, researchers are hopeful that one day PET scans will be able to detect proteins in the brain that are linked to other types of dementia. Examples include TDP-43, which is linked to frontotemporal degeneration, and alpha-synuclein, which is linked to Lewy body dementia.

Single-photon emission computerized tomography (SPECT) Like a PET scan, a SPECT scan uses a radioactive tracer. This imaging test uses a camera to detect the tracer once it's in your body. The camera rotates around your head to create 3D images of your brain. A SPECT scan can show which areas of the brain are more active and which ones show less blood flow.

Spinal fluid tests

A spinal fluid test is typically done to look

AMYLOID PET SCAN

The Food and Drug Administration (FDA) has approved imaging of beta-amyloid with a PET scan. A biomarker of Alzheimer's disease, beta-amyloid is deposited in the brain years before symptoms of Alzheimer's develop.

In this image, a PET scan combined with an amyloid radiotracer shows the amount of beta-amyloid (plaques) in the brain. Bright orange and red colors show areas where the radiotracer has been retained. These areas show where plaques, a hallmark of Alzheimer's disease, are present.

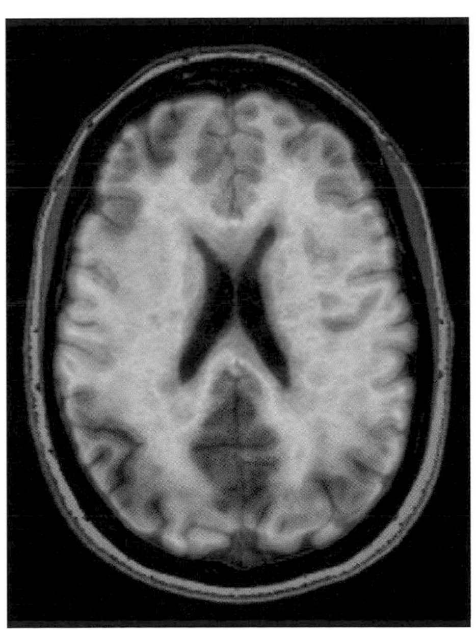

for signs of infection or inflammation in the fluid around the brain and spinal cord. This test can spot a range of diseases, including ones may be treatable.

A spinal fluid test is also used to measure levels of amyloid and tau around the brain and spinal cord. These proteins are biomarkers of Alzheimer's disease. You'll learn more about biomarkers in Part 2.

Amyloid and tau are used to confirm if Alzheimer's disease is causing a person's cognitive impairment or contributing to it. A spinal fluid test is particularly helpful when other tests can't clearly confirm it.

These and other proteins may also be measured when someone seems to have rapidly progressing dementia or in cases of young-onset Alzheimer's disease. A combination of low amyloid and a higher level of tau is the pattern a doctor looks for in the cerebrospinal fluid when diagnosing Alzheimer's disease.

Doctors may also use a spinal fluid test to help determine if something other than Alz-

TAU PET SCAN

Tau is the other hallmark of Alzheimer's disease. Studies suggest that tau deposits in the brain are more closely related to symptoms of Alzheimer's disease than amyloid deposits are. Researchers continue to study the development of tau in the brain in an effort to find characteristics that can be used to help diagnose Alzheimer's disease.

This PET scan highlights tau deposits in the brain. Note that bright yellow, orange and red colors show areas of the brain where tau deposits have developed.

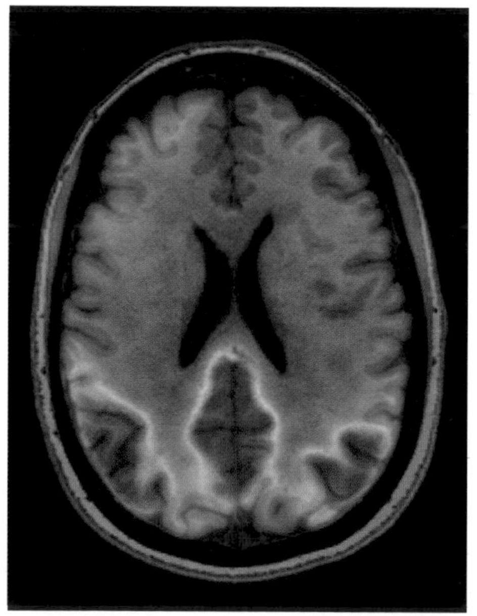

heimer's disease is causing dementia-like symptoms. In the future, a spinal fluid test may be used to decide if someone is a good candidate for medications that may prevent, delay or slow Alzheimer's disease.

Blood test

Researchers are developing a blood test that can detect beta-amyloid in the brain, a hallmark of Alzheimer's disease. Several promising blood tests have been developed and are currently under study. This protein is an early sign of Alzheimer's disease, appearing before cognitive impairment takes place.

Finding beta-amyloid with a blood test could help doctors find Alzheimer's disease in the brain sooner, which may lead to earlier treatment and maybe even prevention. Learn more about the development of a blood test for Alzheimer's in Chapter 20.

RULING OUT OTHER CONDITIONS

In addition to ruling out causes of dementia that may be treatable, a doctor will want to see if symptoms may be caused by something that isn't dementia — but that can still cause memory and thinking changes. These include:

Age-associated impairment

As you get older, you may not be able to learn and retain new information as well as you used to. You also may not process information as quickly as you once did.

This is normal and to be expected. That's because with age-associated impairment, you can still think and learn. It may take longer to manage daily tasks, but this often simply means adjustments, like writing things down that you want to remember or reading instructions a couple of times to complete a form.

Delirium

Delirium affects attention and focus. It may cause you to drift in and out of awareness, making it seem like you have dementia. But delirium is different from dementia. Unlike dementia, which comes on gradually, delirium usually comes on suddenly.

Because delirium and dementia can occur at the same time, it's not always easy to tell the difference between the two. Delirium can last for just a couple of days or for as long as a couple of months. But unlike dementia, delirium is almost always temporary if the cause is identified and treated. Common causes of delirium include infection or medication side effects.

Depression

Depression can produce symptoms similar to dementia. Loss of interest, confusion and lack of focus are all examples. People with depression are generally aware of issues

GUIDELINES FOR NEUROCOGNITIVE DISORDERS

Doctors use the Diagnostic and Statistical Manual of Mental Disorders (DSM-5) to diagnose hundreds of mental health conditions, including disorders like dementia. The criteria is used to guide treatment decisions and determine health insurance coverage. Published by the American Psychiatric Association, this manual is now in its fifth edition.

The DSM-5 outlines three main categories of neurocognitive disorders:

1. Mild neurocognitive disorder
2. Major neurocognitive disorder
3. Delirium

In making a diagnosis, one of the categories will be paired with the condition that's thought to be causing the symptoms. For example, a person may be diagnosed with a mild neurocognitive disorder due to Alzheimer's disease. This reflects a two-step process: first, determine the level of cognitive impairment and its effect on a person's ability to function in everyday life, and, second, find out what's causing the impairment.

While the classifications in the DSM-5 differ from previous editions, little may change in how doctors diagnose Alzheimer's disease. The terms *mild neurocognitive disorder* and *major neurocognitive disorder* are already used by psychiatrists. These terms also match up with the way the terms *dementia* and *mild cognitive impairment* are used in this book.

they may be having with thinking and remembering. This is different from dementia.

With dementia, the person having the symptoms sometimes is not as aware; often, friends and family are the ones who notice and report changes.

Mild cognitive impairment

Some people have problems with memory loss that are noticeable but aren't significant enough to disrupt daily living. Their test results may show some cognitive impairment but not enough to be dementia.

These people may have mild cognitive impairment, which isn't as severe as dementia but is of greater concern than the memory changes of typical aging.

Because mild cognitive impairment makes it more likely that you'll develop dementia in the future, you may need regular testing to check for further cognitive changes.

WHEN TEST RESULTS SIGNAL DEMENTIA

As you've learned, evaluating symptoms to tell whether they're related to dementia is a step-by-step process. Sometimes, symptoms aren't related to dementia at all. But sometimes they are.

The Diagnostic and Statistical Manual of Mental Disorders (DSM-5) is commonly used to diagnose dementia (see page 86). In this manual, dementia is described as a major neurocognitive disorder. According to this criteria, a doctor often says someone has dementia if:

- The person has problems with at least two cognitive functions (see page 50)
- Daily life is disrupted and the person is less able to maintain independence
- Symptoms aren't explained by depression or delirium

Other signals of dementia

A doctor may look for signs of uncharacteristic behavior, like apathy, anxiety, irritability, and inappropriate actions or language. These signs may not be seen as cognitive decline on their own, but they're associated with dementia. They're also often some of the earliest signs that alert family and friends that something may be wrong.

People with dementia may repeat questions or conversations over and over. They may misplace personal items, forget important events or appointments, or get lost on familiar routes. They may have trouble remembering common words or make mistakes when talking or writing. Some people with dementia have trouble recognizing familiar faces or objects. Later on, they may also have trouble using simple tools, like scissors or a fork and knife.

Those affected by dementia may be unaware of memory loss or other problems with how they're thinking. They may make plans that are unrealistic. For example, people with dementia may insist on putting a lot of money into a business they were never interested in before.

People affected by dementia may not observe accepted norms and conventions. They may tell inappropriate or off-color jokes in public and disregard social rules, like being polite, maintaining personal space and keeping one's voice down.

It's important not to jump to conclusions if you or a loved one experiences any of these symptoms — especially if just one of them appears. Remember that dementia is a collection of symptoms (syndrome).

In addition, it's critical not to self-diagnose, either by checking a symptoms list or taking a screening test — the kind found online or at the drugstore. These tests are generally unreliable, and the results can be easily misinterpreted, causing undue worry from a low score or a false sense of security from a high score.

Work with your doctor and the other specialists recommended to you. They're in the best position to make a diagnosis and offer appropriate plans for treatment.

IDENTIFYING THE CAUSE OF DEMENTIA

The various tests and procedures described in this chapter help a doctor reach a diagnosis of dementia. But that's not the end of the story. After diagnosing someone with dementia, a doctor has an even more complex question to answer: What type of dementia is causing these signs and symptoms?

Although different types of dementia have signs and symptoms in common, each type develops in its own ways, with differences that aren't always easy to see. For example, memory loss is a symptom of both Alzheimer's disease and frontotemporal degeneration. But in Alzheimer's, memory loss is often one of the first symptoms to develop. In a common subtype of frontotemporal degeneration, emotional or personality changes typically come first, and memory loss can occur much later.

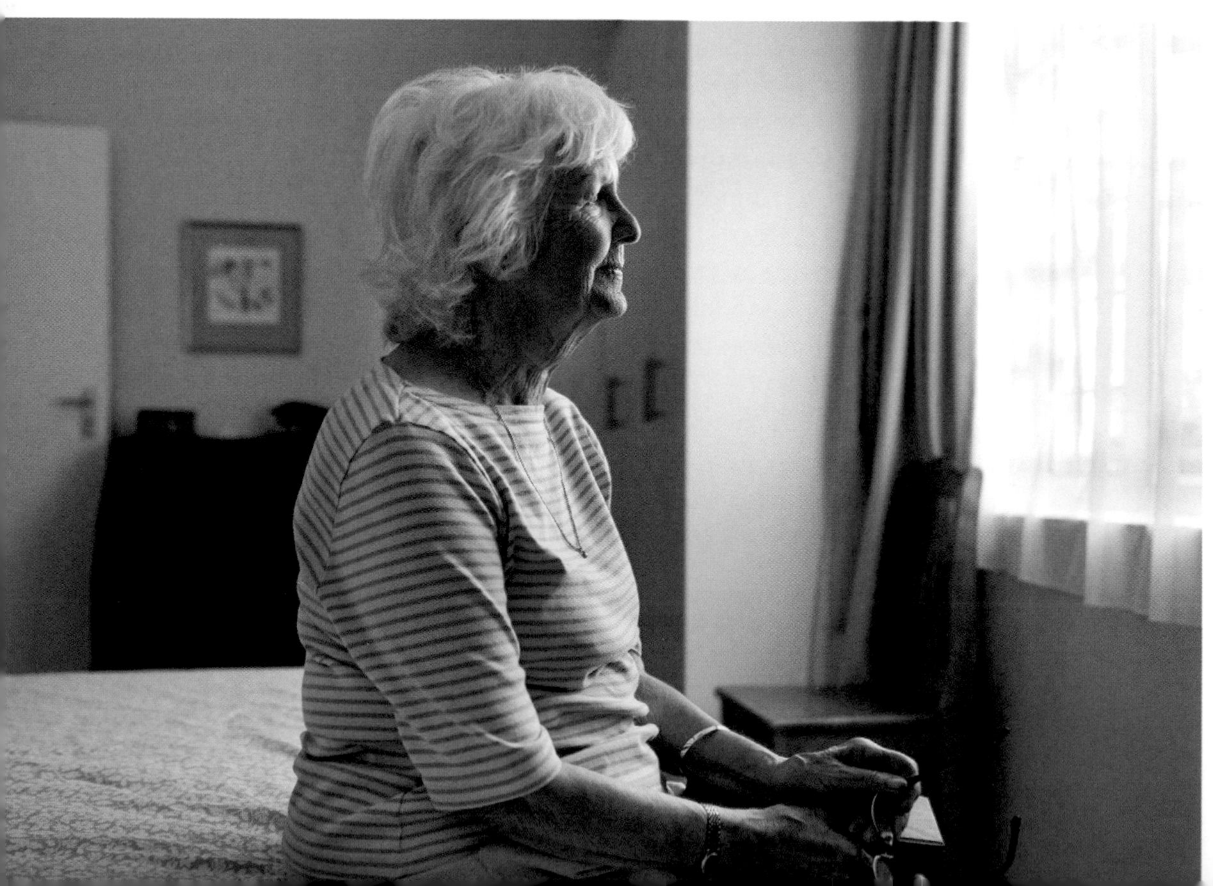

So how can doctors identify what's causing the dementia? In the same way they diagnose dementia in the first place — through a process of evaluation, testing, analysis and comparison. Once again, doctors must look at the signs and symptoms together to narrow the field of possible causes.

Sometimes figuring out what type of dementia is affecting someone is easier than at other times. For example, if strokes are part of the medical history and the doctor can say that cognitive decline started shortly after a stroke, there's a good chance that the type of dementia is vascular, meaning that blood flow to the brain is impaired. Other times, more testing and lab work may be needed before a doctor can say what's causing the symptoms.

Sometimes, even after all the tests have been done, it can be hard to determine what type of dementia is causing someone's symptoms. For example, several common symptoms of Lewy body dementia are the same as those of Alzheimer's disease. The same may be said of common symptoms of vascular cognitive impairment and of Alzheimer's disease.

Adding to the challenge, someone can have several causes of dementia at the same time. For example, most people diagnosed with Alzheimer's disease also have other causes of dementia, including cerebrovascular disease or Lewy body disease.

Even if a doctor can't pinpoint the exact type of dementia, that doesn't change the level of care that's needed. People with dementia and their families can still get treatment for symptoms, seek support and resources, and discuss plans for the future.

It's also important to note that while no two people will experience dementia in the same way, identifying the type of dementia gives families and health care professionals additional information to provide the best care and support.

Compare it to cancer, for example. A person diagnosed with cancer expects to know what type of cancer it is to ensure that it can be treated and that symptoms can be managed in the best way possible. It's no different for people diagnosed with dementia.

HOW A TIMELY DIAGNOSIS CAN HELP

Sarah, age 68, hasn't felt like herself in months. In addition to increasing forgetfulness, she often feels confused and anxious. She needs more help around the house but gets defensive and snaps at friends and neighbors when they try to help her — something she never did before.

Sarah's daughter is urging her to see a doctor, but she's not on board with the idea. She claims that if the family can just be patient for a little longer, she'll work things out and shake off the symptoms on her own. If she were being honest, however, Sarah might admit that she's afraid of going in for medical tests.

COMMON CAUSES OF DEMENTIA

Here are several of the most common symptoms of the most common causes of dementia. You'll learn more in later chapters of this book.

Common causes	Common symptoms
Alzheimer's disease	• Difficulty remembering recently acquired information • Problems with judgment and reasoning • Difficulty carrying out everyday tasks • Trouble applying words and names to people and objects
Lewy body dementia	• Memory, attention and alertness that comes and goes • Seeing and hearing things that aren't real • Movement problems, like walking slowly or shuffling, and rigid muscles • Thinking problems like confusion, poor attention and memory loss • Sleep problems like acting out dreams while asleep
Frontotemporal degeneration	• Personality changes and inappropriate social behavior • Change in dietary preferences, like developing a sweet tooth • Difficulty planning and organizing activities • Trouble using and understanding words • Movement problems like tremors, muscle spasms and lack of coordination
Vascular cognitive impairment	• Slower thinking • Trouble paying attention and concentrating • Not being able to organize thoughts or actions • Difficulty deciding what to do next

Like many other people, Sarah hopes that what she doesn't know won't hurt her. Her daughter assures her that seeing a doctor is the right thing to do.

The truth is that whatever the result — good news or bad news — the doctor will find ways to make Sarah's life easier and ease everyone's concerns. The sooner that Sarah makes an appointment, the better her chances are for getting help.

People often don't recognize a serious medical problem when the signs and symptoms first appear. They may pass them off as a typical part of aging. Or they may see confusion, forgetfulness and mood swings as separate problems instead of drawing connections between them. Some people may be aware that something's going on but are afraid of what they might learn — they'd just as soon not know whether or not they have a serious condition.

It's true that if Sarah is experiencing memory loss, confusion and extreme mood swings, a doctor will very likely consider dementia as a possible diagnosis. But her symptoms may be caused by something else. For example, she may have a treatable condition, like a thyroid disorder, depression or drug interaction. The earlier Sarah makes an appointment, has tests and gets a diagnosis, the more options she'll likely have to improve her symptoms and her quality of life.

For example, the doctor may find that Sarah's problems with memory and household chores are typical for her age. What about her confusion and mood changes? Those could be a result of drug interactions from new medications that she started taking last month. Simply changing the drugs she's taking could help Sarah feel her life rapidly return to normal.

On the other hand, tests may exclude treatable causes and point toward dementia.

Though this diagnosis may be hard to hear, getting this news early may be a good thing. In general, a timely diagnosis can lead to a higher quality of life for the person affected, less stress for family care partners and more time to enjoy the present.

A timely diagnosis can also:

- Provide relief because it provides answers and clarity to concerns and changes.
- Open up access to helpful information, support, resources and services.
- Help someone with dementia continue to live independently, at home, longer.
- Offer someone living with dementia the chance to find new or additional ways of staying connected and engaged by seeking out social groups, clubs and arts organizations that can all be helpful in maintaining quality of life.
- Allow people living with dementia and their families to see cognitive changes as part of the disease process, rather than as personal failings.
- Offer an opportunity to review one's financial situation. This may also be a good time to talk with family and legal experts about topics like care planning,

GETTING THE DIAGNOSIS: QUESTIONS TO ASK YOUR DOCTOR

What type of dementia is it?
Hearing that you have dementia will help you understand what's been causing the changes, but this doesn't tell the whole story. Ask your doctor what's causing the dementia. Alzheimer's disease is the most common cause, but there are other types.

What medications might be helpful?
Only a handful of medications are approved by the FDA to treat Alzheimer's disease, and they're often prescribed to treat other types of dementia, as well. Ask your doctor if any might be appropriate and helpful. Also ask about side effects of medications. Other symptoms associated with dementia, like depression, anxiety and sleep issues, also may be treated with medication. You'll learn about medications later on.

What can I do to live the best life possible with this diagnosis?
After a diagnosis, it's important to focus on planning for the future. It's also important to focus on living the best life possible now. Ask your doctor what you can do to compensate for cognitive changes and improve your overall well-being. This may include things like keeping a calendar, getting regular exercise and staying socially connected. Learn more in Chapter 14.

Should I enroll in research?
Some clinical trials or other research studies may be available for your particular situation. By taking part in research, you can help provide valuable insight into possible treatments, as well as ways to improve care and support. Participating in a clinical trial allows you to:

- Play an active role in your own health care
- Be a part of trials that are testing possible treatments
- Help future generations by contributing to dementia research

Where can I get more information and support?
This book is a good start for information related to dementia; you'll also find additional resources starting on page 390. Your doctor and others on your health care team may also have more information that you'll find helpful.

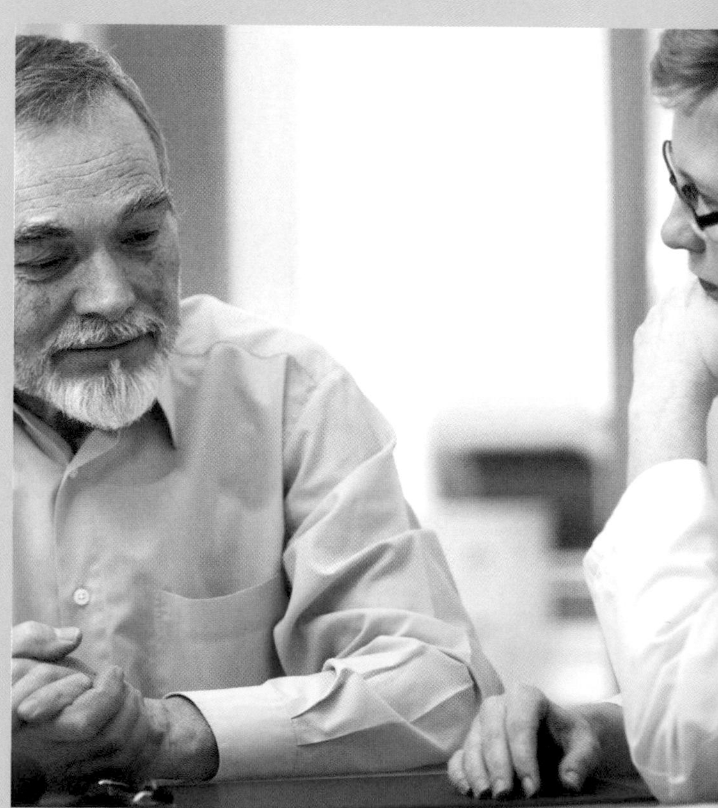

advance directives and arrangements for power of attorney.

After a diagnosis

A dementia diagnosis, whether it's yours or that of a loved one, can be a frightening experience. It's important to give yourself time to work through your feelings and adjust emotionally. You'll learn more about steps to take after a diagnosis in Chapter 13.

Don't be afraid to ask family members, friends and colleagues for help. A doctor, nurse or psychologist can work with you and your family to develop strategies to manage symptoms. Health care workers can help you decide the right time and way to tell others. Resources in your community also may help. A local chapter of the Alzheimer's Association is an example.

Most importantly, take time to learn more about the disease. This book and its list of resources (see page 390) provide a good starting point. Learning about the disease provides explanations for the changes that will happen over time and helps people with dementia and their care partners find ways to live well with dementia.

Each individual is unique, and many people are living with illnesses or conditions. But an illness or condition doesn't define who a person is or determine the quality of an individual's life at any given time. How well people live with dementia depends on the diagnosis, their coping styles, their attitudes, and actions and choices they make. Life goes on after a diagnosis, and people can — and do — live well with dementia.

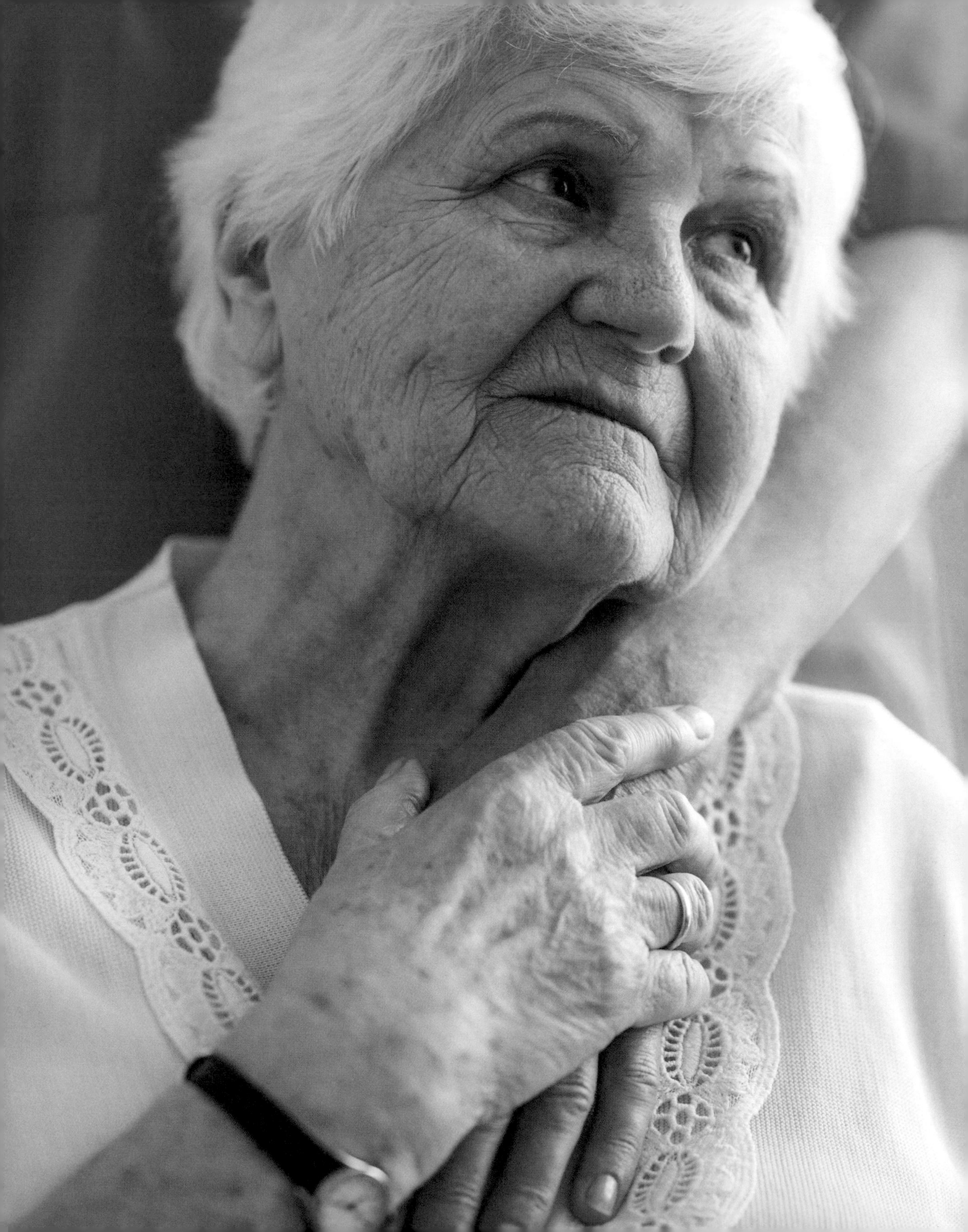

PART 2

Alzheimer's disease

Of the 60 million people around the world living with dementia, two-thirds or more have Alzheimer's disease. Alzheimer's disease is the sixth leading cause of death in the United States and the third most common cause of death for older people.

While these facts may seem to paint a bleak picture, there is hope. First, there's hope in diagnosing Alzheimer's earlier than ever before, before signs and symptoms appear. This offers time and new opportunities for people living with Alzheimer's disease as researchers continue to search for a cure.

In the next few chapters, you'll learn what researchers know about how Alzheimer's disease develops. You'll also learn what's being done to diagnose it more quickly and accurately, allowing people affected by it to live longer, quality lives with this disease.

One exciting development lies in the study of biomarkers — tests used to show a disease, rule out a disease or predict if someone is likely to develop a disease.

Researchers have learned that certain tests can tell if someone has or will develop Alzheimer's disease long before symptoms develop. This breakthrough has led to new ways of looking at Alzheimer's disease and determining who's at risk of developing the cognitive impairment associated with it. You'll learn more about biomarkers in this chapter and then later in this section.

Hope for Alzheimer's lies not just in preventing it entirely, but also in coming up with targeted therapies that can help people maintain their function and enjoy a fulfilling, meaningful life for as long as possible with this disease.

"HOW ALZHEIMER'S IS UNDERSTOOD, DIAGNOSED AND TREATED IS SHIFTING."

CHAPTER 5

The science of Alzheimer's disease

Alzheimer's disease is the most common cause of dementia among adults age 65 and older. Family members and friends see the poignant impact of the disease in someone living with Alzheimer's disease — a gradual loss of intellect and memory, impairment of good judgment, changes in personality, and the inability to perform the tasks of daily living.

Alzheimer's is a neurodegenerative disease. This means nerve cells in the brain lose function and over time will die.

As the cells in the brain stop connecting with each other and die, more of a person's abilities are affected, including memory, language, and the ability to perform calculations or navigate directions. People with Alzheimer's may lose some or all of their ability to communicate, recognize familiar objects, control behavior, and satisfy basic physical urges, like eating or urinating. In the final stages of the disease, they may be bedridden and need others to care for them.

The course that Alzheimer's disease takes can vary, but it often shortens a person's lifespan. Death is generally caused by complications of not being able to move or to eat or drink properly. Pneumonia and other infections and problems with how well blood flows through the body are also factors that lead to death.

In 2011, the U.S. government enacted the National Plan to Address Alzheimer's Disease, in full recognition of this growing health crisis. Its focus is to prevent future cases of Alzheimer's disease and better meet the needs of the millions of American families currently facing this disease.

The National Plan outlines specific goals for meeting some of the most burdensome challenges associated with Alzheimer's disease.

This plan has five goals:

- Prevent and effectively treat Alzheimer's disease by 2025
- Train health care providers and develop new approaches to improve the quality of care
- Expand support for people with Alzheimer's disease and their care partners and families
- Make the public more aware of Alzheimer's disease
- Improve the collection of data to monitor the progress of research

The National Plan to Address Alzheimer's Disease offers a solid framework to deal with this health crisis from both a research and care perspective. For more information about the plan and the progress being made, visit *www.alzheimers.gov.*

This is the first of several chapters in Part 2, which is devoted to Alzheimer's disease. This chapter describes the science behind Alzheimer's disease. It also introduces two of the most common features of Alzheimer's disease: amyloid plaques and neurofibrillary tangles.

BREAKDOWN IN THE BRAIN

Alzheimer's disease affects the brain by killing its most basic components, its nerve cells (neurons). Neurons relay messages within the brain and between the brain and the rest of the body. This process by which Alzheimer's disease destroys neurons is called neurodegeneration. In addition to destroying neurons, Alzheimer's disease also disrupts the communication points (synapses) between neurons. This makes it hard for nerve cells to get messages to each other. How strongly neurons connect to each other also forms the basis of memory in specific areas of the brain, like the hippocampus.

In most people, the first place Alzheimer's disease strikes is the hippocampus. Found inside the brain's limbic system, the hippocampus is the central switchboard for your memory. This is why memory loss is often one of the first symptoms of dementia caused by Alzheimer's. When Alzheimer's disease involves other brain structures, it can also cause disorientation and make it hard to tell where objects or places are in relation to each other.

In addition to the hippocampus, Alzheimer's disease attacks other parts of the limbic system. The amygdala is one example. The amygdala is important for learning and for the emotional part of experiences. From there, the disease spreads to other parts of the brain, including the frontal, parietal and temporal lobes.

The frontal lobes control thinking, planning, organizing, problem-solving, short-term memory and movement. The parietal lobes interpret information involving your senses, like hearing. The temporal lobes process information from your senses and play a

BRAIN CHEMICALS AFFECTED BY ALZHEIMER'S

Chemical	Primary function
Acetylcholine	Attention, memory, thought and judgment
Dopamine	Movement, reward and pleasure
Glutamate	Learning and remote memory
Norepinephrine	Emotional response
Serotonin	Mood and anxiety

role in language and memory storage. By knowing more about the parts of the brain Alzheimer's affects, you can begin to understand the symptoms this disease causes.

As it gets harder and, eventually, impossible for neurons to talk to each other in the brain, other functions become impaired. For example, it becomes harder to make decisions and speak and write.

Gradually, the disease makes it difficult for people to care for themselves and perform tasks they've handled for many years. Some people with Alzheimer's disease also become aggressive and paranoid. That's because Alzheimer's disease ultimately attacks the limbic system, the part of the brain that influences instincts and emotions.

Alzheimer's disease also destroys neurons deep within the brain in an area called the basal nucleus of Meynert. This area is rich in a chemical called acetylcholine (as-uh-teel-KOH-leen). This chemical plays an important role in how memories are formed and recalled. Damage to this area of the brain leads to a sharp drop in the chemical, compounding memory loss caused by damage to other parts of the brain. At the same time, Alzheimer's disease also depletes the brain of other chemicals, including dopamine, glutamate, norepinephrine and serotonin. The chart on page 99 shows the functions affected by low levels of certain chemicals. As Alzheimer's spreads, the size of the brain shrinks (atrophies).

Proteins gone awry

Two classic types of damage seen in Alzheimer's disease are beta-amyloid plaques and tau (pronounced tou) neurofibrillary tangles. Amyloid plaques are large deposits of proteins that make it hard for neurons to communicate with each other. Neurofibrillary tangles come from proteins called tau that have changed shape. They, too, destroy cells in the brain.

In 1907, Dr. Alois Alzheimer published an account of a woman who was paranoid and had severe memory loss. In his report, Dr.

FINDING ALZHEIMER'S DISEASE BEFORE SYMPTOMS APPEAR

How Alzheimer's is understood, diagnosed and treated is shifting. Researchers are studying changes in the brain that happen *before* someone shows signs and symptoms of Alzheimer's disease dementia. The hope is that by spotting these changes earlier, drugs and other interventions may keep the disease from taking hold in the brain. This knowledge may also lead to new treatments for people who already have Alzheimer's disease.

To detect Alzheimer's in its earliest stages, researchers have created a framework of biomarkers to tell if someone has the disease even before the first symptoms begin.

Biomarkers are already used to screen for other conditions, like high blood pressure, high cholesterol, diabetes and cancer. Certain tests are done to show if you have these conditions, even if you're not having any symptoms. The idea is to take the same approach with Alzheimer's, instead of diagnosing the disease only after someone's showing symptoms of it.

Just as blood sugar and A1C testing are used to tell if someone has diabetes, this framework uses known Alzheimer's biomarkers to tell if someone has the disease, even without signs or symptoms. According to this framework, positron emission tomography (PET) scans and cerebrospinal fluid tests for the hallmark proteins of Alzheimer's would detect whether someone has Alzheimer's disease based only on the presence of both amyloid and tau proteins in the brain.

It's important to note that the presence of amyloid and tau proteins doesn't guarantee that someone will develop the cognitive symptoms of the disease. Some people with these protein deposits never develop cognitive decline. This is not much different from

Alzheimer said he found a heavy buildup of plaques and tangles in the woman's brain when he examined it after her death.

Plaques and tangles are seen in other forms of dementia, too. In fact, they can even develop in people who don't have any symptoms of dementia at all. But people with Alzheimer's dementia have far more plaques and tangles and often have them at an earlier age.

Plaques Plaques are large clumps of proteins and other pieces of cells that can't be absorbed into the body. They're found between and around living nerve cells. The plaques seen in Alzheimer's disease are made mostly of the protein beta-amyloid. Bits of matter from cells and other proteins are also mixed in.

Beta-amyloid is a small piece of a larger protein called an amyloid precursor protein

having a cardiac computerized tomography (CT) scan that detects plaque buildup in the heart that leads to a stiffening of the arteries (atherosclerosis). This is a sign of coronary artery disease even if the person has never had a heart attack.

From there, magnetic resonance imaging (MRI) may be used to detect neurodegeneration. This is done to help measure the severity of the disease. For example, an MRI may show if the hippocampus — a part of the brain that's important for memory — is shrinking. This allows researchers to identify an individual who has evidence of amyloid and tau in the brain but also evidence of neurodegeneration (shrinking in the hippocampus). This additional piece of information is important because researchers have found that people whose memory declines most quickly have abnormalities in all three biomarkers — amyloid, tau and neurodegeneration.

Finding a specific combination of biomarkers in the brain may change how Alzheimer's disease is diagnosed, offering more options to address it earlier than ever before. Research is already showing that this framework can accurately predict memory decline in people without dementia.

Researchers will continue to test and refine this framework. Studies are currently being done to see if other types of tests can help predict who will develop Alzheimer's disease.

This framework provides a common language for researchers to exchange ideas. Although it's important to remember that this framework is currently not for use in doctors' offices, the hope is that someday, it will be a tool that helps doctors detect Alzheimer's early, before signs and symptoms appear, and offer treatment that can reduce and even prevent its effects.

WHAT AN AMYLOID PLAQUE LOOKS LIKE

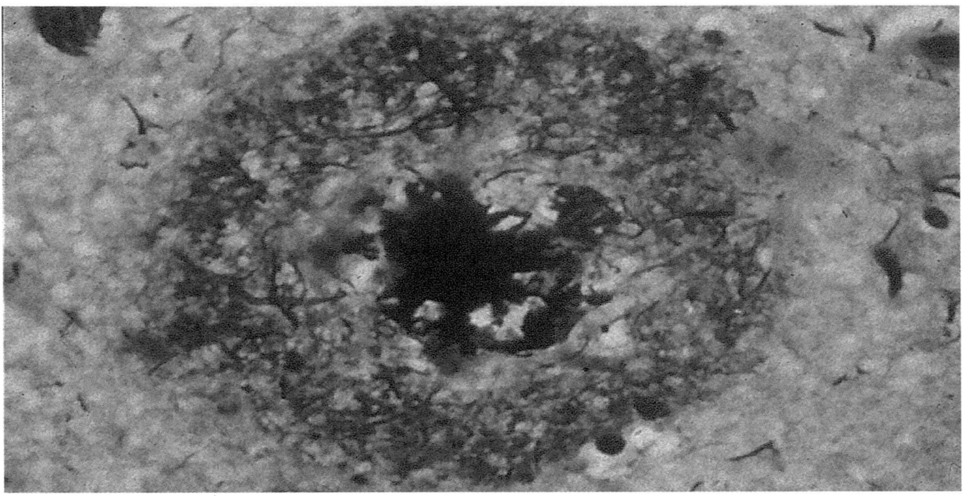

The dark, irregular spot in this microphotograph is the dense core of an amyloid plaque in brain tissue. The discoloration around the core shows inflammation in the brain, which causes cells in the brain to die.

(APP). Other proteins cut this larger protein into smaller sections. Some of the sections of APP stay inside brain cells and others move outside of them. When the larger protein is cut, beta-amyloid is one of the pieces it produces. See how this process unfolds in the illustration on the right. Certain processes remove these proteins from the brain.

Everyone has APP and the fragments it creates, but certain processes can make it more likely for deposits of these proteins to form in the brain, either because too many of these proteins are being made or because the brain isn't removing enough of them. And because beta-amyloid is stickier than other proteins, they're more likely to form clumps and harden into plaques.

Scientists think that these plaques disrupt communication between brain cells and activate immune cells that trigger harmful inflammation. Researchers have found that smaller clumps of beta-amyloid are also

FORMATION OF PLAQUES

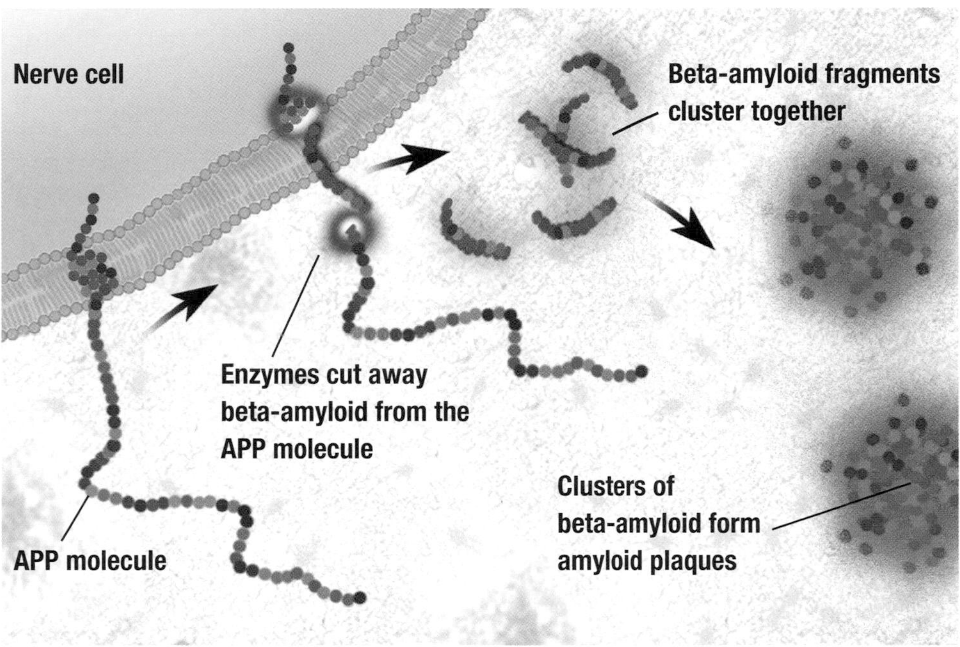

Plaques are dense deposits of protein and cell material in the brain. Plaques are a hallmark sign of Alzheimer's disease. They form outside of brain cells.

The formation of plaques starts with a large protein called an amyloid precursor protein (APP). Everyone has this protein. APP gets cut into smaller pieces, but some of these pieces, called beta-amyloid, are sticker and more toxic than other pieces.

In Alzheimer's disease, either too much beta-amyloid is produced or not enough of it is removed from the brain. In either case, the pieces of beta-amyloid build up and clump together. Eventually, these clumps harden into plaques.

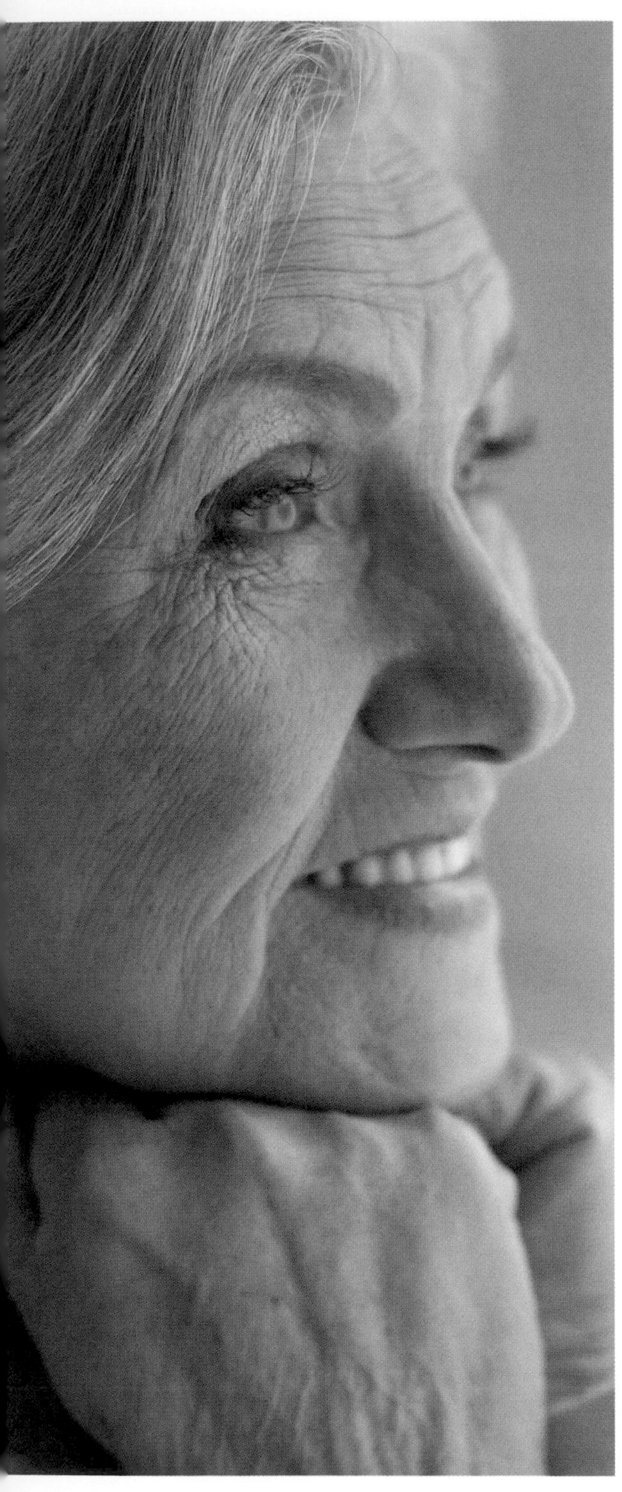

toxic to brain cells. All of these changes cause brain cells to die.

How do scientists know that this process is taking place in the brain? Here's one reason: Scientists have found that with rare, inherited forms of Alzheimer's, changes to genes almost always increase the production of beta-amyloid. This leads to earlier and more abundant plaques in the brain.

The abnormal processing and buildup of beta-amyloid in the brain seems to happen early on in late-onset Alzheimer's, the more common form of the disease. Imaging tests used to see deep inside the living brain show that these deposits may develop many years or even decades before any signs or symptoms appear. Changes in the levels of beta-amyloid can also be seen in spinal fluid decades before symptoms appear in Alzheimer's disease.

Scientists have started to refer to this early stage, where there are no noticeable symptoms but there are biomarkers of both plaques and tangles in the brain, as preclinical Alzheimer's disease.

Stages of toxicity. Beta-amyloid fragments pass through several stages before they form a plaque. A growing body of research suggests that the fragments may be more toxic in some stages of plaque formation than in other stages.

At first, a few beta-amyloid fragments clump together but are still fairly easy to dissolve and remove from the brain. In this stage they're called oligomers (OL-ih-go-murz). When several oligomers join together, the clumps get larger and stickier. From there, they form long, slender chains of amyloid fragments. These chains keep growing in size and density until they form the hard, insoluble plaques seen in Alzheimer's.

For a long time, scientists believed that it was the fully developed amyloid plaques that caused neurons to die. But as more evidence is uncovered about how plaques form, some scientists are starting to rethink this. They argue that beta-amyloid is most toxic during the earlier oligomer stage — *before* plaques have formed.

The researchers believe that oligomers attack and destroy the brain's synapses — the narrow spaces that neurons must bridge so they can communicate with each other and form memory. The damage to the synapses results in memory loss and other cognitive impairments.

According to this theory, by the time large plaques have formed, the beta-amyloid fragments may have already lost some of their toxicity and the insoluble clumps are merely inactive masses, or "litter" of the disease process. However, it's also possible that beta-amyloid fragments lead to toxicity in the brain as they grow and accumulate.

Not by beta-amyloid alone? Although researchers continue to expand and refine what's known about the mechanisms that cause Alzheimer's, some aspects aren't clearly understood.

On one hand, tests reveal that some people have a large amount of beta-amyloid in their brains but suffer little damage to the neurons. These individuals remain cognitively sound throughout their lives. On the other hand, tests show that some people may have normal levels of beta-amyloid in their brains but still show measurable damage to the brain.

This brings up several questions. Can nerve cells in the brain get destroyed even without high levels of beta-amyloid in the brain? Do other processes have to take place for nerve cells in the brain to become damaged and for dementia to develop? Are some people more able than others to resist damage from beta-amyloid, so much so that they live a long life without noticeable changes in how the brain works?

Researchers think that people who have cognitive impairment but don't seem to have much beta-amyloid in their brains may be on a pathway toward dementia, but not the kind that's caused by Alzheimer's disease.

Amyloid has been studied in other ways, too. For example, because amyloid is involved in genetic forms of Alzheimer's disease, many clinical trials have focused on therapies that reduce amyloid in the brain. However, these approaches have been met with mixed results. This is leading some researchers to wonder if amyloid is truly toxic and if other therapies should be used instead. Researchers who believe amyloid is harmful, however, counter this thought,

HOW TANGLES FORM

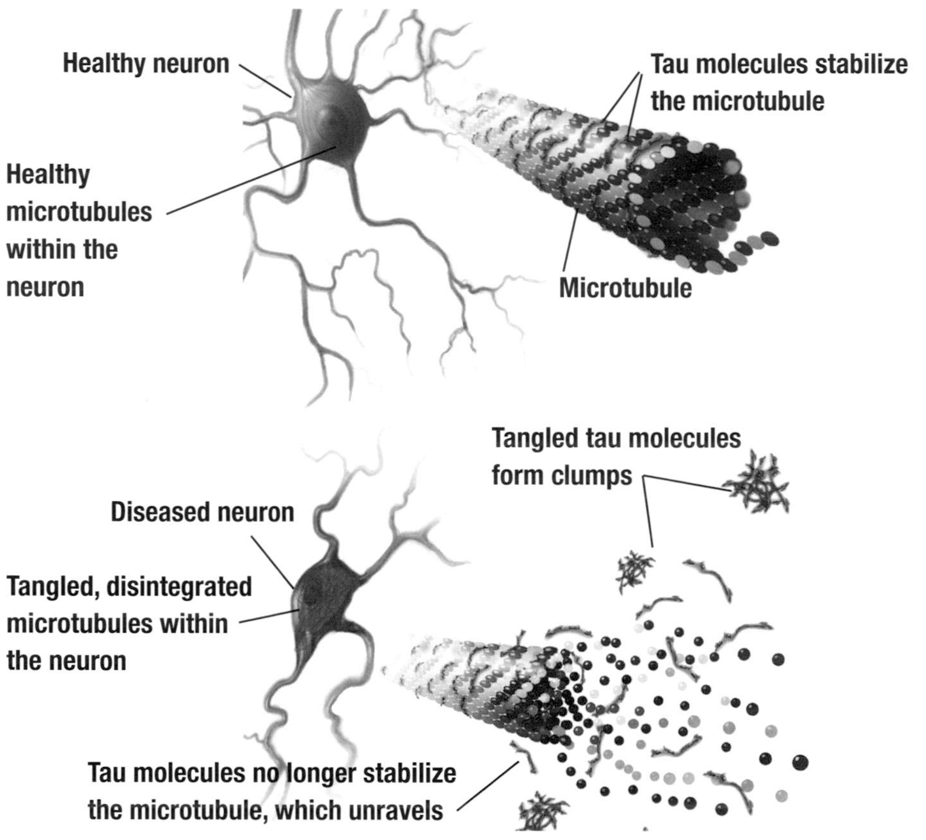

Microtubules are a basic part of a nerve cell (neuron). They look like long, skinny cylinders. They maintain a cell's structure and transport materials within a cell. Tau is a protein that helps support microtubules, a type of cell structure that supports many different functions, like transporting proteins.

In Alzheimer's disease, the chemical makeup of tau changes. This causes the tau to destabilize the microtubules. In turn, the structure of the cell collapses. From there, the pieces of tau clump together within the cell and form tangles, a hallmark sign of Alzheimer's disease.

proposing that the people in these studies didn't receive treatment early enough for it to be helpful. Treating people before symptoms develop, they argue, would make a difference. This kind of strategy, often referred to as prevention, is being tested in clinical trials.

At the same time, researchers know that Alzheimer's disease is complex. This may be another reason why therapies that target beta-amyloid haven't been clearly helpful. With this in mind, more than one therapy may be needed to address beta-amyloid, as well as other processes involved in Alzheimer's disease. This is much like how certain infections and types of cancer are treated with more than one approach.

These are just some of the issues scientists are working to resolve so a clear outline of the disease process can be established.

Tangles Neurofibrillary tangles are the other abnormal structure seen in Alzheimer's disease. Tangles happen inside a nerve cell (neuron). They're caused by the abnormal buildup of a protein called tau. Tau helps uphold a cell's structure. But in Alzheimer's disease, this protein undergoes changes that alter it and cause it to malfunction. Instead of stabilizing a cell's structure like it's supposed to, strands of this protein unravel and clump together. In turn, they form tangled masses inside the neuron. See how this happens on the left page.

These tangles prevent nutrients and messages from getting where they need to in the brain. This leads to a breakdown in how well the neurons in the brain work.

Tangles and plaques seem to be firmly intertwined in how Alzheimer's disease develops. However, scientists are still learning their exact role. For example, the number of tangles in the brain is more closely linked to the timing and severity of neurodegeneration (brain shrinkage) and dementia symptoms than is the number of plaques. Some researchers think this is because a buildup of beta-amyloid happens before or causes tau to build up. However, what happens between beta-amyloid and tau is still under study.

CONTRIBUTING FACTORS

Although plaques and tangles are the prominent features of Alzheimer's — and ones that have been studied most — many scientists feel that research on the disease is only beginning.

The current thinking is that Alzheimer's, like many other diseases, is caused by many factors that are as varied as your genes. Lifestyle and your body's ability to adapt to age-related changes and to other diseases play roles, too. Here are several factors that may contribute to or are linked to Alzheimer's disease.

Genetics

While some genes determine what eye color or hair color you'll have, other genes predict

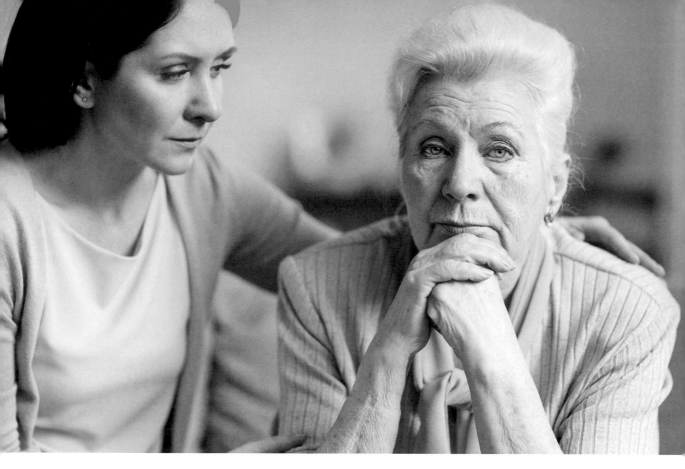

how likely you are to get a condition like Alzheimer's disease.

Young-onset Alzheimer's genes Three genes make it more likely that you'll develop young-onset Alzheimer's disease, a form of the disease with symptoms often developing before age 65.

These three genes are the amyloid precursor protein (APP) gene and two presenilin genes, presenilin 1 (PSEN1) and presenilin 2 (PSEN2). All three genes are involved in changing the production of beta-amyloid. These mutations are very rare.

Mutations of these genes cause too much beta-amyloid to be produced. This causes plaques to form that kill nerve cells in the brain. This is what leads to symptoms of the disease that get worse and worse over time.

Symptoms of young-onset Alzheimer's disease are similar to the late-onset form, but nonmemory symptoms are more likely, and seizures are more likely to develop at some point.

A parent with one of the known mutations has a high chance of passing it on to a child — each child has a 50% chance of getting the

IS GENETIC SCREENING HELPFUL?

Screening kits are available to detect genetic changes linked to young-onset and late-onset forms of Alzheimer's disease, but specialists don't routinely recommend genetic testing.

If someone has symptoms of young-onset Alzheimer's disease (which typically affects people younger than age 65) and has a strong family history of young-onset dementia, screening for the young-onset familial Alzheimer's mutations in APP, PSEN1 and PSEN2 genes may be useful. Before testing, it's best to talk to a genetic counselor. In addition, there's a common genetic risk factor for late-onset Alzheimer's disease known as the e4 allele of the apolipoprotein E (APOE) gene. Screening for the APOE e4 allele doesn't have much clinical value at this time, however. Having it doesn't guarantee you'll get Alzheimer's disease, and not having it doesn't mean you won't. For these reasons, in addition to the fact that there's no preventive therapy available, genetic testing for APOE isn't recommended outside of research settings.

gene and developing the disease. However, some people with young-onset Alzheimer's don't have mutations in these genes. This means that young-onset Alzheimer's may have other causes that haven't been found yet.

Genes that predict late-onset Alzheimer's
Late-onset Alzheimer's disease, the most common form, usually starts after age 65. The gene most often linked to it is apolipoprotein E (APOE). Before this gene was linked to Alzheimer's disease, it was known in the medical community for its role in carrying blood cholesterol throughout the body. There are three major variants of this gene, named e2, e3 and e4. It's the e4 variant that makes Alzheimer's more likely. You get one copy of the APOE gene from your mother and one from your father. If one of these copies is of the e4 variant, you have an increased risk of Alzheimer's disease. If you get the e4 variant from your mother and your father, your risk is even higher.

It's also possible that people with the e4 variant may develop Alzheimer's several years earlier than those who don't have it. For people with the e4 variant, the risk of Alzheimer's seems to peak around age 70.

It's important to note that having the e4 variant of the APOE gene doesn't guarantee that you'll develop Alzheimer's. And if you don't have it, you may still develop Alzheimer's disease.

It's not entirely clear how the e4 variant increases Alzheimer's risk. Research shows that this form of the APOE gene slows down the clearance of beta-amyloid from the brain. It also seems to make beta-amyloid stick together more quickly. It may also affect how blood vessels work and how the brain responds to inflammation, both of which are related to the development of Alzheimer's disease. At the same time, one of the other APOE variants — e2 — actually *reduces* the risk of Alzheimer's disease. How this happens is still under study.

A number of other genes have also been linked to late-onset Alzheimer's disease. Many of these genes were identified in large studies, and researchers are still learning about their roles in the development of Alzheimer's. More research is underway to identify other genes that may be involved in Alzheimer's disease.

Here are just some of the genes that may be involved in Alzheimer's disease:

ABCA7. Although its exact role isn't clear, some variants of ABCA7 seem to be linked

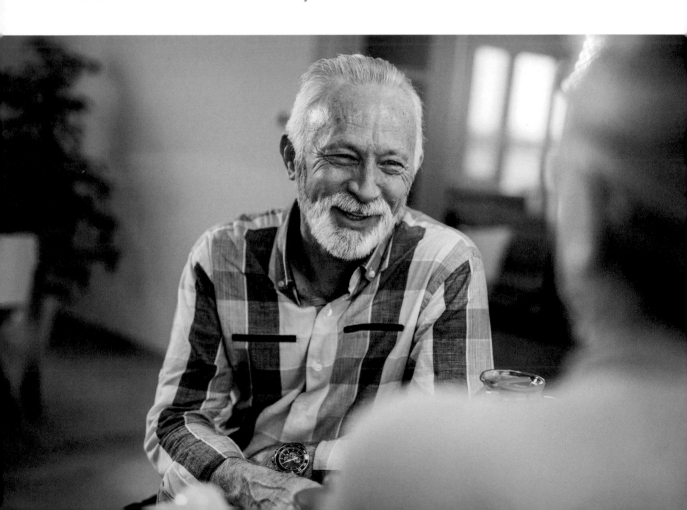

to a higher risk of Alzheimer's disease. Researchers think it may have something to do with the gene's role in how the brain uses cholesterol and breaks down APP.

CLU. This gene is involved in removing beta-amyloid from the brain. As you've already learned, beta-amyloid is believed to be central to the development of Alzheimer's disease. Problems with this gene may lead to too much beta-amyloid in the brain.

CR1. When this gene produces too little protein, it can contribute to inflammation in the brain. Inflammation may be a factor in the development of Alzheimer's disease. This gene has also been linked to how APP is broken down.

PICALM. This gene helps keep neurons in the brain communicating with each other. This communication, as you've learned, is important to keep nerve cells functioning and to help memories form in the brain. PICALM is also thought to be involved in how APP is broken down in the brain.

PLD3. Although scientists don't know much about the role of PLD3 in the brain, it's been linked to a higher risk of Alzheimer's.

SORL1. This gene plays an important role in producing beta-amyloid, among other processes. Some of its variants are also linked to Alzheimer's disease risk.

TREM2. This gene is involved in the brain's response to inflammation. Rare variants in this gene are associated with a higher risk of Alzheimer's disease. Other genes associated with Alzheimer's risk are also involved in inflammation.

Oxidative stress

Oxidative stress happens when structures within a cell, called mitochondria, get damaged. Mitochondria are a cell's energy factory. Damage causes mitochondria to produce too many free radicals.

Free radicals form naturally when you exercise and your body turns food into energy. Your body can also get exposed to free radicals from sources in the environment, like cigarette smoke, air pollution and sunlight. Too many of these molecules can overwhelm a cell and damage it. This damage is often caused by a process known as oxidative stress.

Experts think oxidative stress plays a role in many diseases. Signs of oxidative stress have been found in the brains of people with Alzheimer's disease, particularly in later stages. It may also play a role in other forms of dementia.

What causes oxidative stress? Normal aging may cause a buildup of free radicals, as can various disease-related factors. Evidence also suggests that the formation of amyloid plaques and inflammation may play roles.

There are also indications of oxidative stress in the earliest stages of Alzheimer's disease. This has led some researchers to question if

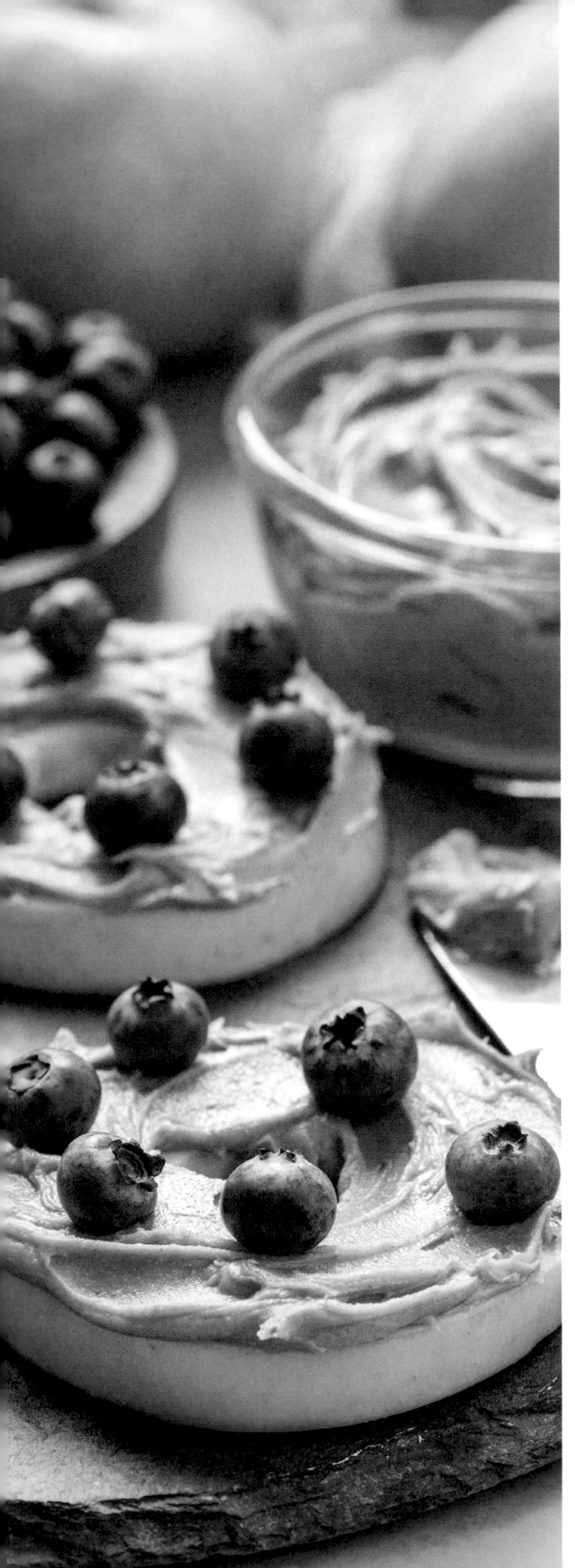

stress may cause plaques and tangles to form. Some argue that plaques and tangles may form to protect the body from the stress. Other researchers think that a chronic state of low-level oxidative stress, combined with other factors, may be enough to trigger damage to the brain's neurons.

Regardless of whether oxidative stress causes neuron damage or is the result of it, most researchers agree that it plays a part in the disease process.

Are there ways to combat oxidative stress and prevent it from causing damage that may lead to dementia? Maybe. Foods rich in antioxidants, including several types of nuts, nut butters, fruits and vegetables may be helpful. In some studies, vitamin E has shown promise. But not all research shows that it offers benefits. In addition, there are concerns about taking high doses of vitamin E; taking too much may cause bleeding and increase the risk of dying. For these reasons, taking vitamin E as a supplement isn't recommended.

Inflammatory response

Inflammation and its links to Alzheimer's disease have been mentioned several times in this chapter. But what is inflammation, exactly, and how does it work?

Inflammation is your body's natural protective response to injury. It may involve pain, swelling, heat and redness of the inflamed area of the body. Alzheimer's disease is linked to a low level of chronic inflammation in the brain.

What causes inflammation to happen in the brain? Even as amyloid plaques develop between neurons, immune cells called microglia work to clear damaged neurons, dead cells and other waste products from brain tissue. Scientists think that the microglia see plaques as foreign substances and try to destroy them. This triggers inflammation.

Properly functioning microglia are needed to clear toxic substances like beta-amyloid and dead cells from the brain. If microglia can't do their job or can't do it well, these toxic substances can build up in the brain, causing cells in the brain to die. At the same time, if microglia stay activated for too long, this can lead to chronic inflammation in the brain, which can also damage brain cells.

Researchers think that different types of manipulation may be needed for the brain's immune response at different stages of Alzheimer's disease. It's possible that the immune system may benefit from a gentle boost in the earlier stages. After chronic or long-term inflammation sets in, the immune system may benefit from a reduction in activity. The timing and types of these immune system-based approaches are being studied.

Vascular brain injury

As one of the largest, busiest organs in the body, the brain depends on a vast network of blood vessels to feed it the oxygen and nutrients necessary to operate successfully. Blood vessels also help remove waste, including beta-amyloid. The brain relies heavily on the heart to pump enough blood for its needs.

Over time, the brain's system of blood vessels starts to look like the rest of an aging body. Arteries in the brain become more narrow and less elastic, and some get clogged with fatty deposits. New capillary growth — offshoots from the main arteries — slows down. The heart may not pump as well as it used to. As a result, the brain doesn't get as much blood, and the blood that does arrive may not flow as well as it once did.

The wear and tear of age also takes a toll on the blood vessels in the brain, leading to tiny injuries, inflammation and oxidative stress. Conditions like high blood pressure, a buildup of fats, cholesterol, and other substances in the artery walls (atherosclerosis) and head trauma can add to these effects.

It's possible that a faulty, aging system of blood vessels in the brain may set the stage for neurons in the brain to get damaged and die. For example, many studies show that people who are at risk of heart disease in midlife — those with high blood pressure, high cholesterol and obesity, for example — are more likely to have cognitive impairment and dementia later in life.

It's also important to note that Alzheimer's disease and any kind of disease that reduces

DEMENTIA DUE TO ALZHEIMER'S

This line graph compares the cognitive decline that happens with typical aging with the decline that happens in someone with Alzheimer's disease.

Alzheimer's may start when a person is in his or her late 50s or early 60s, even without noticeable physical signs of the disease. Over time, signs and symptoms — mostly memory issues — start to make it difficult to perform everyday tasks. Eventually, cognitive impairment is significant enough that the person is diagnosed with dementia due to Alzheimer's disease.

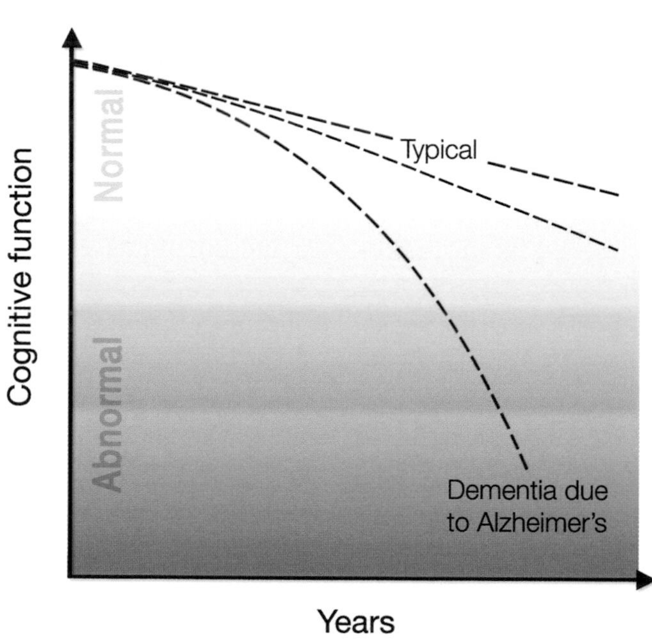

blood flow to the brain (cerebrovascular disease) often occur together. Examples of cerebrovascular disease include strokes and ministrokes, both of which can cause brain injury and dementia.

People with severe blood vessel disease often have beta-amyloid, and people with Alzheimer's disease also have cerebrovascular disease.

How one condition affects the other is under study. One theory is that beta-amyloid helps prevent toxic materials from spreading into the brain. But when there are chronic issues with the blood vessels in the brain — whether it's from heart disease or a head injury — too much beta-amyloid builds up, choking out small blood vessels and leaving behind free-floating fragments. It's at this stage that beta-amyloid deposits become harmful, scientists say.

It also seems that beta-amyloid can affect how the blood vessels in the brain work. For example, it may cause the blood vessels in the brain to leak.

A number of studies are exploring how to address the connection between Alzheimer's disease and blood vessel health. Can high blood pressure drugs used now help people with Alzheimer's disease or reduce the risk of it developing in the first place? What's the connection between heart disease and Alzheimer's? Are there drugs that can target that connection and prevent Alzheimer's from occurring? These are just some of the questions researchers are seeking to answer.

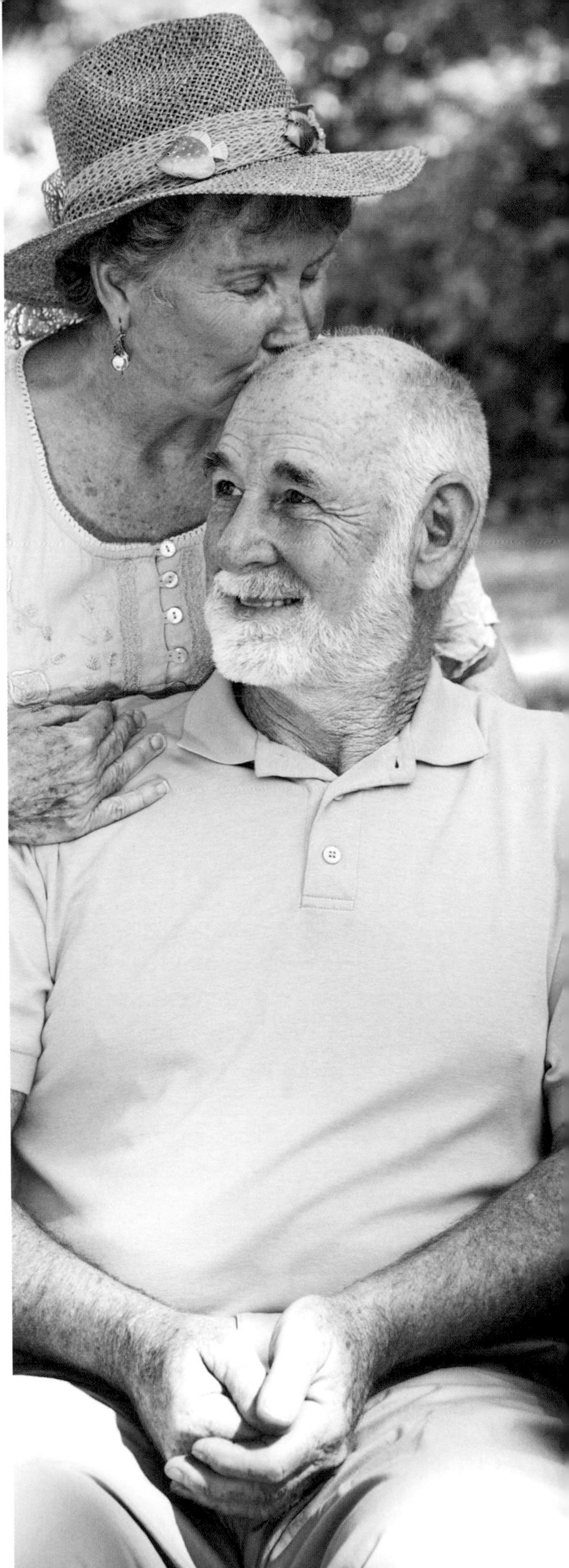

Despite this possible relationship, many studies suggest that with Alzheimer's disease and cerebrovascular disease, one doesn't directly make the other one worse. Instead, one may add to the other; in other words, someone with both Alzheimer's disease and cerebrovascular disease will have more cognitive impairment than someone with the same amount of Alzheimer's disease alone.

Diabetes

Diabetes and Alzheimer's disease may be connected, but this relationship is still under review. Some research suggests that having diabetes makes it more likely that you'll develop dementia at some point, but not all researchers agree.

Diabetes can cause damage to the body, including to blood vessels. That makes it a risk factor for vascular dementia. Because many people with diabetes have the hallmark brain changes of both Alzheimer's disease and vascular dementia, some researchers think that each condition makes damage from the other condition worse. Diabetes may also increase the risk of mild cognitive impairment — and make it more likely that mild cognitive impairment will transition to dementia.

While diabetes damages blood vessels in the brain and this can increase the risk of dementia, autopsy studies haven't shown a direct relationship between diabetes and the hallmark amyloid and tau deposits of Alzheimer's disease. As they continue to study the link between dementia and diabetes, researchers are seeking to find ways to capitalize on this connection and come up with treatment for both conditions.

One option is the use of insulin to treat Alzheimer's disease. Early research suggested that when taken as a nose spray, insulin may be able to improve memory and help preserve cognitive function in people with early Alzheimer's disease or mild cognitive impairment. However, more recent trials showed that insulin taken as a nose spray showed no benefit for people with mild cognitive impairment or Alzheimer's.

Investigation is ongoing as researchers try to better understand the link between diabetes and Alzheimer's and learn more about ways to prevent and treat both conditions.

PROTECTIVE FACTORS

More and more research suggests that while many factors may increase your risk of dementia, there also may be ways that you can help prevent it.

Many studies show that a number of lifestyle habits — exercising, eating a diet rich in fruits and vegetables, engaging in mentally stimulating activities, and staying socially connected — may reduce your risk of developing dementia.

Whether these daily habits act against the basic disease mechanisms of Alzheimer's or whether they build a reserve of brain capacity that can be accessed when other areas of the brain become damaged is still under study. You'll read more about possible protective measures, as well as the latest research around them, later in this book.

THE ALZHEIMER'S EXPERIENCE

As you've learned, dementia isn't a disease, but a syndrome — a collection of signs and symptoms. In the next chapter, you'll read about how doctors diagnose Alzheimer's based on its signs and symptoms.

Each person's experience with Alzheimer's is unique. It doesn't come on at the same age for every person who has it. How severe it is and how quickly it progresses will also vary. Many factors influence how Alzheimer's progresses, including age, physical health, family history, and cultural and ethnic backgrounds. However, some patterns are common in Alzheimer's. Doctors have been able to use these patterns to describe stages in terms of how Alzheimer's develops.

In this book, three stages are used to characterize dementia due to Alzheimer's disease: mild, moderate and advanced. One stage differs from another in terms of how a person thinks, acts and is able to perform basic tasks. These stages are relatively general in nature, meaning that they may not fit every individual's situation exactly. Some signs and symptoms may appear throughout the disease, not just one stage. Others may never develop for some people. You'll learn more about these stages in the next chapter.

How long someone will live with Alzheimer's varies, as well, and compared to past estimates, people are often able to live longer with Alzheimer's than they did in the past. On average, people with Alzheimer's disease live between three and 11 years after they're diagnosed — but others live for 20 years or more.

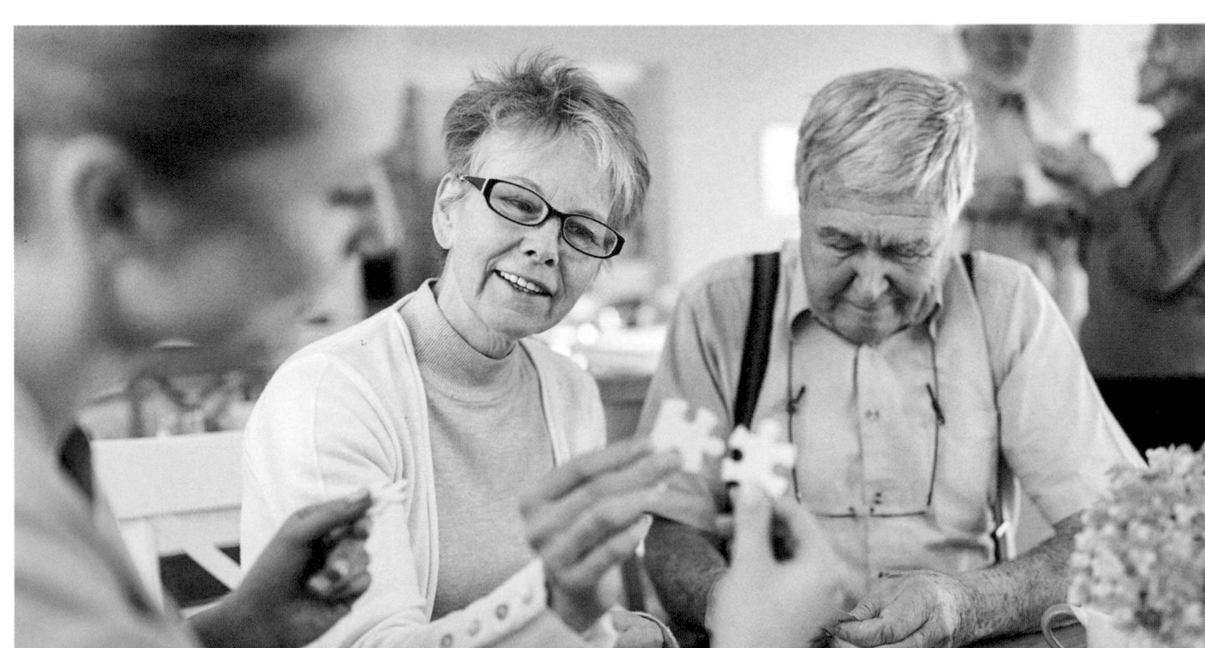

“GETTING AN ALZHEIMER’S DIAGNOSIS EARLY ON — ONCE SYMPTOMS HAVE STARTED, BUT THEY’RE STILL MILD — OFFERS SEVERAL ADVANTAGES.”

CHAPTER 6

Diagnosing Alzheimer's disease

Years ago, people with dementia due to Alzheimer's disease typically were diagnosed after its signs and symptoms had already begun to drastically alter their quality of life and ability to live independently.

Then in the 1990s and early 2000s, it became recognized that individuals with Alzheimer's disease develop mild cognitive impairment first. As you learned in Chapter 2, mild cognitive impairment is when an individual has a clear change in cognition — typically memory — but can still function normally in everyday activities.

Since then, advances have been made that allow the hallmark proteins of Alzheimer's disease to be measured in people while they're still living. With these advances, experts now know that the biological underpinning of Alzheimer's disease starts well before the first memory problem appears — an estimated 15 years before the onset of symptoms. This is referred to as the preclinical stage, when Alzheimer's disease is taking shape in the brain but hasn't started to cause symptoms.

Experts don't yet know exactly how long someone can have the biological features of Alzheimer's disease in the brain before they start showing symptoms. Some people, in fact, may have the hallmark plaques and tangles of Alzheimer's disease taking shape in their brain, yet never develop Alzheimer's disease dementia. Currently, preclinical Alzheimer's disease is characterized only in clinical trials or research studies, not in a doctor's office.

If you're experiencing memory loss, you may wonder if your symptoms are part of natural aging or if they're a sign of the mild cognitive impairment or mild dementia stage of Alzheimer's disease.

In turn, this leads to a question that many people struggle with: Is it helpful to know that Alzheimer's is developing in your brain, as symptoms start to appear, if there's no approved treatment that can stop it or slow its progress?

The short answer is yes.

Getting an Alzheimer's diagnosis early on — once symptoms have started, but they're still mild — offers several advantages. For one, a diagnosis offers the chance to take medication that can lessen symptoms, like memory loss, for a period of time. An early diagnosis allows the person and family to associate the cognitive changes with the disease rather than to personal failings, which can bring a sense of relief. Receiving a diagnosis gives families the opportunity to understand the disease, know what to expect, and learn how to adapt, cope and gain access to resources. All of this can reduce stress and feelings of regret later on.

An early diagnosis also empowers the person to be part of decision-making and planning and offers the possibility to participate in clinical trials of potential new treatments.

In this chapter, you'll learn what steps a doctor takes to diagnose Alzheimer's disease. You'll also learn what experts know today about how Alzheimer's progresses over time.

DETECTING COGNITIVE IMPAIRMENT DUE TO ALZHEIMER'S DISEASE

Dementia, as you've learned, isn't a disease. It's a syndrome — a collection of signs and symptoms that signal impairment in a person's ability to think, reason, and interact with his or her environment (cognitive impairment). These signs and symptoms lessen a person's ability to live independently.

When a person first visits a doctor because of persistent memory problems or difficulty thinking through things, the doctor will likely recommend a variety of tests to determine whether the person's symptoms are related to a neurodegenerative disease, like Alzheimer's disease, or to something else, like a stroke, delirium or another medical issue. These tests are described in depth in Chapter 4.

Most commonly, older people experience dementia because of a brain disorder that progressively destroys the brain's nerve cells by targeting their pathways throughout the brain (neurodegenerative disorder). Among the many different neurodegenerative disorders, Alzheimer's disease most commonly causes dementia.

Is Alzheimer's disease the cause of dementia?

If a person's signs and symptoms are confirmed as dementia, the next step is figuring out what's causing it. Keeping in mind that Alzheimer's is the most common cause of

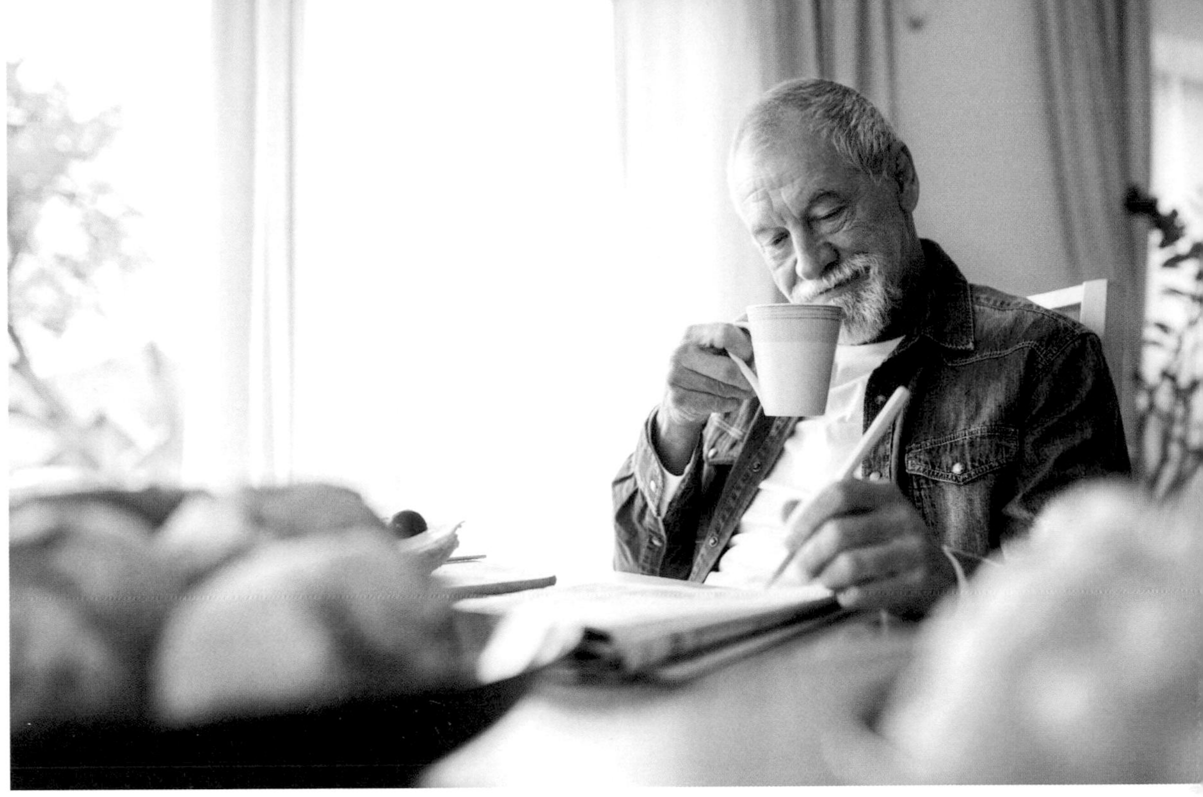

dementia, a doctor will look for specific clues that differentiate Alzheimer's disease from other diseases and conditions that can cause dementia. These clues may show up in a person's past medical history, medication list or physical exam, or in the results of laboratory and brain imaging tests.

A doctor looks for several signs and symptoms to tell if Alzheimer's disease might be causing dementia. They include:

Slow onset and gradual progression of symptoms Alzheimer's disease and other neurodegenerative diseases start out slowly and gradually get worse over time — to the point where they interfere with a person's usual activities.

A sudden onset of symptoms, on the other hand, might be an indication of something else, like a stroke or medication side effect. Symptoms that come on quickly over several weeks may be a sign of a prion disorder like Creutzfeldt-Jakob disease or an autoimmune condition.

Noticeable memory loss Memory loss — especially forgetting recent events — is a classic sign of Alzheimer's disease. It's usually the most prominent feature at first.

Other signs and symptoms, which tend to occur along with memory loss or later in the course of the disease, include:

- Visual-spatial difficulties
- Language difficulties

- Problems with reasoning, judgment and organizing tasks, thinking abstractly, managing time, and solving problems (executive function skills)
- Behavior changes

If a person's initial signs and symptoms are more related to personality or behavior changes, rather than memory problems, another neurodegenerative disorder — such as frontotemporal degeneration — may be causing the dementia. Or if a person experiences hallucinations early on, Lewy body disease may be the cause.

Mental status issues A doctor may conduct a brief mental status test to assess memory and other thinking skills. Trouble remembering three to five words after a delay of five minutes is common in people with Alzheimer's disease dementia.

Longer forms of neuropsychological testing (see page 75) may offer additional details about mental function. These tests may be particularly helpful when symptoms are mild. They're also important for establishing a starting point to track the progression of symptoms in the future.

Normal neurological exam A person with Alzheimer's generally tests normal on functions like strength, balance, reflexes and sensory skills. These are all skills that are assessed during a neurological exam (learn more in Chapter 4). A person with signs of parkinsonism based on this test may have a different cause of dementia, like Lewy body disease.

Normal lab results Blood tests are used to rule out possible causes of dementia-like signs and symptoms, like a thyroid disorder or a vitamin B12 deficiency.

A person with Alzheimer's disease typically shows no sign of metabolic problems that might be contributing to dementia.

Imaging tests show signs of brain tissue loss In someone with Alzheimer's disease, there's no specific pattern of atrophy (shrinking) in the brain. However, an MRI often shows atrophy of the medial temporal lobe, a part of the brain involved in memory. Specifically, an MRI of someone with Alzheimer's typically shows atrophy of the hippocampus, the brain's central switchboard for information storage and recall.

In general, how severe a person's symptoms are corresponds with the degree of shrinkage seen on an MRI. Other anatomical irregularities, like shrinking in the parietal lobe or decreased thickness of the cerebral cortex, also may provide signs of Alzheimer's-related decline. If there's no damage to the hippocampus but dementia is present, this may be an indirect clue that Lewy body disease is the cause. On the other hand, if brain tissue loss occurs mostly in the frontal or temporal areas, then frontotemporal degeneration may be suspected.

If after a full evaluation a person fits this general profile and no other disease or condition can explain the symptoms, the doctor will say that this person likely has dementia due to Alzheimer's disease.

When outward clues aren't clear

Sometimes, a person doesn't fit the typical profile of Alzheimer's disease. Signs and symptoms that come on more quickly than expected, aren't related to memory, or that occur in younger individuals are examples.

In cases like these, additional tests that measure biological markers (biomarkers) in the brain or in the fluid around the brain and spinal cord (cerebrospinal fluid) can help confirm or rule out the diagnosis.

Many of these tests are used mostly in research settings or teaching hospitals for now. But in the future, doctors and researchers hope that biomarker tests will be used routinely to confirm a diagnosis of Alzheimer's and detect it before symptoms begin.

A person who's mid-career, in her 50s, offers an example of when biomarker tests might be helpful. Perhaps this person is experiencing cognitive impairment that's been confirmed by mental status and neuropsychological testing. However, a diagnosis still isn't certain even after an MRI and standard lab tests. Because the likelihood of Alzheimer's disease in a 50-year-old is low, biomarker tests can help confirm or rule out Alzheimer's disease as the cause of this person's cognitive problems. In turn, an accurate diagnosis may allow this person to start the appropriate treatment and proceed to make certain life decisions.

Biomarker tests include:

Cerebrospinal fluid tests Samples of the fluid around the brain and spinal cord can be taken with a spinal tap and tested for specified levels of amyloid and tau proteins. Abnormal levels of these proteins have been shown to indicate the presence of Alzheimer's disease. A low amount of amyloid with a higher level of tau is typical of Alzheimer's disease.

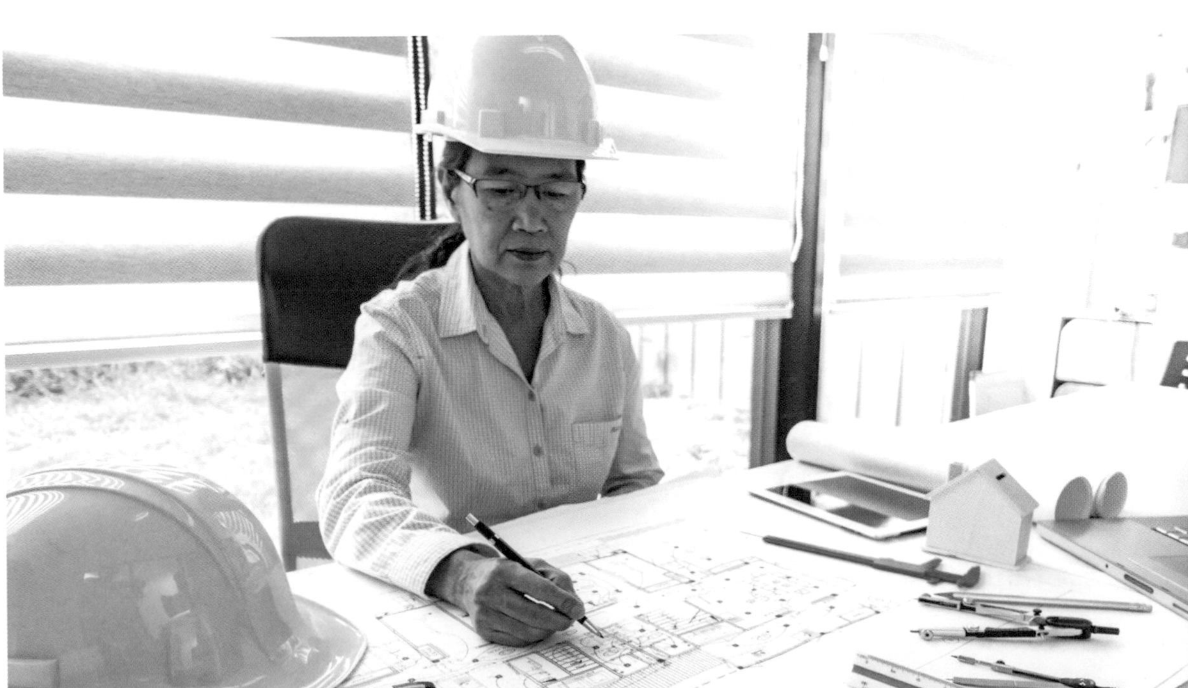

Fluorodeoxyglucose-PET scans This type of PET scan highlights areas where the brain isn't using glucose as it should. In medical terms, this is known as decreased glucose metabolism.

Glucose is the primary source of energy for brain cells. This test compares patterns of low glucose metabolism, which can help show differences between different neurodegenerative disorders. This type of PET scan is particularly helpful for distinguishing Alzheimer's disease from other causes of dementia. If a doctor can't tell which disorder is causing symptoms after a routine exam, this test may be helpful.

Amyloid and tau positron emission tomography (PET) scans These scans use a radioactive tracer to measure the amount of amyloid or tau buildup in the brain. This, in turn, confirms the presence of amyloid in the brain, a hallmark sign of Alzheimer's disease.

A PET scan that doesn't show a specific amount of amyloid or tau may be used to rule out Alzheimer's. However, a positive scan — one that shows increased amounts of amyloid and tau — doesn't necessarily rule out the presence of other diseases, in addition to Alzheimer's disease.

Both of these tests are used mostly in research settings. Amyloid PET scans are available at some medical centers, but they're rarely used by doctors in a health care setting. Tau PET scans are used strictly for research.

Is a definitive diagnosis needed?

In the vast majority of cases, a clinical diagnosis of Alzheimer's disease dementia can confidently be made with a basic dementia evaluation. When certainty is needed, a more definitive diagnosis may be made using biomarker tests (CSF amyloid and tau tests or an amyloid PET scan). After death, tissue samples obtained at autopsy that reflect the plaques and tangles characteristic of the disease can confirm a diagnosis. In the future, when treatments are available that can slow or stop the disease, a definitive diagnosis will become more important.

STAGES OF ALZHEIMER'S DISEASE

People with Alzheimer's vary in how they experience the disease. It may develop at different ages in different people, and symptoms may be worse for some than they are for others. These differences can be influenced by many factors, including physical health, family history, and cultural and ethnic backgrounds.

Alzheimer's disease is recognized as a continuum that may be divided into roughly five stages: preclinical Alzheimer's disease, mild cognitive impairment due to Alzheimer's disease, mild dementia due to Alzheimer's disease, moderate dementia due to Alzheimer's disease and severe dementia due to Alzheimer's disease.

These five stages can help you understand what may happen as the disease progresses.

WHAT IF MY PARENT HAS ALZHEIMER'S DISEASE DEMENTIA?

Many times, people wonder about their risk of developing Alzheimer's disease if one or both parents or a sibling develop it.

Keep in mind that when it comes to developing Alzheimer's disease, the most important risk factor is age. The lifetime risk of developing Alzheimer's disease dementia is between 10% to 15%. People who have a parent or sibling with Alzheimer's dementia are about two times more likely to develop it, compared with those without a family history — so they're still more likely *not* to get Alzheimer's disease at some point. Your risk increases if both of your parents had Alzheimer's disease dementia or if one of your parents developed Alzheimer's disease at a young age.

Learning that a parent has dementia offers opportunities, however. This is where taking steps to keep your brain healthy as you age becomes important (learn more in Chapter 19). Or, you may take part in research focused on understanding genetics of Alzheimer's or treatment trials focused on preventing Alzheimer's.

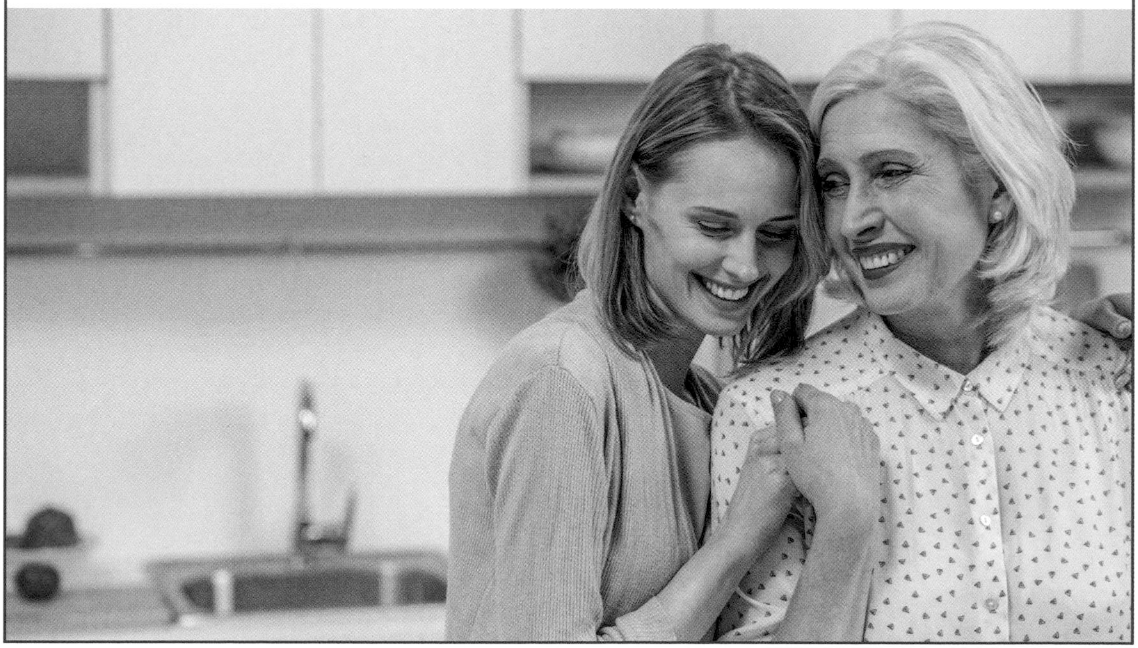

These stages are only rough generalizations, however. In fact, the first stage is of concern mostly for researchers because symptoms aren't a factor.

It's also important to note that symptoms that appear in the mild cognitive impairment stage don't affect a person's ability to live independently.

Some people may never get past the preclinical or mild cognitive impairment phase. Others do progress, however, and are generally diagnosed in the mild dementia stage. For some, symptoms may worsen slowly. For others, symptoms become severe within a few years. Each person's experience with Alzheimer's and its symptoms, and when they appear, will vary.

STAGES OF DEMENTIA DUE TO ALZHEIMER'S

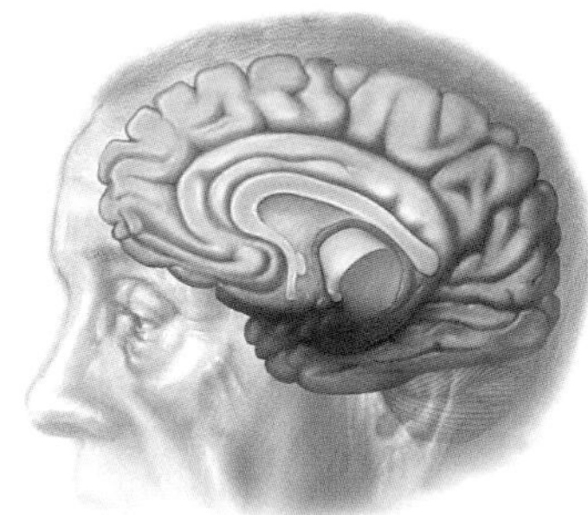

Mild

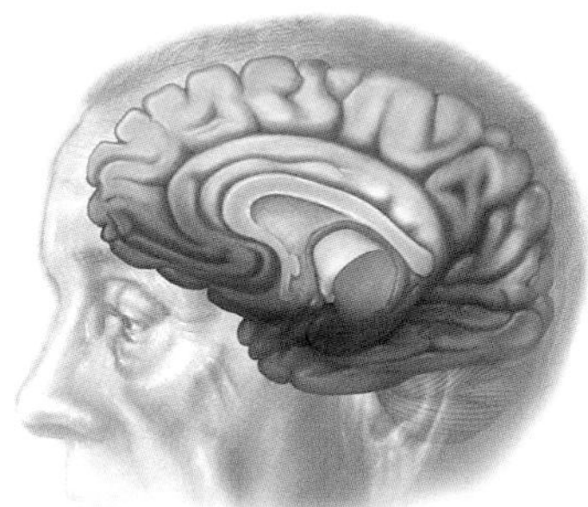

Moderate

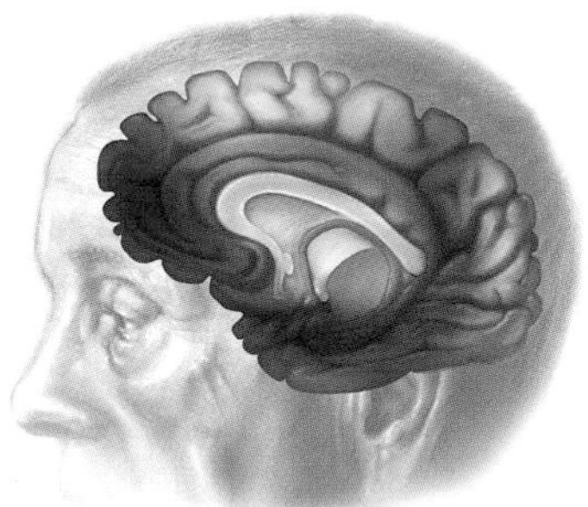

Severe

Alzheimer's destroys the brain's most basic component, the nerve cell (neuron). When mild symptoms appear, they're due to neuron loss in the area of the hippocampus that spreads to the amygdala (see purple shading). In the disease's moderate stage, nerve cell damage spreads into the cerebral cortex.

In typical Alzheimer's disease that starts with memory loss, the areas related to motor skills, sight, hearing, smell, taste and touch aren't as affected. However, as the disease progresses, even these areas may be affected — especially in the severe stage.

Preclinical Alzheimer's disease

Studies suggest that the biological process of Alzheimer's disease begins long before symptoms are noticeable. This preliminary stage is often referred to as preclinical Alzheimer's disease. This is when changes are taking place in the brain but symptoms aren't obvious. Researchers are actively looking into how long this stage lasts. They think it may range between 15 and 25 years.

Preclinical Alzheimer's disease is signaled only by the presence of abnormal biomarkers, amyloid and tau. The presence of amyloid *without* tau is referred to as Alzheimer's pathological change. This means that a person has some Alzheimer's-related changes in the brain, but not enough changes to qualify for Alzheimer's disease.

Mild cognitive impairment due to Alzheimer's disease

In the mild cognitive impairment stage, a person has developed mild changes in the ability to think and remember, but these changes aren't significant enough to affect work or relationships yet.

Someone with mild cognitive impairment may have memory lapses when it comes to information that's usually easily remembered, like conversations, recent events or appointments. Being unable to remember these types of information represents a change for the person.

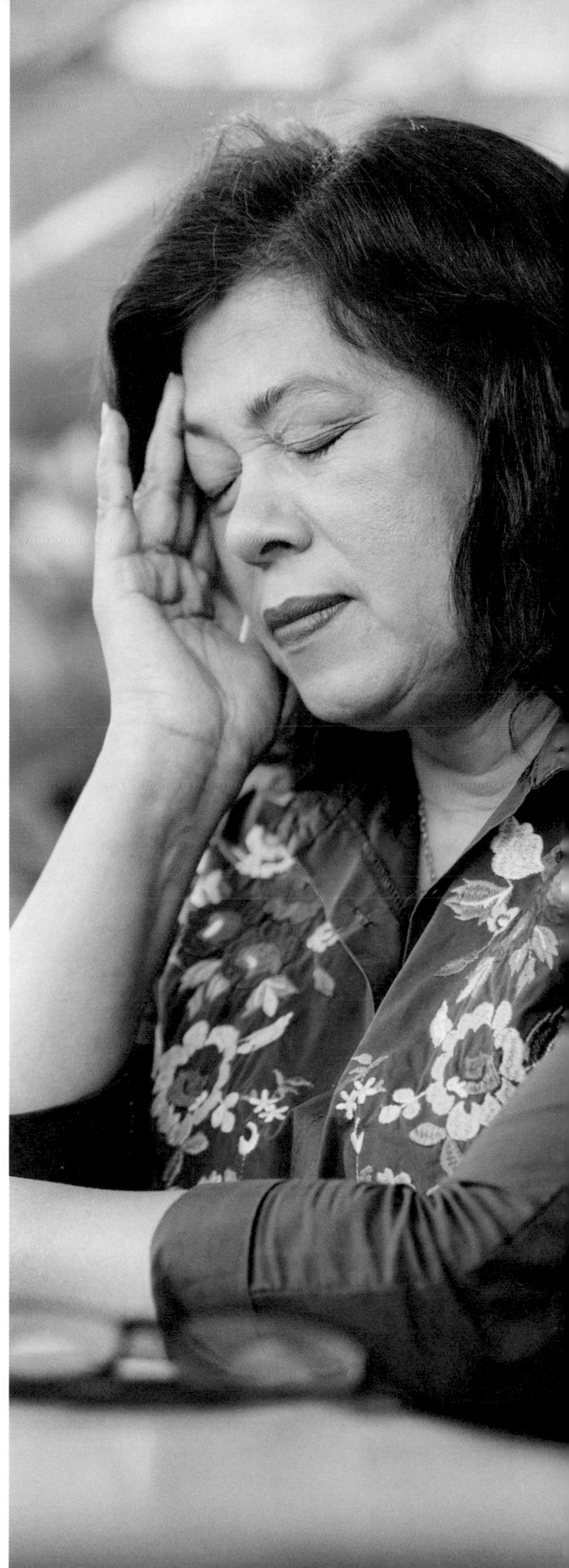

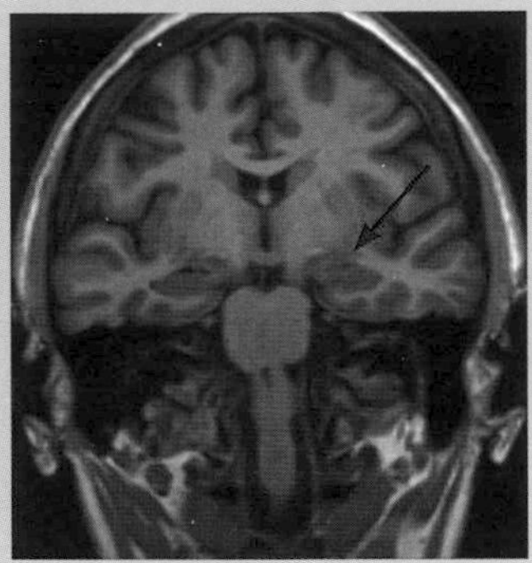
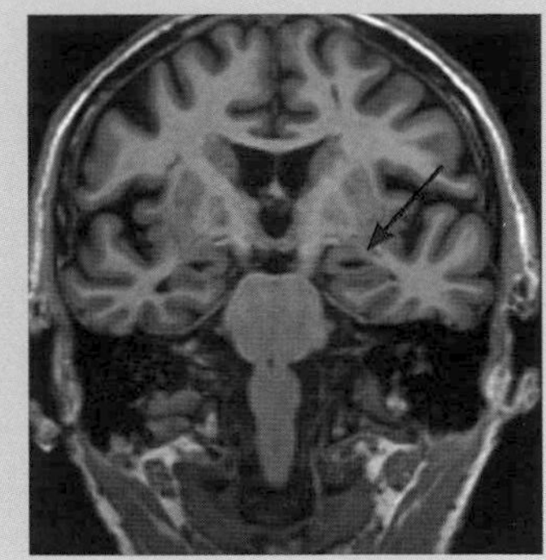
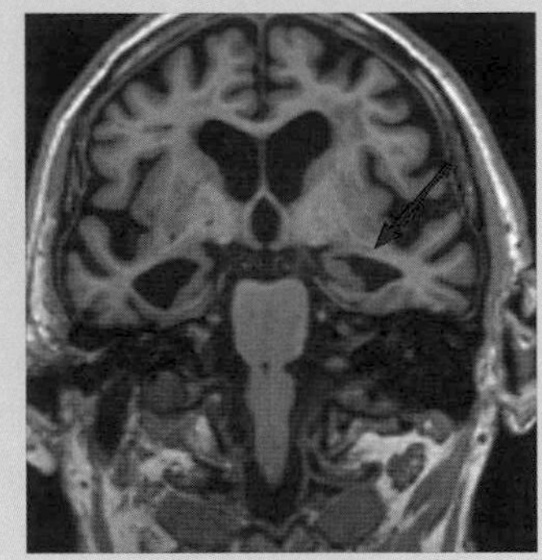

This series of coronal MRIs represents the pattern of brain atrophy known as the "AD signature" in three 70-year-old individuals.

The left image is the brain of a person who is still cognitively normal. The center image is of a person diagnosed with mild cognitive impairment. The right image is a person diagnosed with Alzheimer's. In addition to the loss of overall brain mass, the red arrows highlight shrinkage of the hippocampus. The hippocampus, which is associated with memory processing and retrieval, is one of the earliest brain structures affected by Alzheimer's.

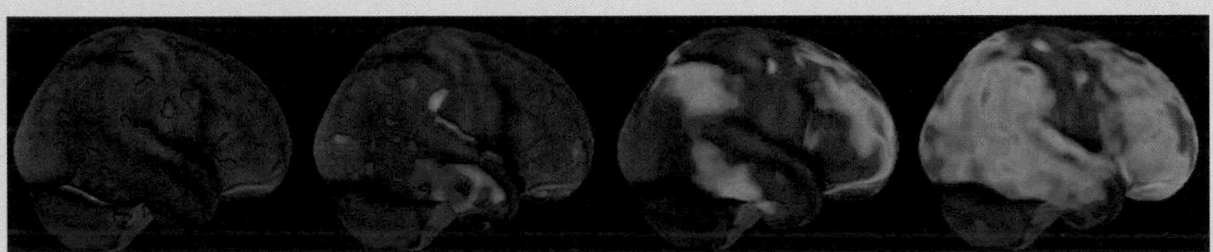

These glucose PET scans show the progression of hypometabolism from a brain that is cognitively normal (left) to a brain with mild cognitive impairment (second from the left), a brain with mild dementia (second from the right) and then moderate dementia (right). Hypometabolism means that certain chemical processes in the brain have slowed down. A scan that's primarily black and blue means metabolism is relatively normal. Colors that range from green to yellow, orange or red show metabolism levels that are progressively lower. These kinds of changes may become evident only at the end of the preclinical stage, when subtle cognitive changes are just beginning to develop.

People with mild cognitive impairment may also have trouble judging how much time is needed for a task, or have difficulty correctly judging the number or sequence of steps needed to complete a task. The ability to multitask and make sound decisions can also become harder.

Not everyone with mild cognitive impairment has Alzheimer's disease. The same procedures used to identify preclinical Alzheimer's disease can help determine if mild cognitive impairment is being caused by Alzheimer's disease or by something else.

Mild dementia due to Alzheimer's disease

Alzheimer's disease is often diagnosed in the mild stage, when it becomes clear to family and doctors that a person is having significant trouble with memory and thinking that impacts daily functioning. In the mild Alzheimer's dementia stage, people may experience:

Memory loss for recent events Individuals may have an especially hard time remembering newly learned information and ask the same question over and over.

Difficulty with problem-solving, complex tasks and sound judgment Planning a family event or balancing a checkbook may become overwhelming. Many people experience lapses in judgment, such as when making financial decisions.

Difficulty organizing and expressing thoughts Finding the right words to describe objects or clearly express ideas becomes increasingly challenging.

Changes in personality People may become subdued or withdrawn — especially in socially challenging situations — or show uncharacteristic irritability or anger. Reduced motivation to complete tasks also is common.

Getting lost or misplacing belongings Individuals have increasing trouble finding their way around, even in familiar places. It's also common to lose or misplace things, including valuable items.

Moderate dementia due to Alzheimer's disease

During the moderate stage of Alzheimer's disease, people become more confused and forgetful and begin to need more help with daily activities and self-care.

In the moderate stage of Alzheimer's disease, a person may:

Show increasingly poor judgment and deepening confusion Individuals lose track of where they are, the day of the week or the season. They may confuse family members or close friends with one another, or mistake strangers for family. They may wander, possibly in search of surroundings that feel more familiar.

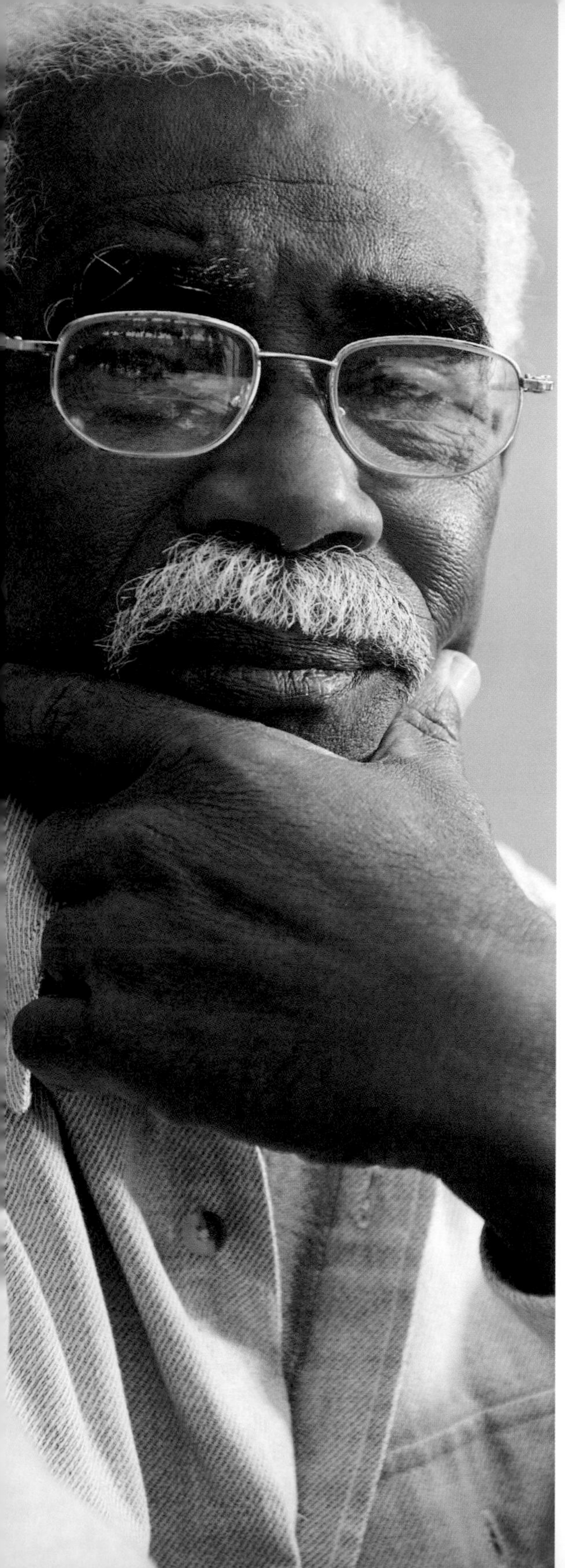

These difficulties make it unsafe to leave those in the moderate Alzheimer's stage on their own.

Experience even greater memory loss People may forget details of their personal history, such as their address or phone number, or where they attended school. People in this stage of dementia due to Alzheimer's disease may repeat favorite stories or create stories to fill gaps in memory.

Undergo significant changes in personality and behavior It's not unusual for people with moderate Alzheimer's disease to develop unfounded suspicions. For example, they may become convinced that friends, family or professional caregivers are stealing from them or that a spouse is having an affair. Others may see or hear things that aren't really there. Individuals often grow restless or agitated, especially late in the day. Some people may have outbursts of aggressive physical behavior.

Need help with some daily activities Assistance may be required with choosing the right clothing for an occasion or the weather and with bathing, grooming, using the bathroom and other self-care. Some individuals occasionally lose control of their bladder or bowel movements.

Severe dementia due to Alzheimer's disease

In the severe (late) stage of Alzheimer's disease, mental function continues to decline, and the disease has a growing impact on movement and physical capabilities. In this stage, people generally:

Experience a decline in physical abilities A person may become unable to walk without help, then unable to sit or hold up his or her head without support. Muscles may become rigid and reflexes abnormal. Eventually, a person loses the ability to swallow and to control bladder and bowel functions.

Lose the ability to communicate coherently An individual can no longer speak coherently, although he or she may occasionally say words or phrases.

Require daily assistance with personal care This includes total assistance with eating, dressing, using the bathroom and all other daily self-care tasks.

How quickly Alzheimer's disease stages progress

The rate of progression for Alzheimer's disease varies widely. On average, people with Alzheimer's disease dementia live between three and 11 years after diagnosis, but some live with Alzheimer's disease dementia for 20 years or more.

Pneumonia is a common cause of death because impaired swallowing allows food or beverages to enter the lungs, where an infection can begin. Other common causes of death include dehydration, malnutrition, falls and other infections.

CONCURRENT CAUSES OF DEMENTIA

It's not uncommon for Alzheimer's disease to occur at the same time as other disorders that cause dementia. This can make it difficult for a doctor to make a diagnosis.

Because treatment options may vary, a doctor will carefully study all of the signs and symptoms and perform various tests in hopes of distinguishing between Alzheimer's and another cause of dementia. Here are several common causes of dementia that may occur at the same time as Alzheimer's.

Vascular brain damage

Based on autopsy reports, most people with Alzheimer's disease also have blood vessel (cerebrovascular) disease, like a stroke or damage to the blood vessels in the brain. A doctor may use the terms *vascular cognitive impairment* or *vascular dementia* to describe these changes.

Lewy body disease

Approximately 15% of those with Alzheimer's disease dementia also have Lewy bodies. Research estimates that 50% to 80% of the nearly 1 million people with Parkinson's disease may experience dementia.

Lewy bodies are abnormal protein deposits in the brain that progressively destroy neurons and disrupt communication between cells in the brain. Lewy bodies occur in some people with Alzheimer's disease, highlighting the fact that for most people with dementia, more than one disease is causing their cognitive decline. For more on dementia with Lewy bodies, see Chapter 10.

Parkinson's disease

Some people with Alzheimer's develop Parkinson's disease. Parkinson's disease is a movement disorder. It affects nerve cells in parts of the brain that control muscle movements. It's characterized by limb stiffness, tremors, difficulty with walking and speech impairment.

Parkinson's disease is also associated with Lewy body deposits in the brain, particularly in the structures of the brain that are important for movement. These Lewy bodies can occur with or without coexisting Alzheimer's disease changes. This suggests a close but still undetermined relationship among all three disorders.

OTHER CONDITIONS THAT CAN ACCOMPANY ALZHEIMER'S

Often, certain conditions may develop at the same time as Alzheimer's. The signs and symptoms of these conditions can make it more difficult for a doctor to make a diagnosis. They may also make cognitive decline worse or cause it to worsen more quickly.

The fact that many of these conditions are treatable emphasizes the importance of getting an early diagnosis. Conditions that commonly coexist with Alzheimer's include depression, anxiety and sleep disorders. Here's more on each.

Depression

Research suggests that up to 40% of people with Alzheimer's dementia experience significant depression at some point. It's especially common during the early stages when social isolation, diminishing mental and physical abilities, and loss of independence occurs. While brief periods of discouragement and apathy are understandable, prolonged sadness is not.

Although it's common for depression and Alzheimer's disease dementia to coexist, scientists aren't sure of the exact relationship between the two. Studies indicate that chronic feelings of sadness or worthlessness may be linked to the awareness of mental decline — despite the fact that many people with Alzheimer's lose insight into their behavior early in the disease process.

Other research has found that the biological changes caused by Alzheimer's may make depression more likely. Some studies suggest that the symptoms of depression, like apathy and lack of motivation, may be among the earliest signs of Alzheimer's.

What's clear is that depression strongly affects quality of life for someone living with Alzheimer's disease, as well as for the person's loved ones. In addition to the emo-

The Alzheimer's Association offers an online tool at *www.alzheimersnavigator.org* to help people living with Alzheimer's create and organize action plans addressing a variety of issues.

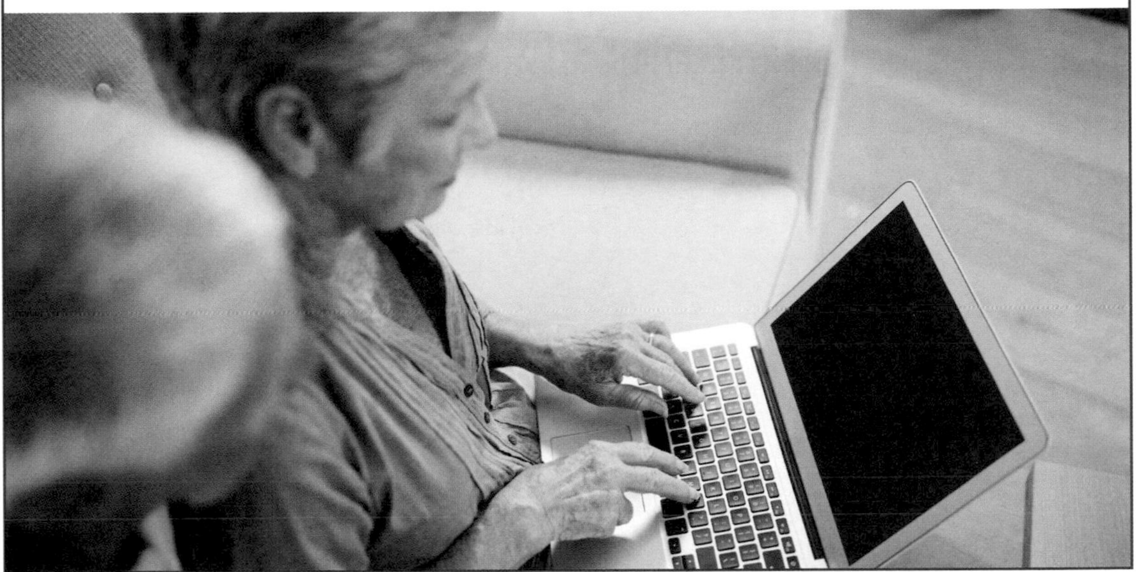

tional problems it causes, depression can lead to weight loss and physical frailty. Depression is associated with earlier placement in assisted living and nursing homes, greater disability in the performance of daily living skills, and physical aggression toward caregivers. Depression in a person with Alzheimer's also increases the chances of depression in caregivers.

Diagnosing depression in a person with Alzheimer's can be especially challenging. This is due, in part, to the person's growing inability to describe how he or she feels. With this in mind, experts encourage anyone involved in the daily life of the person with Alzheimer's to take part in doctor visits to provide a more complete picture of the person's moods.

Counseling and nondrug therapy can be helpful, especially for people with mild depression. A licensed mental health professional can help a person with Alzheimer's develop daily routines and find enjoyable activities to take part in. A therapist can also help care partners learn problem-solving and coping skills that can help with symptoms.

Antidepressants can help relieve severe symptoms of depression. In particular, the

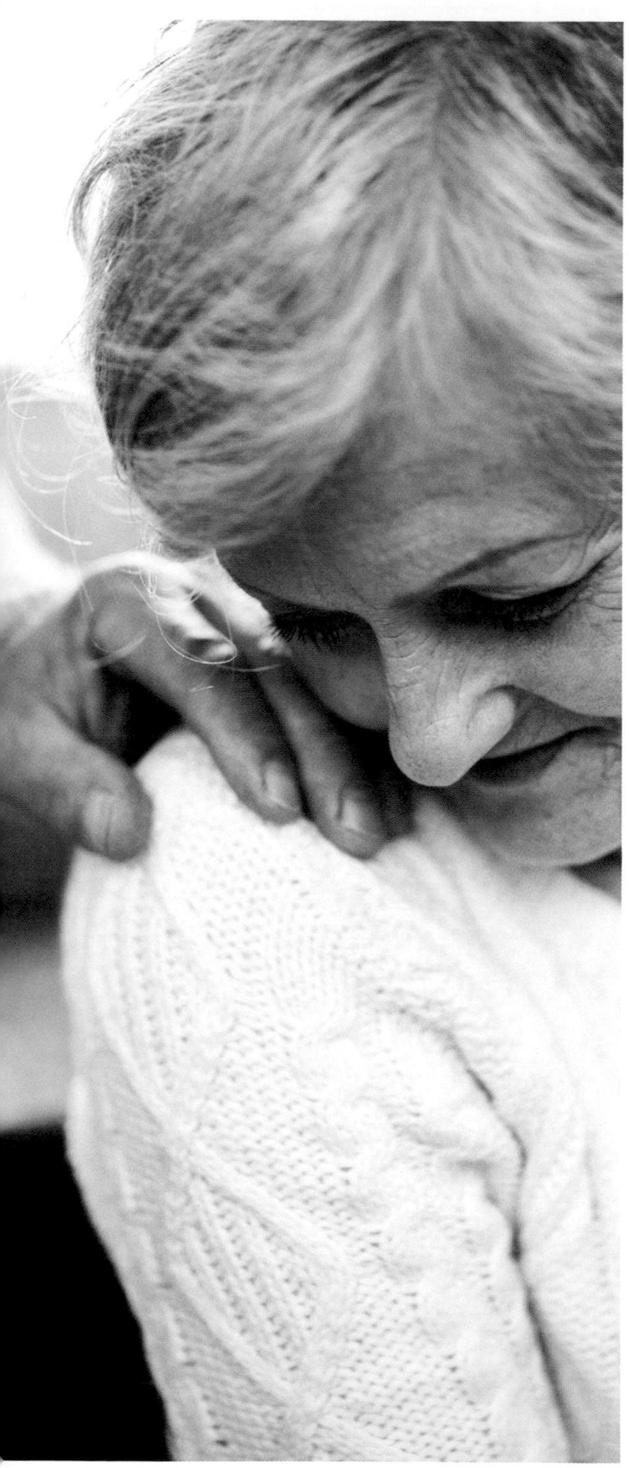

most commonly prescribed antidepressants, selective serotonin reuptake inhibitors (SSRIs), are effective, and most people have few issues with taking them.

Anxiety

Symptoms of anxiety — fearfulness, restlessness, agitation, apprehension, fidgeting or pacing, excessive worry, and even anger — are common among people with Alzheimer's, especially early on, such as during the mild cognitive impairment stage.

In addition, anxiety and depression often occur at the same time. It's not hard to imagine how someone whose memory — of the past, of how to do routine tasks, of familiar faces and places — is failing would frequently feel anxious and insecure.

Anxiety is associated with some challenging behaviors that may occur with Alzheimer's. These include agitation, wandering, inappropriate behavior, hallucinations, verbal threats and physical abuse. These behaviors can lead to a move to a nursing home or other residential care community. Treating the anxiety with medication, as well as addressing psychosocial needs and environmental triggers, may improve these symptoms. In turn, this can reduce stress and fatigue for the care partner.

Treatment for anxiety generally includes strategies to address and understand the root cause of the behavior. A common method is to identify the behavior that's causing concern, find out what may be causing it, and adapt the person's environment to minimize his or her discomfort. See Chapter 17 for more on behavioral strategies.

If anxiety symptoms are severely disruptive, a doctor may prescribe short-term doses of medications like SSRIs to ease some of these signs and symptoms.

Sleep disorders

Disturbed sleep patterns are common among people with Alzheimer's, particularly in later stages. These disturbances take many forms. Some people may sleep more than they ever did before — up to 16 hours a day. Others may sleep less, perhaps only two to four hours at night. Plus, the cycle of sleep and wakefulness may be reversed between night and day. Restlessness and nighttime wandering are also common.

Factors that may contribute to excessive sleeping include medication side effects, metabolic problems and boredom. On the other hand, anxiety and depression can contribute to insomnia, as can lack of daytime physical activity, too much napping, certain medications and the excessive intake of stimulants such as caffeine.

People with Alzheimer's dementia often have altered sleep patterns, and there are likely many factors behind this. For example, they typically experience more and longer awakenings, as well as a decrease in REM sleep — that period of sleep when the brain is very active. The body's circadian rhythms, which act as an internal clock to help regulate sleep, are also disrupted by Alzheimer's and may lead to sleep problems. The rhythms may become delayed or muted, leading to increased activity at night compared to the day (sundowning). People with Alzheimer's are also less likely to have exposure to environmental factors that can help regulate circadian rhythms, such as bright light.

Helping a person with Alzheimer's maintain a routine, participate in meaningful activities daily, monitor napping and caffeine intake, increase physical activity, and maintain a reasonable bedtime (not too early) may improve sleep patterns.

Other sleep disorders that commonly affect people with Alzheimer's include restless legs syndrome, sleep apnea and periodic limb movements during sleep. People with Alzheimer's may snore loudly and experience episodes of snorting or gasping, a creepy-crawly sensation in their legs (especially at night), or nightmares.

These signs and symptoms should be discussed with a doctor. Successfully treating a sleep disorder can improve cognition, mood and quality of life. Sleep disturbances often affect a bed partner's sleep patterns, as well, making it important for a care partner to find alternate ways to get rest.

"THESE TWO FORMS OF ALZHEIMER'S DISEASE DEMENTIA ARE ADDRESSED TOGETHER BECAUSE THERE'S CONSIDERABLE OVERLAP BETWEEN THE TWO."

CHAPTER 7

Atypical and young-onset Alzheimer's dementia

Some types of Alzheimer's don't quite fit the typical profile of the disease. These atypical variations are less common than typical Alzheimer's dementia — they affect about 15% of the total number of people with Alzheimer's disease dementia.

It can be challenging to tell if someone has an atypical form of Alzheimer's. That's because the first signs that appear are usually things other than memory loss, like trouble with language, vision or sequencing tasks like cooking. When nonmemory symptoms are the first to appear, it may take longer for someone to be diagnosed with Alzheimer's disease.

A living diagnosis of atypical Alzheimer's has become more common recently because of advances that allow doctors to check for biomarkers of Alzheimer's disease. Biomarkers can be measured with brain imaging and in the fluid that surrounds the brain and spinal cord (cerebrospinal fluid). These biomarkers measure the hallmark proteins of Alzheimer's disease: amyloid and tau.

Another important form of Alzheimer's is young-onset Alzheimer's. This happens when people develop signs and symptoms of Alzheimer's, including memory loss, much earlier than most people with Alzheimer's — before age 65.

Young-onset Alzheimer's disease accounts for about 5% to 6% of all cases of Alzheimer's disease. About 200,000 Americans are living with young-onset Alzheimer's disease. Of them, around 1 in 10 has familial Alzheimer's. This means the disease is caused by specific genetic mutations that cause Alzheimer's disease.

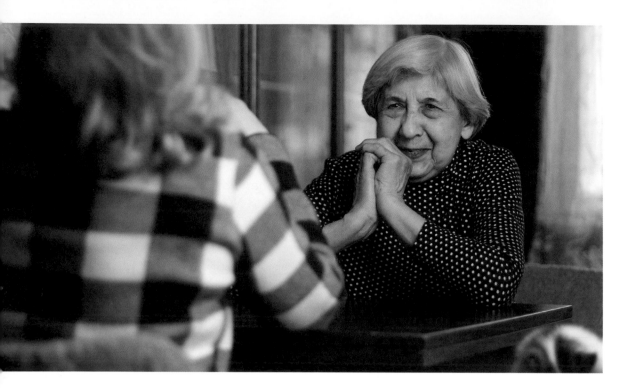

This chapter addresses both atypical and young-onset Alzheimer's disease dementia These two forms of Alzheimer's dementia are addressed together because there's considerable overlap between the two. While atypical Alzheimer's disease dementia tends to occur in younger people, it also affects people over age 65. Similarly, people with young-onset Alzheimer's disease frequently have atypical symptoms, but typical symptoms of Alzheimer's disease are more common.

ATYPICAL ALZHEIMER'S

You might sometimes hear atypical forms of Alzheimer's referred to as nonamnestic Alzheimer's. Nonamnestic means not related to memory. Most Alzheimer's is amnestic, which means the main issue is memory loss.

The most common forms of atypical Alzheimer's disease affect language (logopenic variant primary progressive aphasia), vision and spatial perception (posterior cortical atrophy), and behavior or executive thinking skills (behavioral/dysexecutive Alzheimer's). These conditions are less common than typical Alzheimer's dementia, so it's difficult for researchers to assemble studies with enough participants to show reliable patterns in how a disease progresses or what therapies are most helpful. Here's more on what's known about these three conditions.

Logopenic variant primary progressive aphasia

Janice is 54 years old. For the past couple of years, she's noticed that it's harder for her to find words in the middle of a conversation. She's also noticed that it's harder to pronounce words and follow and repeat more complex sentences.

Most of Janice's test results were normal. However, a language exam given to her by her doctor uncovered problems with word finding, pronunciation and repetition. Brain imaging tests showed abnormalities in the parts of the brain involved in language. Janice was diagnosed with logopenic variant primary progressive aphasia.

What is it? Logopenic variant primary progressive aphasia (lvPPA) is most commonly considered an atypical form of Alzheimer's, but it can also be placed in other categories.

For starters, it can be categorized as a syndrome called primary progressive aphasia. Primary progressive aphasia affects how well you understand and express language. It's caused by brain damage from neurodegeneration.

You'll learn about three types of primary progressive aphasia in this book. LvPPA is the only one strongly associated with Alzheimer's disease. The other types generally fall under the category of frontotemporal degeneration.

But lvPPA is also seen as a form of Alzheimer's disease because it involves the same hallmark plaques and tangles found in the brain of someone with typical Alzheimer's disease.

Put another way, the signs and symptoms of lvPPA are different from those seen in typical Alzheimer's — at least at first. However, what causes the symptoms — plaques and tangles — is the same as what causes typical Alzheimer's disease. In lvPPA, the tangles tend to occur in the language network. This is why it causes problems with language.

Not all cases of lvPPA are due to Alzheimer's disease. Rarely, the damage is due to changes in the brain that are more like what happens in frontotemporal degeneration.

What are the symptoms? People with this form of Alzheimer's disease are gradually less able to find words when speaking. As a result, they may pause or talk around a word, especially when they need to be specific or use an unfamiliar word.

They may also make errors with sounds when they speak. As a result, they may leave out or substitute letter sounds. They may say *bing* instead of *bring* or *that* for *sat*. They also have trouble repeating long or complex sentences.

The ability to remember, think and reason stays fairly stable early on. They can usually remember the meanings of words, for example, even if they can't find the right word. They're also able to use proper grammar. Not much is known about the course of the disease, but memory may be impaired to some degree eventually.

How is it diagnosed? A visit with a doctor is typically scheduled when language becomes impaired enough that a person or his or her family and friends notice.

A doctor will likely take a detailed history of the language problems, along with any other signs, like memory loss or behavioral changes. A doctor may also do tests that measure speech, language comprehension and skills, recognition and naming of objects, recall, and other factors.

From there, a doctor may suggest a visit with a speech-language pathologist. This specialist can assess speech and language issues and help determine if they're being caused by lvPPA or something else.

Brain scans like magnetic resonance imaging (MRI) scans can show if there's shrinking in certain areas of the brain. MRI can also show which area of the brain might be affected. MRI can also rule out strokes, tumors or other conditions that affect brain function.

Tests that show brain function, like positron emission tomography (PET) scans, may be used to uncover glucose metabolism problems. Glucose PET scans usually aren't needed unless a doctor isn't certain of the diagnosis after a routine evaluation and imaging tests are done. PET scans measuring beta-amyloid or tau are typically used in the research setting to measure the hallmark proteins of Alzheimer's.

Occasionally, the fluid around the brain and spinal cord (cerebrospinal fluid) is checked for beta-amyloid or tau. These are the proteins that make up plaques or tangles. A doctor may use this test if a diagnosis isn't clear after routine tests are done.

People diagnosed with primary progressive aphasia may not know whether the disease is a form of Alzheimer's until later on, when other areas of the brain are affected, resulting in additional signs and symptoms.

How is it treated? No treatment can cure lvPPA or stop its progression. However,

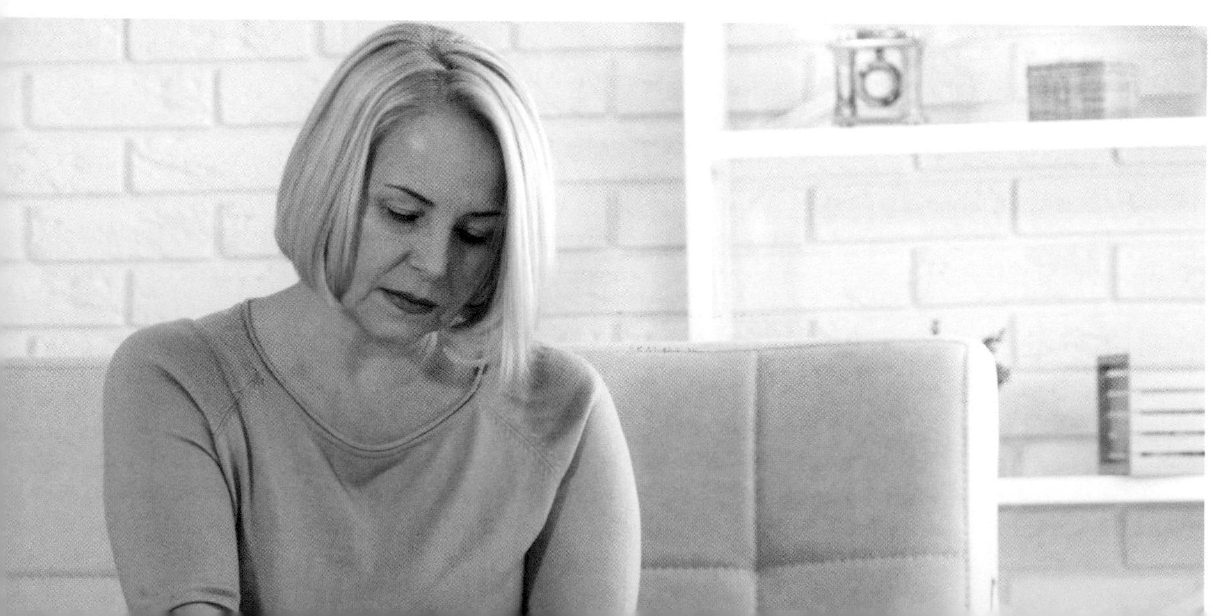

working with a speech-language pathologist, focusing primarily on ways to make up for lost language skills, can be helpful. Speech and language therapy can help a person manage the condition and may slow the progression of symptoms.

Cholinesterase inhibitors, like donepezil, galantamine and rivastigmine, may help with symptoms in some people with lvPPA, especially as memory problems appear later on. Chapter 8 offers detailed information on these medications.

If you're caring for someone with lvPPA, the following tips may help:

- Have the person carry an identification card and other materials that can help explain the syndrome to others.
- Give the person time to talk.
- Speak slowly in simple, adult sentences and listen carefully.
- Avoid communicating from a distance.
- Reduce background noise to help with communication.
- Use gestures, when helpful, to complement what you're saying.
- When needed, choose a different word to help with understanding.
- Instead of asking, "What?" restate what you heard and understood and ask for clarification when you need it.

Posterior cortical atrophy

Sarah is 62 years old and has developed vision problems. She's having trouble reading, and her ability to find where she is going has decreased. The results of an eye exam were normal. But over the course of the next several months, her vision problems worsen, and she now needs more help carrying out daily activities.

She often can't reach objects with her hands, and she needs help getting dressed. Cognitive tests and imaging point to posterior cortical atrophy.

What is it? Posterior cortical atrophy is a collection of nervous system symptoms marked by a gradual loss in a person's ability to purposefully process visual information. This difficulty is caused by shrinking (atrophy) of the back (posterior cortical) part of the brain. This is the region responsible for vision and spatial reasoning. The hallmark plaques and tangles of typical Alzheimer's disease are the most common cause of this damage. But it can also be caused by corticobasal degeneration (see Chapter 9) or other brain disorders. Over time, memory and thinking abilities (cognitive skills) may decline.

What are the symptoms? People with posterior cortical atrophy often have trouble reading, judging distances, and recognizing objects and familiar faces. Difficulty with stairs is common. They may have trouble getting dressed or using a fork or a toothbrush. Before being diagnosed, they may have trouble driving because staying within the lines and seeing at night are difficult. It may even be difficult to navigate familiar surroundings without bumping into things.

Most people with posterior cortical atrophy start to experience symptoms in their 50s or

SPEECH THERAPY FOR LOGOPENIC VARIANT PRIMARY PROGRESSIVE APHASIA

Speech therapy can maximize independence in communication and lessen frustration caused by communication issues.

One of the biggest sources of frustration is being unable to come up with a specific word. Speech-language therapists use an approach involving repetition to help. They work with the person living with dementia and the person's care partner to identify the words that cause the biggest challenges. These words are said over and over again. Reading or writing the word also can sometimes help. This type of repetition has been shown to help people remember the names of these items.

Practicing talking around a word is another strategy that can help someone who's having trouble finding the right word to say. This strategy involves describing an item when you can't come up with the word for it. "You peel it, it's yellow, you find it in the kitchen, it's a fruit" is a way for people with dementia to say that they're asking for a banana.

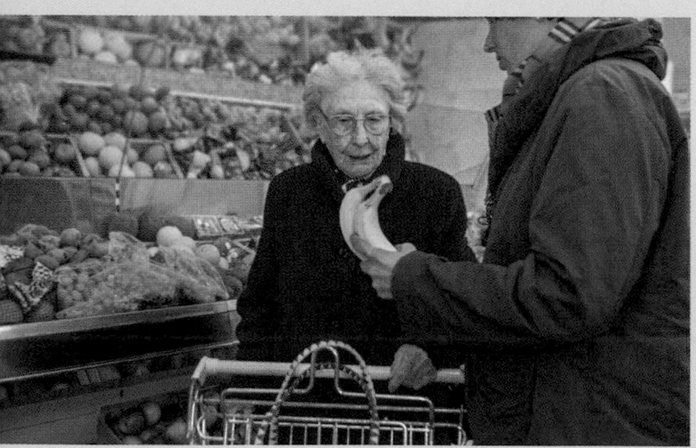

Speech-language therapists can also help identify how much information someone with dementia can process. This helps care partners learn the best way to give information.

For example, someone with dementia may be able to follow a series of simple instructions, like "Grab your shoes, hat and coat, and meet me by the door," but not instructions that include a lot of extra information, like, "We have to be at the restaurant in 20 minutes. We're leaving from the back door in five minutes, but it's cold outside; before we go, you need to dress for the weather. Get your hat, coat and boots first."

Later in the disease, gauging preferences is still important, but limiting choices becomes more helpful. Instead of asking, "Would you like coffee, tea, juice, water or milk?" you might ask, "Would you prefer something hot or cold to drink?"

Speech-language therapy can also be used to support memory challenges as they develop. Building a visual schedule or developing a planner to keep track of day-to-day events are examples. Picture books of people and places can help prepare for events or talk about the past.

A speech-language therapist can help assess communication breakdowns and identify ways to address new or worsening challenges as they arise.

early 60s. As the disease progresses, they may start to have trouble with functions controlled by other nearby areas of the brain, like performing calculations and spelling. Problems with memory, insight and judgment usually don't appear until later on.

How is it diagnosed? Because posterior cortical atrophy causes vision problems, people with this disorder often see an eye doctor first. Some people even have surgery to correct visual issues, like having cataracts removed, only to find that it doesn't help them see better. That's because the problem is in the brain, not the eye. Other times, vision tests don't offer any answers.

An eye doctor may suspect that the problem is in the brain, and refer someone to a doctor who specializes in the brain and nervous system (neurologist) or a doctor that takes

MORE ABOUT PET SCANS

Throughout this chapter, you'll read about PET scans that are used to diagnose Alzheimer's disease. Here's a little more background on two types that may be used.

A fluorodeoxyglucose (FDG) PET scan may be used to look for changes in glucose metabolism in certain areas of the brain. Reduced glucose metabolism is often a sign that brain networks aren't functioning as they should. This test helps tell the difference between Alzheimer's disease and frontotemporal degeneration, which you'll read about in Chapter 9. These two types of dementia affect different parts of the brain. This test may also help a doctor tell the difference between other causes of young-onset dementia, including dementia with Lewy bodies.

Amyloid PET is a test that can spot amyloid deposits in the brain. This can help confirm a diagnosis of Alzheimer's. While this is a promising imaging test and it's approved for use by the Food and Drug Administration, it currently isn't used widely in doctor's offices due to its high cost. It's important to note that not all newer tests, like amyloid imaging, are covered by insurance.

care of visual issues related to the brain (neuro-ophthalmologist). From there, a neurologist will ask for a detailed account of symptoms and will likely test the person's cognitive skills.

The neurologist will likely rule out other possible causes of the symptoms first. This may mean having blood tests to check for a vitamin deficiency or thyroid disorder, or brain scans to check for a tumor or stroke, like those in a typical cognitive evaluation.

Neuropsychological tests (see Chapter 4) also may be helpful; they may pinpoint a problem with visuospatial skills. In everyday life, these problems can affect your ability to judge the height of a step or find your way around familiar places.

An MRI is likely to show shrinking in the part of the brain used for vision and spatial reasoning, and a PET scan may show low levels of glucose metabolism in these areas. These tests may help confirm a diagnosis.

WHAT POSTERIOR CORTICAL ATROPHY LOOKS LIKE

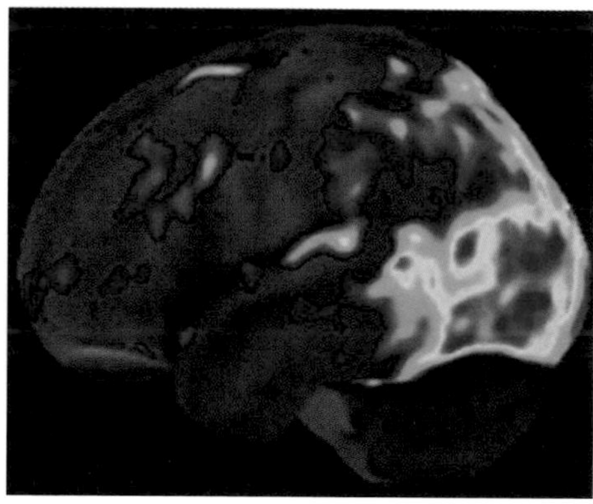

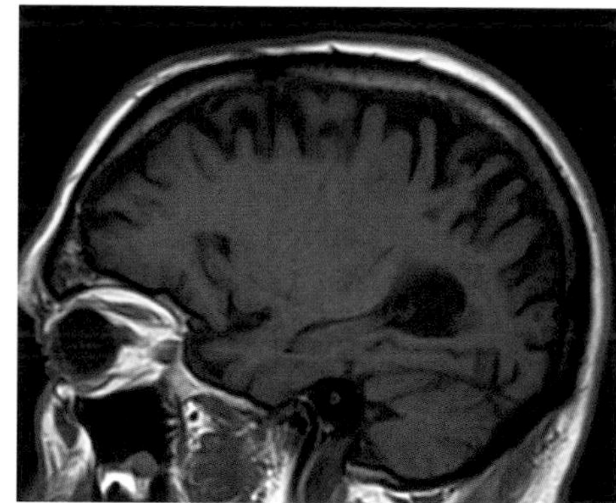

The left image is a PET scan showing posterior cortical atrophy. Colored areas show areas of damage to the brain. Dark blue areas are affected the least, while red shows areas of the brain that are most affected. This PET scan shows damage to the areas of the brain responsible for vision and spatial reasoning. The MRI on the right shows the same brain. The dark area toward the back of the brain shows shrinking (atrophy) in the same area.

How is it treated? Although posterior cortical atrophy can't be cured, these options can minimize the impact of the disease.

Adaptive equipment. Equipment designed to help those who live with low vision or blindness can help those with posterior cortical atrophy. Examples might include a walking cane, voice recorder or talking watch. Downloading audiobooks or podcasts onto a digital audio device, like a smartphone or tablet, can be helpful when reading is difficult. (See page 146.)

Smartphone apps that use the phone's camera to identify colors, read texts, describe scenes and even recognize people can all be useful — but the interface may be visually confusing. A simple smartphone with large buttons and good contrast may be helpful.

Disease education. It can be helpful for people with posterior cortical atrophy and their loved ones to understand the differences between posterior cortical atrophy and *typical* Alzheimer's.

For example, a person with posterior cortical atrophy may not be able to pick up a cup of coffee, but can still have a conversation about current affairs or remember day-to-day events, like appointments and items on a grocery list. Focusing on strengths is essential. It can help reduce stress and anxiety for everyone.

Cognitive behavioral therapy. A person with posterior cortical atrophy retains memory and thinking skills for much of the disease course, which can make it hard to accept the loss of other skills, like driving or reading. People with posterior cortical atrophy often report feelings of guilt, anger and frustration when they have to depend on others.

Cognitive behavioral therapy (CBT) can help a person who has posterior cortical atrophy develop positive coping skills, such as challenging negative thought and behavior patterns and learning relaxation techniques. CBT can also help caregivers.

Medications. Although cholinesterase inhibitors like donepezil, galantamine and rivastigmine are used mostly to help with memory issues, they may help with symptoms of posterior cortical atrophy, as well. Chapter 8 offers more information more detailed information on these medications.

Behavioral/dysexecutive Alzheimer's disease

Roger is 63 and has noticed years of declining productivity at his job. Some days, he realizes he's spent the whole day staring at his computer without doing work. He has also been having trouble staying organized and is experiencing memory problems. Those close to him say it seems like he can't complete tasks properly.

On tests, Roger has problems with organizing tasks, managing time, solving problems and thinking abstractly (executive function). Imaging tests that show shrinkage in the brain suggest that Roger has behavioral/dysexecutive young-onset Alzheimer's disease.

WHEN SEEING IS DIFFICULT

Early signs of posterior cortical atrophy often include vision problems that make it hard for the brain to interpret what the eyes are seeing. This can make it hard to read, recognize objects and faces, tell time, judge distance, drive, and navigate surroundings. An occupational therapist experienced in dealing with low vision can help find ways to compensate for these vision issues. Ask your doctor for a referral. In the meantime, here are three strategies that might help:

Contrast. Good lighting and high contrast make it easier for a person to distinguish letters and shapes. Avoid busy patterns. Use contrasting colored markers, tape, paint or fabric to make items such as the following stand out:

- Written words on paper
- Light switches
- Doors, windows and railings
- Steps
- Rugs
- Throws and pillows on furniture
- Place mats and dishes
- Cutting boards and cooking utensils
- Appliances
- Toilet seats, tub edges and grab bars
- Drawer handles

Consistency. Maintaining a consistent location for regularly used items can minimize the effort needed to find things. For example, milk goes in the right hand refrigerator door, keys on the side table, pens in the left hand drawer and jacket in the hall closet. Avoid moving furniture or appliances, and keep clutter to a minimum. Organize closets and drawers in a system that simplifies identification. For example, color-code drawer handles for different types of clothing. Use wallets with several compartments to keep various money denominations separate. Fold bills so the large, bold number on the bottom right corner is plainly visible. Have a specific pocket for each credit card.

Texture. Use texture and memory to make objects more easily identifiable. Coins can be identified by running a finger around the edge of the coin. Pennies and nickels are smooth; quarters and dimes have ridges. Use a safety pin or a button sewn to clothing to identify the inside of clothing, as well as the front, back, top or bottom. Use locator (tactile) dots or bumps to mark common settings on a microwave, an oven dial or a TV remote control.

Take time to survey your surroundings and let yourself think outside of the box. What changes would make it easier to engage in daily activities without an overreliance on vision? Allow room for creativity to find a solution that works for you.

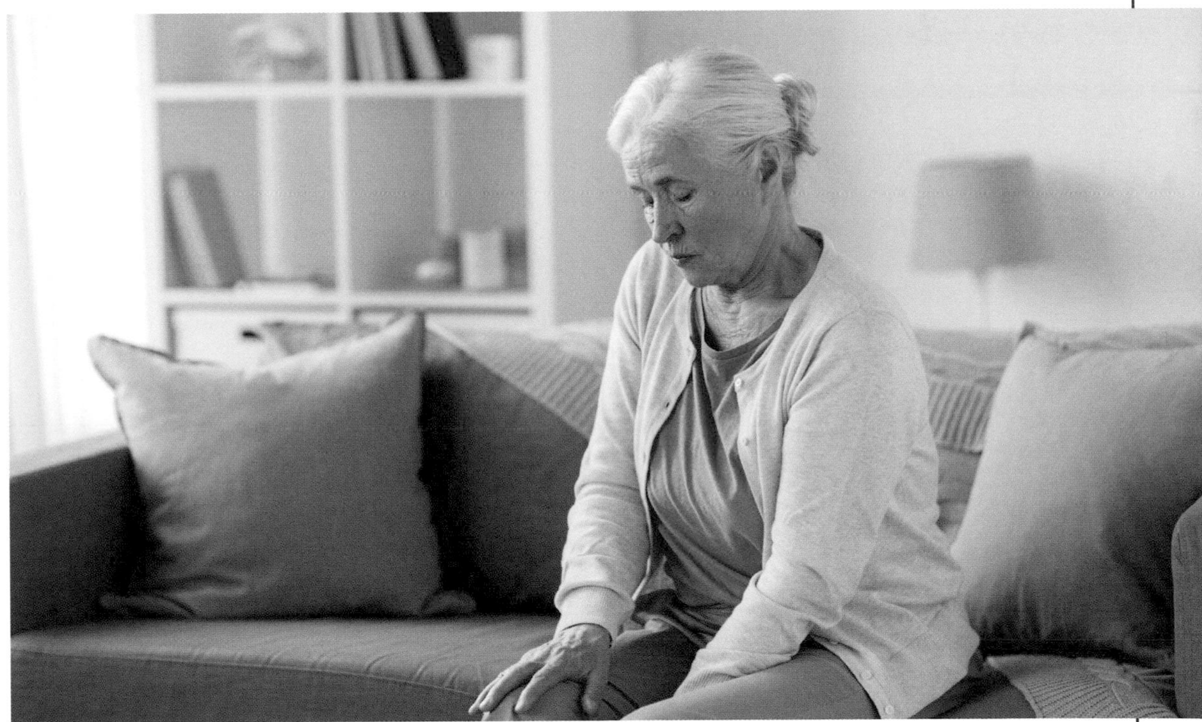

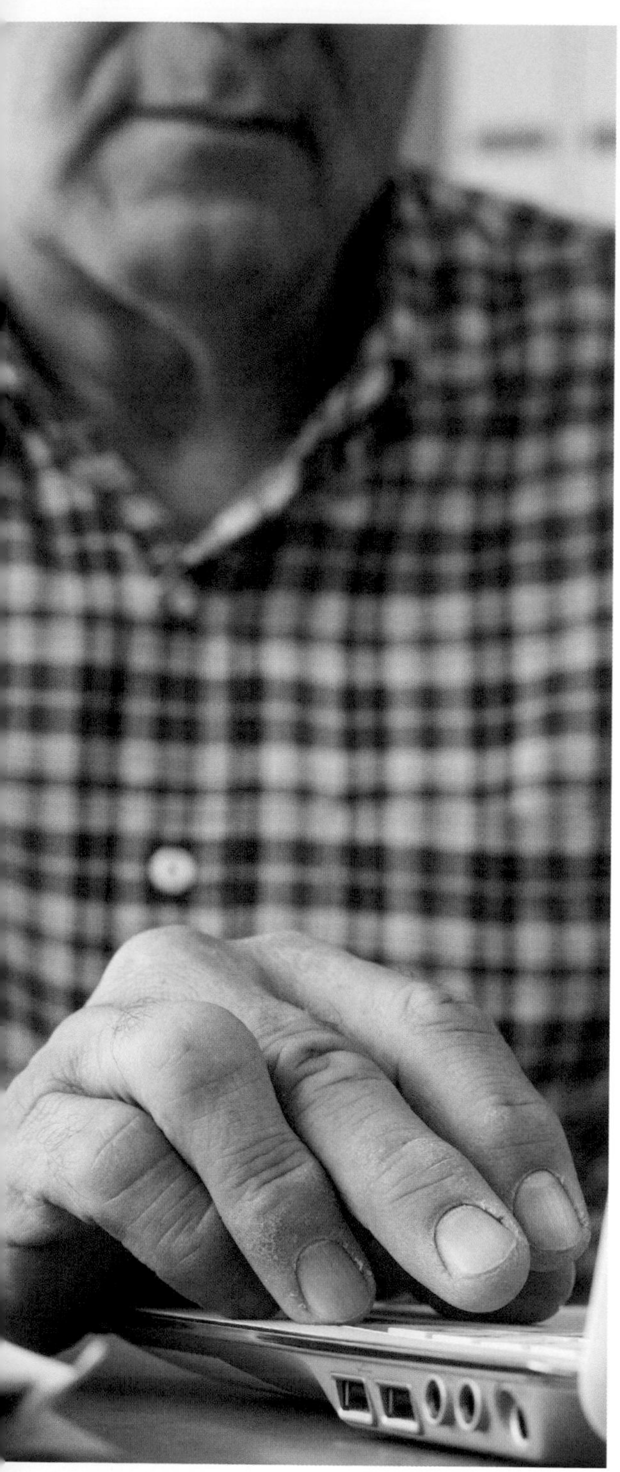

What is it? Behavioral/dysexecutive Alzheimer's disease is sometimes called frontal variant Alzheimer's disease, but behavioral Alzheimer's and dysexecutive Alzheimers are actually two different disorders. There are enough differences in symptoms and the changes in the brain to tell the difference between behavioral and dysexecutive Alzheimer's disease.

Behavioral Alzheimer's disease is a very rare subtype of atypical Alzheimer's disease. Its signs and symptoms include changes in personality, behavior and language. These signs and symptoms are similar to those of behavioral variant frontotemporal dementia (bvFTD), which causes shrinkage in the frontal and temporal lobes of the brain.

In dysexecutive Alzheimer's disease, people have trouble with higher order thinking skills, like planning and focusing.

Some have a combination of behavioral and dysexecutive Alzheimer's disease, which is why they're sometimes lumped together. On average, people with behavioral/dysexecutive Alzheimer's tend to develop symptoms when they're younger than age 65, but symptoms can appear anywhere from the early 40s to the early 80s.

What are the symptoms? In most people, the first symptoms involve problems with higher order thinking (executive skills). It may be harder to focus, stay on task, plan ahead, prioritize, understand other ways of thinking and regulate emotions.

Early on in dysexecutive Alzheimer's disease, someone may have trouble following recipes, using a remote control or doing more than one thing at a time at work. This type of Alzheimer's affects younger people who are still working, and they may be disciplined or demoted because they can no longer perform the high-level tasks of their jobs. They also often have trouble performing purposeful actions even though they have normal muscle strength and tone.

People with behavioral Alzheimer's often begin to show a lack of concern or initiative (apathy), along with memory problems. They are less likely to fixate on putting things in their mouths and engage in repetitive, compulsive behaviors compared with those with bvFTD. In general, people with behavioral Alzheimer's have fewer behavioral symptoms than people with bvFTD do, as well as less anxiety, irritability and agitation.

How is it diagnosed? Even for experts, it can be difficult to tell the difference between behavioral/dysexecutive Alzheimer's and bvFTD. However, there are key differences.

With behavioral Alzheimer's disease, for example, apathy tends to be a primary symptom. And unlike people with bvFTD, those with behavioral Alzheimer's disease are less likely to have obsessions or compulsions with food.

Differences between behavioral/dysexecutive Alzheimer's and bvFTD can also be found with these tests.

Brain imaging. Researchers are looking into patterns of changes in the brain that show if someone's behavioral symptoms are being caused by Alzheimer's disease or bvFTD. For example, PET scans used by researchers that detect amyloid and tau in the brain have been able to show if someone has Alzheimer's disease or frontotemporal dementia.

Spinal fluid testing. Sometimes, a spinal tap is used to test the fluid around the brain and spinal cord (cerebrospinal fluid). This is occasionally done to distinguish Alzheimer's disease from frontotemporal dementia.

Cognitive testing. People with behavioral/dysexecutive Alzheimer's disease tend to do worse on memory tests than those with bvFTD do. Early on, they may have trouble with sequences, like following a recipe or other directions. Also, they don't have the range of abnormal behaviors usually found in people with bvFTD.

In general, the combination of cognitive and memory problems with behavioral issues that are minimal to moderate helps doctors tell the difference between behavioral/dysexecutive Alzheimer's disease and bvFTD.

How is it treated? As with other forms of Alzheimer's, there is no cure. Not much is known about specific therapies for behavioral/dysexecutive Alzheimer's. A doctor may recommend certain medications to help with behaviors. Selective serotonin reuptake inhibitors (SSRIs) may be used to treat symptoms of depression.

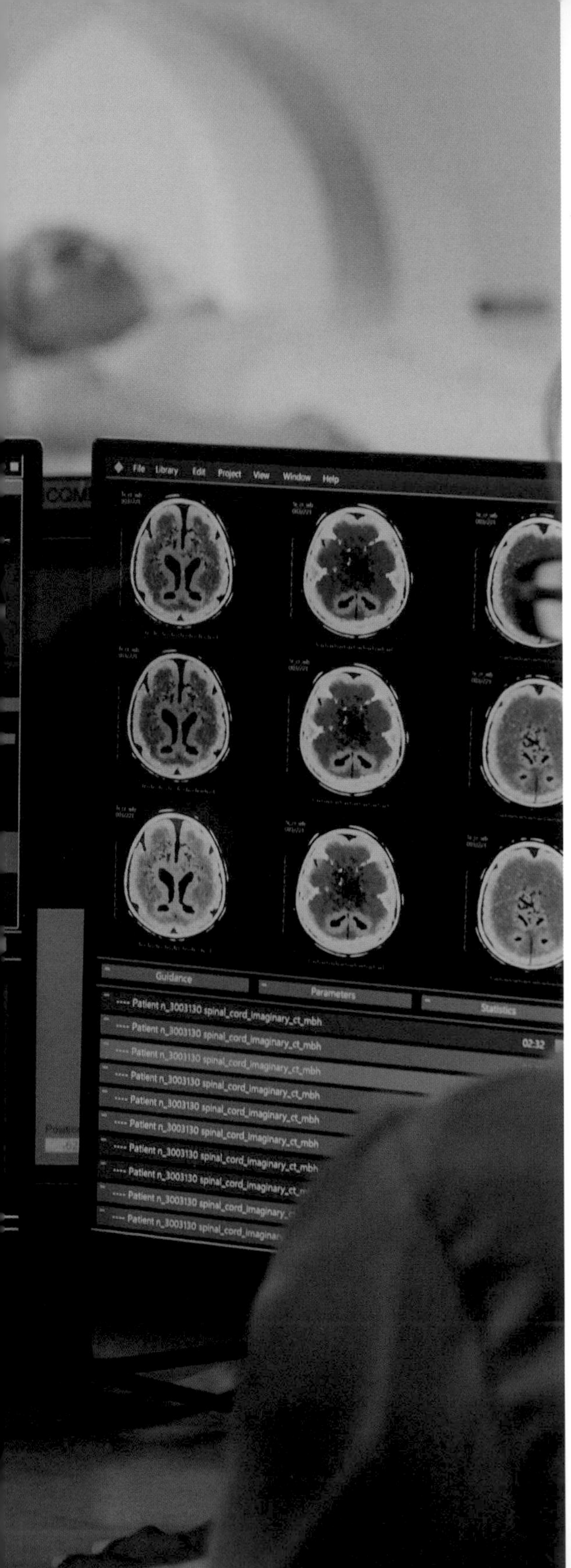

Cholinesterase inhibitors — drugs that target memory, like donepezil, galantamine and rivastigmine — may also help manage symptoms. Learn more in Chapter 8.

YOUNG-ONSET ALZHEIMER'S

Young-onset Alzheimer's is technically defined as an Alzheimer's diagnosis before the age of 65. Yet young-onset Alzheimer's differs significantly from the late-onset form in several other important ways, too.

For example, research suggests that young-onset Alzheimer's disease is more aggressive than the late-onset form. In addition, people with young-onset Alzheimer's are more likely to carry two apolipoprotein E (APOE) e4 alleles, a genetic combination known to increase a person's risk of Alzheimer's and decrease the age of onset. In comparison, as you'll recall, carrying one APOE e4 allele is associated with late-onset Alzheimer's disease. People who develop young-onset Alzheimer's are also more likely to have a history of traumatic brain injury.

Symptoms may develop as early as a person's 40s and 50s, but it can take people with young-onset Alzheimer's longer to get a diagnosis than it takes older adults. Symptoms may be attributed to more-common causes of cognitive problems at midlife, like stress, menopause or depression. This can lead to an incorrect diagnosis and ineffective treatment. Because the disease occurs at a younger age, people diagnosed with young-onset Alzheimer's face additional challenges, including loss of work, financial instability and concerns about raising a family.

As you learned earlier, people diagnosed with young-onset Alzheimer's are more likely to also have atypical forms of Alzheimer's. Unlike the typical memory problems associated with late-onset Alzheimer's, initial symptoms of young-onset Alzheimer's may involve problems with language, vision, behavior or executive skills. Between one-fifth and two-thirds of people with nonfamilial (sporadic) young-onset Alzheimer's have an atypical form of the disease.

Diagnosing young-onset Alzheimer's

Because Alzheimer's occurs less often in younger adults, doctors may recommend the following broader range of tests to rule out other, more common conditions. This means the diagnostic process can take longer than it may with an older adult.

Medical history A doctor usually starts by taking an extensive medical history, detailing what areas of cognition seem to be the most affected, like memory, language or learning.

It's usually helpful to have a family member or close friend present during the appointment — someone who's familiar with the changes the person has experienced. Because young-onset Alzheimer's disease may have a genetic component, a doctor may ask about the person's family history — whether other family members have been diagnosed at a young age with dementia.

Physical and cognitive exams A careful physical assessment may yield clues about what's causing symptoms. Sometimes, diseases that affect the entire body also affect the brain and can cause cognitive impairment. Other diseases that affect the brain and spinal cord, like inflammatory and autoimmune disorders, as well as strokes and seizures, can mimic dementia. These need to be ruled out, too.

A doctor may also look for neurodegenerative diseases outside of Alzheimer's disease, like frontotemporal dementia, Parkinson's disease and dementia with Lewy bodies.

Cognitive and behavioral exams Tests that assess thinking skills or mood and thought content also are helpful. These tests are especially helpful when their results match up with information family members offer.

Cognitive tests can check for problems with memory, language, name recall and other related skills. People evaluated for problems with thinking skills are also usually screened for depression, which can cause issues with thinking and memory. Neuropsychological tests like those you read about in Chapter 4 also may be included.

Blood tests These tests help rule out vitamin or mineral deficiencies, as well as infections or thyroid problems.

Brain imaging and other tests MRI is usually the first imaging test used, and it can help rule out a tumor or stroke. This test can also show brain shrinkage in certain areas, a sign of neurodegenerative disease like Alzheimer's. An MRI shows problems with the blood vessels in the brain (cerebrovascular disease), which also can cause dementia.

When the diagnosis isn't clear, additional tests may be needed, especially in younger people with problems related to thinking and memory. These may include testing the fluid around the brain and spinal cord (cerebrospinal fluid) with a spinal tap to check for amyloid and tau proteins, a hallmark of Alzheimer's disease. A combination of low levels of amyloid and higher levels of the tau in cerebrospinal fluid is the pattern most often linked to Alzheimer's disease.

Genetic testing If someone is showing signs of dementia at an early age and another close family member has already been diagnosed with young-onset Alzheimer's, genetic testing may be considered.

But screening for Alzheimer's-linked mutations in people who have no symptoms and no family history of young-onset Alzheimer's disease isn't recommended. If there is a family history of young-onset Alzheimer's disease, family members with no symptoms will find it helpful to meet with a genetic counselor, to talk through the pros and cons of genetic testing.

If you have young-onset Alzheimer's linked to one of the three genes or carry a form of these genes without symptoms, talk to your doctor about taking part in a research study. By studying the young-onset form of Alzheimer's, researchers hope to learn more about the causes and progression of the disease and develop new treatments.

The Dominantly Inherited Alzheimer Network (DIAN) study, for example, is focusing on individuals with genetic forms of Alzheimer's disease. It consists of observational studies and clinical trials. You may want to learn more about this study if you have a parent or relative with a mutation in the PSEN1, PSEN2 or APP gene or if two generations of your family have Alzheimer's disease that started before age 60.

Managing symptoms

Medications that treat symptoms of other types of Alzheimer's disease may be used to manage symptoms of young-onset and atypical Alzheimer's as well. Cholinesterase inhibitors, like donepezil, galantamine and rivastigmine, and the drug memantine are examples. Learn more in Chapter 8.

Coping with young-onset Alzheimer's

Alzheimer's disease has a tremendous impact at any age. But people with the young-onset form of Alzheimer's may face unique challenges.

First, they may face stigmas and stereotypes about the disease. Due to their young age,

A FAMILIAL THREAD

Most people with young-onset Alzheimer's have what's known as sporadic Alzheimer's. That means it has no genetic cause. But many people with young-onset Alzheimer's do have a genetic mutation that's linked to development of the disease.

Here are the three most common genetic mutations:

- **Presenilin 1 (PSEN1)** This is the most common known cause of genetic young-onset Alzheimer's. People with this mutation are guaranteed to develop Alzheimer's. Half of people with this mutation have symptoms by age 43.
- **Presenilin 2 (PSEN2)** Alzheimer's involving this mutation is more rare. Those who carry this gene have a 95% chance of developing Alzheimer's, which means up to 5% of people who carry it won't ever develop symptoms of Alzheimer's. People who have this mutation generally develop symptoms at a slightly older age than those with the PSEN1 gene. Most are age 50 or older.
- **Amyloid precursor protein (APP)** Up to 15% of inherited Alzheimer's is caused by a mutation in the APP gene. More than 30 mutations in this gene have been linked to Alzheimer's development. These mutations guarantee that the disease will develop at some point. Half of people with this genetic mutation experience symptoms by age 49.

These genetic mutations usually cause more-typical signs of Alzheimer's early on, like memory loss. On the other hand, familial forms of Alzheimer's can also produce less-common signs, like problems with muscle control, seizures and problems with walking. Together, these three genes account for Alzheimer's in less than 1% of people with the disease.

people with the disease may encounter friends and family who deny or question the diagnosis. People with young-onset Alzheimer's may lose relationships or jobs as a result of this misunderstanding rather than being identified as medically ill or disabled. They may also face a loss of income if they are diagnosed while still working.

Here are some ways to address a young-onset Alzheimer's diagnosis.

Work Consider how a young-onset Alzheimer's diagnosis may affect your ability to work.

Here are several steps to take:

- Talk to your doctor about whether you can continue to work. An occupational therapist can help determine whether there are parts of your job you can continue and whether reducing work hours is an option. Learn more about occupational therapy on page 168.
- Explore benefits offered under the Americans with Disabilities Act, Family and Medical Leave Act and COBRA.
- Familiarize yourself and your spouse, partner or caregiver with your benefits, and find out whether an employee assistance program is available.

You'll learn more about ways to approach the workplace in Chapter 13.

Tips for partners After a loved one's diagnosis of young-onset Alzheimer's, spouses or partners often feel a sense of fear and sadness as they face an uncertain future, a changing relationship and an unexpected role as a caregiver. Try to:

- Talk openly about what kind of help you need from each other. Communicate about changes you're experiencing and ways in which your needs also may have changed. Don't be afraid to ask for help.
- Seek out and discuss with your partner what support and resources you need now and may need in the future. Keep a folder of resources you may need as the disease changes.
- Continue living your life as fully as you can. This includes doing activities that you and your partner enjoy, realizing

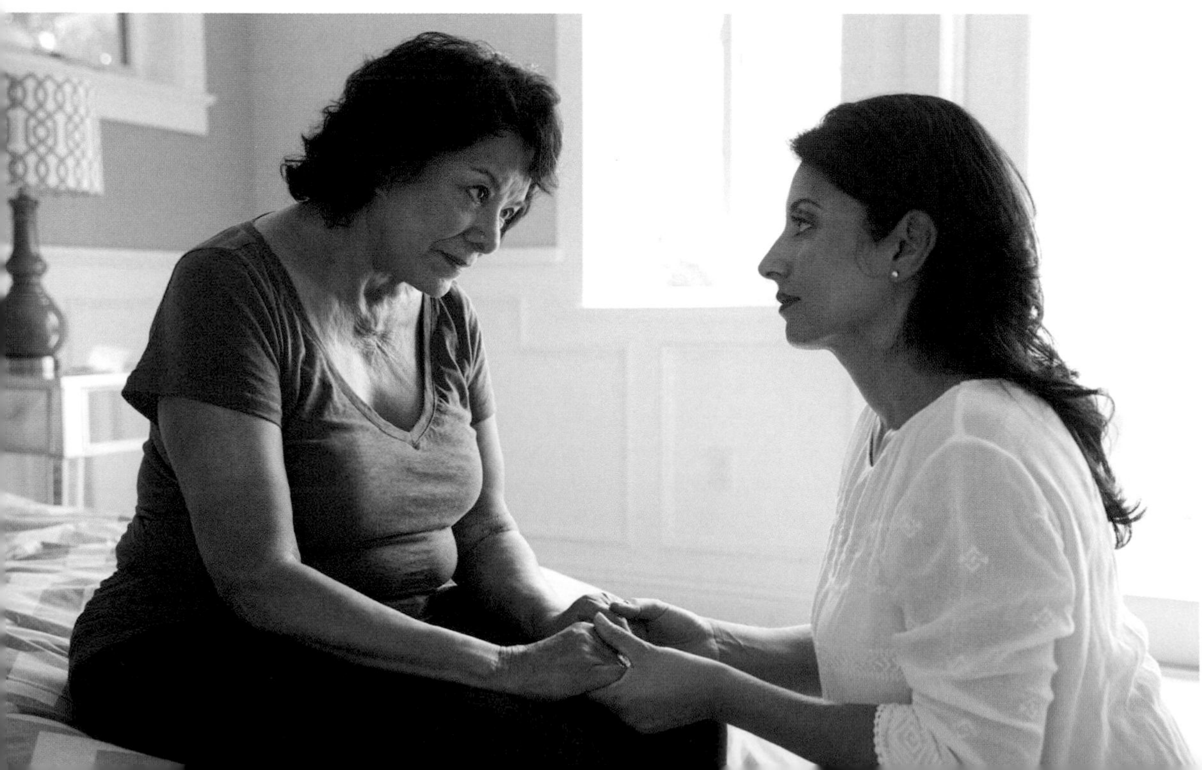

that some adaptations may be needed.
- Find a counselor who works with couples facing issues you feel challenged by, such as intimacy, sexuality and changing roles in the relationship.

You'll find other strategies for care partners later in this book.

Involving children A diagnosis of young-onset Alzheimer's can be difficult for children, who may not understand. Children may become angry or withdrawn or react in any number of ways. Try to:
- Talk with your children honestly about what's happening. If you aren't sure what to say, invite your children to ask questions. This can gauge their level of understanding and guide the conversation. Ask what they're noticing and feeling.
- Look for a support group for children and seek out counseling. Inform your child's school counselor and social worker about your condition.
- Remind children that their parent or loved one is still a person. Reassure them that it's not the fault of the person with dementia, and that they can't help or control what they do.

Learn more about ways to talk with children about dementia in Chapter 13.

Financial issues People with young-onset Alzheimer's dementia often have to quit working, and this loss of income is a serious concern. Finances may be even more affected if a spouse or partner also quits working to care for the person living with dementia. Some medical benefits and many social-support programs may not provide help unless the person with Alzheimer's is older than age 65. Younger people may need special waivers to get into such programs.

Here are several steps to take:
- Talk with a financial planner and an attorney to plan for future financial needs.
- Meet with a social worker to discuss what benefits may be available to you.
- Ask about benefits available through your employer.
- Explore the benefits available through Social Security, Medicare or Medicaid.
- Organize financial documents and make sure your spouse or partner understands and can manage your family's finances.
- Review resources available through the Alzheimer's Association *(www.alz.org).*

Key elements of Alzheimer's care are education and support. These are especially crucial given the unique challenges of young-onset Alzheimer's. Getting connected to services, like support groups, can help you identify resources, gain a deeper understanding of what the future entails and learn ways to adapt.

For more information on strategies for coping with a diagnosis, see Chapter 13.

"A NUMBER OF STRATEGIES CAN HELP PEOPLE WITH ALZHEIMER'S LIVE TO THEIR FULLEST CAPACITY AND MAINTAIN INDEPENDENCE FOR AS LONG AS POSSIBLE."

CHAPTER 8

Treating Alzheimer's disease

Scientists are searching intently to find a cure for Alzheimer's disease. Every day, they're developing and testing new approaches and methods that may stop or slow its progress, or possibly even prevent it entirely. But for now, no treatment can halt Alzheimer's or change its course.

Treatment strategies currently in use are focused instead on easing signs and symptoms. You may wonder what the point of treatment is if it can't offer a cure.

The truth is, a lot can be accomplished.

Treatment can make symptoms less severe. It can also improve quality of life. It can help maintain memories, reduce anxieties, raise spirits, relieve health concerns, encourage alertness during the day and foster quality sleep at night. That's a lot to offer.

Treatment strategies for Alzheimer's disease most often involve a combination of medications and other therapies. Some medications have been designed to treat physical changes in the brain, while others help with memory and can address distressing behaviors.

A number of strategies can help people with Alzheimer's live to their fullest capacity and maintain independence for as long as possible. You'll read about them in this chapter.

GOALS FOR TREATMENT AND CARE

Living with Alzheimer's disease dementia can challenge anyone's courage, fortitude, patience, creativity and adaptive skills. The level of stress can be high and the demands challenging for the person living with Alzheimer's, a care partner, family and friends. Dealing with a host of complex issues requires trust and honesty.

The one constant you can depend on is change. Symptoms may change, fluctuate, go away or intensify. In response, treatment and care must be adapted or refined. What worked in the milder stages of Alzheimer's may no longer be as effective for more-moderate and advanced stages.

Just as important is the need for a team effort. The most effective approach involves care among a group of people. This includes a doctor, specialists like a physical or occupational therapist, nurses, social workers, friends, family, and, most important, the person living with Alzheimer's dementia.

This background lays the foundation for the first step in choosing Alzheimer's care: deciding what's most important.

When faced with a disease that has no cure, many people want to feel relief from symptoms and live as long as possible. Medical treatment is often the focus.

But people living with dementia and their care partners often want something different. In fact, for more than 80% of people living with dementia and their care partners, what they want isn't related to medical treatment at all.

Instead, quality of life and support are their highest priorities. Quality of life and care partner support mean something unique to every individual, and what they mean changes over time. This makes goal-setting a valuable process and a tool that can help at every stage. Goal-setting helps people living with dementia and their care partners decide what's important now and plan for the future.

Early on, for example, being able to take part in daily life — including work — may be the priority. Then over time, goals may shift. Mobility, managing certain symptoms and relieving care partner stress may become more important later on. Ultimately, a good end-of-life experience is the focus.

For someone living with Alzheimer's, examples of goals may include physical safety, being able to live at home, avoiding hospital stays, and getting mental stimulation and physical activity. For care partners, goals may include maintaining good health, managing stress and minimizing family conflict.

In general, goals fall under the broad categories of managing symptoms and living well. You'll learn more about living well in Parts 4 and 5 of this book. The rest of this chapter is devoted to managing symptoms.

MEDICATIONS FOR COGNITIVE SYMPTOMS

Medications used to treat the cognitive (thinking) symptoms of Alzheimer's demen-

ACETYLCHOLINE: THE THOUGHTFUL MESSENGER

Acetylcholine is one of the body's primary chemical messengers (neurotransmitters). It controls muscles, attention, sleep, heart rate and muscle activity.

In the 1970s, neuroscientists learned that acetylcholine drops dramatically in people with Alzheimer's disease. Since then, they've learned that the level of acetylcholine in the brain relates directly to how severe dementia is. The lower the level, the more severe the symptoms. This evidence has led to the development of medications designed to boost acetylcholine levels, or at least keep this chemical from decreasing.

Although scientists still don't know exactly what role acetylcholine plays in thinking and memory, most agree that it's involved in what's called ***selective attention***. Selective attention refers to the way the brain filters incoming information, processing some messages while ignoring others. These tasks are essential at the start of the memory process. Some researchers also think that not having enough acetylcholine may affect how well people can recall information stored in their memory.

tia can't cure the disease or slow it down as of yet. However, they can help make thinking and memory issues more manageable.

Medications commonly prescribed for Alzheimer's disease dementia can help with memory loss, confusion, poor judgment, lack of concentration and many other cognitive symptoms.

While these drugs don't work for everyone, they're designed to help keep the brain's communication network working as well as it can for as long as it can. Here's more on the most common medications used for cognitive symptoms of Alzheimer's disease.

Cholinesterase inhibitors

Alzheimer's disease depletes a chemical in the brain called acetylcholine. Important for learning and memory, this chemical helps messages get from cell to cell in the brain. A drop in this chemical makes it harder for messages to get where they need to go in the

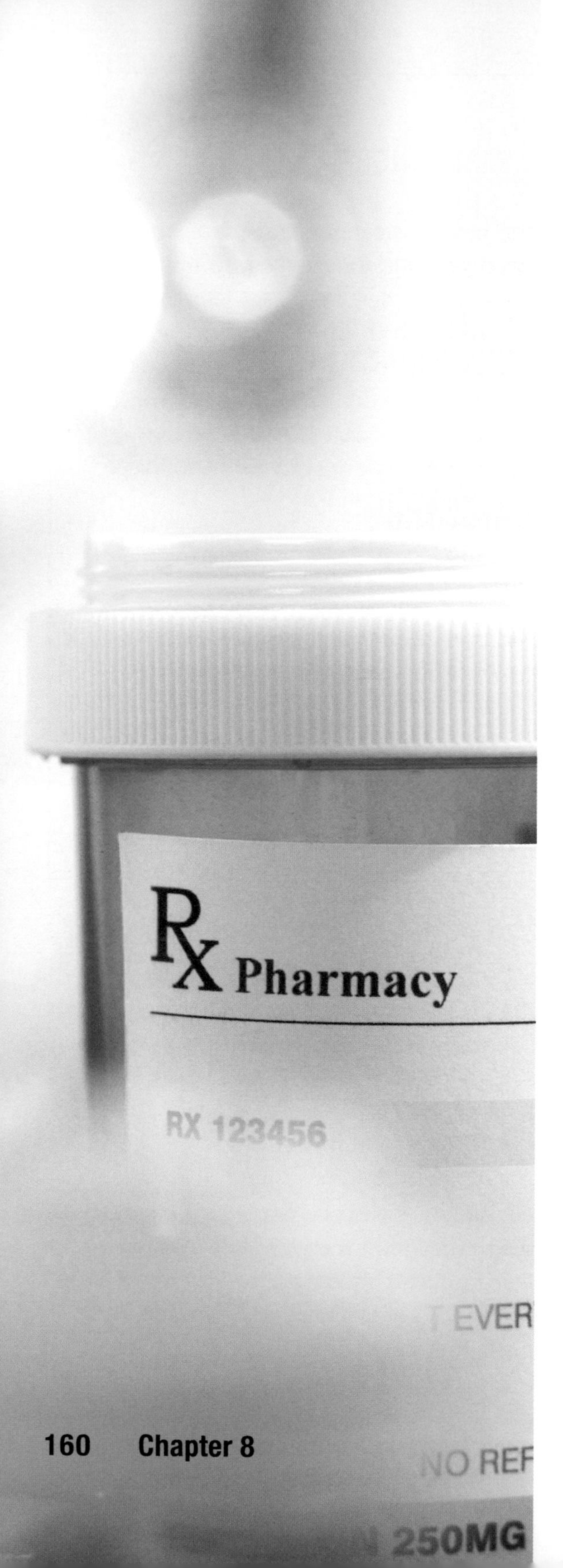

brain. Cholinesterase (koh-lin-ES-tur-ays) inhibitors are drugs that help keep acetylcholine from breaking down. In turn, these drugs support communication in the brain. This helps delay learning and memory problems.

These drugs play a valuable role in managing the disease during the mild to moderate stages. They not only can stabilize memory, judgment and attention, but may also help with agitation and depression.

As the disease progresses into advanced stages and memory and thinking problems worsen, however, these drugs may not help as much. Whether or not to use this medication in advanced stages is a decision best made with a doctor.

These medications all cause several similar side effects. Although they're generally well tolerated, they can cause stomach upset, nausea, vomiting, loss of appetite and diarrhea. They may also disrupt sleep and cause vivid dreams and nightmares.

Taking these drugs with food can help lessen stomach upset and related side effects. Starting with a low dose and working up to a higher dose also can help. People with a slow heart rate (bradycardia) may need to talk with a heart specialist (cardiologist) before taking these drugs.

People who have problems with electrical signals in their heart, like heart block, should also talk to a cardiologist first. They may not be able to take these drugs.

Donepezil (Aricept), rivastigmine (Exelon) and galantamine (Razadyne) are the three cholinesterase inhibitors most commonly prescribed.

Donepezil (Aricept) Approved to treat all stages of Alzheimer's, this is the oldest cholinesterase inhibitor still in use. Many doctors prefer to prescribe this drug because it's a pill, which makes it easy to take, and it's needed just once a day.

The starting dose is 5 milligrams (mg) a day. From there, as long as it's well tolerated, it may be increased to 10 mg a day after four to six weeks. A 23-mg dose is available, but it's not widely recommended because it may increase side effects without major added benefit.

Studies show that people with Alzheimer's who took 10 mg of donepezil a day for six months were able to think and remember a little better than were people who took an inactive pill (placebo). Donepezil has also been shown to help with daily activities. In smaller doses, the side effects of this drug are generally mild.

Rivastigmine (Exelon) This drug is used for mild or moderate Alzheimer's disease. It works in the same way donepezil does.

This drug can be taken twice a day as a pill, but it's also available for severe Alzheimer's as a skin patch that can be worn on the chest, back or upper arm. Because the patch seems to work as well as the pill and may lessen stomach issues, it's often the preferred way to take this medication. The patch can irritate the skin, though, so it's important to rotate where on the body the patch is placed.

Galantamine (Razadyne) Like rivastigmine, galantamine is used for mild or moderate Alzheimer's disease. This drug is taken as a pill or solution twice a day or as an extended-release capsule once a day. Its dose is increased gradually to no more than 12 mg twice a day. It's been shown to help with memory and thinking skills.

People taking a cholinesterase inhibitor often wonder if the medication is doing any good. They may be tempted to stop taking it if they don't see results right away. These drugs are designed to maintain cognitive functions, and this isn't something that's always easy to self-check and assess.

Some experts suggest taking this type of drug for about six months before deciding whether or not it's helping. A combination of tests is often used to assess how well these medications help with thinking and remembering. It's important to note that some people who stop taking these drugs notice a dramatic drop in functional ability.

How long someone should take a cholinesterase inhibitor isn't known. Usually, treatment lasts until the symptoms of dementia become severe enough to offset any benefit from taking the medication. But at least one of these drugs — donepezil — has been studied long enough to show that its effects persist even into the advanced stages of Alzheimer's disease.

Currently, there's no evidence to suggest that one cholinesterase inhibitor is better than another. Based on personal preference, a doctor may switch prescriptions at some point for someone who has an adverse reaction to one of the drugs or can't tolerate a drug's side effects.

Cholinesterase inhibitors are also sometimes used for people with mild cognitive impairment whose main symptom is memory loss. However, these drugs aren't FDA-approved for this use and aren't recommended for routine treatment of mild cognitive impairment.

To date, there's no proof that these drugs can keep mild cognitive impairment from progressing to dementia.

NMDA antagonists

Memantine (Namenda) is approved for treating Alzheimer's disease in the United States. It's become the second most widely used drug after donepezil (Aricept) to treat Alzheimer's disease.

Memantine is an N-methyl-d-aspartate (NMDA)-receptor antagonist. It regulates the activity of glutamate — a chemical messenger involved in memory and learning. Memantine also acts on nerve cells (neurons) that use glutamate to get messages to and from different parts of the brain.

Without glutamate, new memories can't be formed in the brain. But too much glutamate causes problems, too. As cells die in Alzheimer's disease, their stores of glutamate are released. This causes there to be too much glutamate in the brain. In turn, more cells in the brain die. It's a vicious cycle, and memantine helps prevent it.

Memantine is used to treat moderate to severe Alzheimer's disease. There's not much evidence that it can help people with mild Alzheimer's disease. It can help people maintain their ability to handle daily tasks by treating memory loss, confusion, and problems with thinking and reasoning.

The drug is usually started at a low dose and increased to 20 mg a day (10 mg twice a day). An extended-release capsule of 28 mg, taken once a day, is also available.

Memantine is usually well tolerated, but occasional side effects may include dizziness, headaches, confusion and agitation. In people who have side effects, dizziness happens most often.

Because cholinesterase inhibitors and memantine differ in how they work, they're sometimes used together. Some research has shown that this combination helps improve symptoms.

Dietary supplements

The number of herbal mixtures, vitamins and dietary supplements that are promoted

CAN THE MEDITERRANEAN DIET HELP?

Although taking fish oil supplements doesn't seem to help with Alzheimer's symptoms, following a diet that includes fish may.

Eating fish is one component of the Mediterranean diet, a way of eating that's based on the traditional cuisine of countries along the Mediterranean Sea. Following the Mediterranean diet involves:

- Consuming vegetables, fruits, whole grains, nuts and healthy fats, particularly olive oil
- Eating fish, lean, skinless poultry, beans and other legumes each week
- Having only moderate portions of dairy products
- Limiting intake of red meat
- Drinking a glass of wine a day

The Mediterranean diet has been shown to help prevent dementia; you'll learn more about this in Chapter 19. But it can also help treat dementia symptoms.

Some research suggests that following a Mediterranean diet can help slow the progression of Alzheimer's disease, especially when it's paired with regular physical activity, social engagement and mentally stimulating activities. It can also help preserve thinking-related skills. This style of eating has also been linked to less agitation and improved quality of life in people with Alzheimer's disease. It may also help people with this type of dementia live longer.

Researchers think the balance of nutrients in the Mediterranean diet are key, with its ratio of healthy fats from a variety of sources. It may be the interaction of the diet's components — at a molecular level — that helps preserve thinking function with age.

NONDRUG THERAPY FOR COGNITIVE SYMPTOMS

Aside from medications, memory aids can help a person with Alzheimer's disease cope with cognitive loss and maintain a degree of independence. Writing down information and keeping it somewhere visible, along with well-placed clocks and calendars, are all examples. A list of the day's activities, including specific instructions for tasks like using a coffee maker and preparing food also can help, particularly in the early stages of the disease. Other examples include making a list of important phone numbers, labeling drawers with their contents, and labeling the doorways to different rooms (for example, "bathroom" and "bedroom"). Learn more in Chapter 14.

For a care partner, reassurance may be the most important thing you can provide. If the person living with Alzheimer's gets worried about a family member who is no longer living, for example, it's often more comforting to reassure him or her that everything is OK rather than to insist on the person accepting reality. You'll find more information for care partners in Part 5.

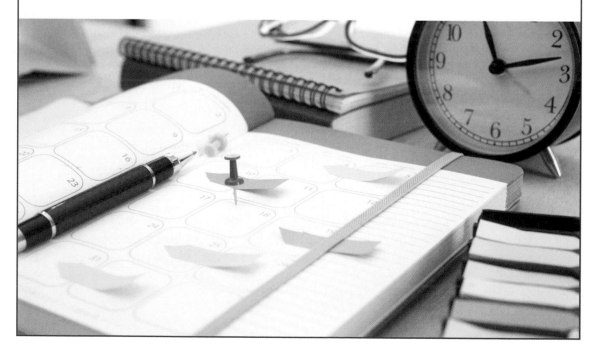

for cognitive health is growing every day. Unfortunately, these over-the-counter remedies offer more hype than hope.

Of the many vitamins and supplements that have been tested in clinical trials, none has shown any benefit for thinking and memory. Supplements studied include fish oil, curcumin and ginkgo. Some studies suggest vitamin E may be helpful, but this remains controversial.

Before taking any herbal medicines, nutritional supplements or vitamins, talk to your doctor. Supplements promoted for cognitive health can interact with drugs prescribed for Alzheimer's disease or other health conditions. In addition, claims about the safety and effectiveness of supplements aren't based on the rigorous scientific research that drugs go through before the FDA approves them.

MEDICATIONS FOR PSYCHOLOGICAL SYMPTOMS

Later in this chapter, you'll learn about nondrug strategies that can help with the many symptoms related to Alzheimer's. While much of what you'll read about can help alleviate symptoms of anxiety and depression, these strategies aren't always enough. Sometimes, medication is used along with nondrug strategies to manage certain behaviors.

As with treatment for cognitive symptoms, these medications can't cure or slow the progression of Alzheimer's disease, but they can help make behavioral symptoms more manageable.

Unfortunately, no single medication can treat all of the behavioral symptoms associated with Alzheimer's. And, although medications may be of some benefit, they're generally not used first. That's because these drugs can make cognitive impairment worse. In addition, their side effects may be more severe in older adults.

It's best to work with a doctor to weigh the pros and cons of taking these drugs. In general, it's recommended that they're used only when they're needed, for a short period of time, alongside nondrug approaches.

Cholinesterase inhibitors, which you read about earlier, are designed to help with cognitive symptoms — but they may help with behavioral symptoms, too. If a person with Alzheimer's isn't already taking a cholinesterase inhibitor, a doctor may recommend one before prescribing any of the medications that follow.

Antidepressants

Like anxiety, depression is common in Alzheimer's disease dementia. Depression can worsen problems with thinking and make daily living skills more challenging, leading to greater dependence on a care partner.

People with Alzheimer's often find it easier to cope with changes caused by the disease

NONDRUG STRATEGIES FOR BEHAVIORAL SYMPTOMS

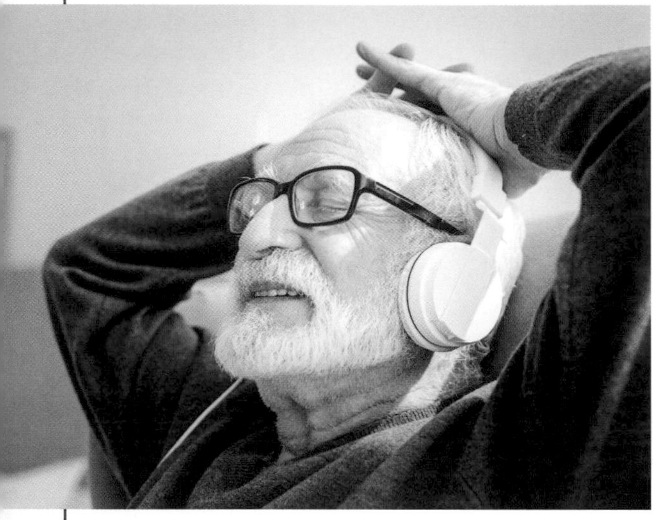

Before considering medication to address a behavioral symptom, these strategies may help. If medication is prescribed, it will likely work best when used along with these approaches.

- Consider your approach. This includes your body language and tone of voice. Communicating in a respectful way that preserves a person's sense of autonomy, self-worth and self-esteem can reduce behavioral symptoms like anger and agitation.
- Reassure the person in a calm voice. Let the person know you care. Validate what the person is expressing. For example, you may say, "I can see you are angry. I am here for you and I care."
- Consider the environment. Sometimes the environment can be too stimulating. Consider sounds, noise level and activity. Assess lighting to help with confusion and restlessness.
- Consider the task. If a task is too difficult or confusing, reactions like irritability or agitation are common. Simple adjustments include offering one-step requests, providing extra time to complete a task or demonstrating how to complete a task.
- Recognize that the root cause of most distress is an unmet psychosocial or emotional need. People need to feel respected and worthy, and have a sense of choice and control.
- Employ empathy. Try to see the situation from the view of the person with dementia. If you were in their shoes, you might respond in the same way.

Learn more about other nondrug strategies starting on page 168.

when they feel less depressed. To this end, drug therapy is often advised for people with Alzheimer's and depression.

The first antidepressants a doctor will prescribe for someone with depression and Alzheimer's are selective serotonin reuptake inhibitors (SSRIs). These medications have a low risk of side effects and drug interactions.

Some SSRIs can block the effect of acetylcholine. As you learned earlier, this chemical messenger controls muscles, attention, sleep, heart rate and muscle activity. People with Alzheimer's disease already have less acetylcholine in their brains. Other side effects may include sleep problems, nausea, weight gain, drowsiness, dizziness, blurred vision, constipation and dry mouth.

A doctor will start these medications at a low dose and then increase the dose gradually while watching closely for side effects.

It's important to be careful with citalopram (Celexa) and escitalopram (Lexapro). These drugs may interact with Aricept and cause heart rhythm problems. Other SSRIs like sertraline (Zoloft) may be prescribed instead. Other antidepressants, like venlafaxine (Effexor XR) or bupropion, also may be used.

Anti-anxiety drugs

Anxiety is common in Alzheimer's disease dementia. A person living with Alzheimer's may get upset in certain situations or feel the need to move around and pace.

Just as anxiety can have many causes, many strategies can help soothe it. A calm environment, exercise and movement, and avoiding bright lights and loud noise are examples. But sometimes, these measures aren't enough. That's when a class of drugs known as anxiolytics may be considered. These medications are generally recommended for occasional or short-term use only and are used for anxiety, restlessness, verbally disruptive behavior and resistance.

Anxiolytics include lorazepam (Ativan) and diazepam (Valium). These medications are often avoided for people with cognitive impairment because they can make confusion worse and increase the risk of falls. Side effects include sleepiness, confusion and memory problems, and trouble swallowing. There is also a risk of generating even more agitation. Some SSRIs, which are used to treat depression, may also help with anxiety. Lexapro is an example.

Antipsychotics

These medications may be prescribed for people with dangerous or extremely challenging behaviors, like aggression, delusions, hostility and hallucinations, but they're rarely prescribed because of significant potential side effects.

Antipsychotics are divided into two groups: conventional and atypical. Both groups work by blocking certain neurotransmitter receptors, particularly dopamine, in hopes of regulating the emotions. Newer atypical antipsychotics are often used because they generally cause fewer side effects than conventional antipsychotics.

The decision to use an antipsychotic medication must be considered carefully. Older adults with dementia who take these drugs have a higher risk of heart problems and death. The Food and Drug Administration requires these medications to carry a black box warning label about these risks, as well as a reminder that they're not approved for treating dementia symptoms.

In addition, atypical antipsychotics can raise blood glucose levels to abnormally high levels, which can lead to diabetes. Some experts recommend regular screening for diabetes in people who take atypical antipsychotics.

Antipsychotics may be helpful for some people in limited situations after the risks have been discussed with a doctor. They should only be used for the shortest time possible to help with severe agitation and aggressiveness that pose a danger to the person with Alzheimer's dementia or to others. Antipsychotics shouldn't be used to sedate or restrain someone with Alzheimer's disease dementia, and their use should be reevaluated regularly.

Commonly prescribed antipsychotic drugs include olanzapine (Zyprexa), risperidone (Risperdal) and quetiapine (Seroquel).

Mood stabilizers

Mood stabilizers (some of which are used for seizures) are also sometimes used to treat hostility or aggression. These drugs aren't often recommended, however, because there's not much evidence to support their effectiveness for Alzheimer's. In addition, side effects, like sedation, can be severe.

These drugs include lithium (Lithobid), valproic acid, divalproex sodium (Depakote) and lamotrigine (Lamictal).

THERAPIES AND DAILY LIVING STRATEGIES

Despite its challenges, dementia doesn't automatically take away someone's abilities. People with dementia can still do the things they could do before they were diagnosed. And with the help of various strategies and interventions, these abilities can be preserved longer.

Research is starting to shed light on the ways people living with dementia can maximize their quality of life and even achieve higher levels of well-being. Here's what researchers know about the approaches that are helping people with Alzheimer's disease dementia live well.

Occupational therapy

Helping people do what they need and want to do in their daily lives is the goal of occupational therapy. An occupational therapist assesses abilities and recommends changes that can help someone living with dementia do things safely and effectively. This may mean adapting to changes brought on by dementia.

An occupational therapist helps with making changes to the environment, recommends equipment or devices that can help with the activities of daily living, and teaches problem-solving strategies and other skills, including ways to get better sleep.

It's the combination of strategies — rather than any one on its own — that seems to help people with dementia maintain their independence most. Occupational therapists also provide education and training for care partners.

Although occupational therapy may not slow the decline in function that comes with Alzheimer's disease dementia, it can help people with Alzheimer's continue to perform the activities of daily living and engage with life in meaningful ways.

Physical therapy

Physical therapy helps reduce the risk of falls, improves mobility and helps a person perform the activities of daily living.

Physical therapists work with people who don't move as well because of a medical condition like Alzheimer's disease. They develop a plan that's focused on physical

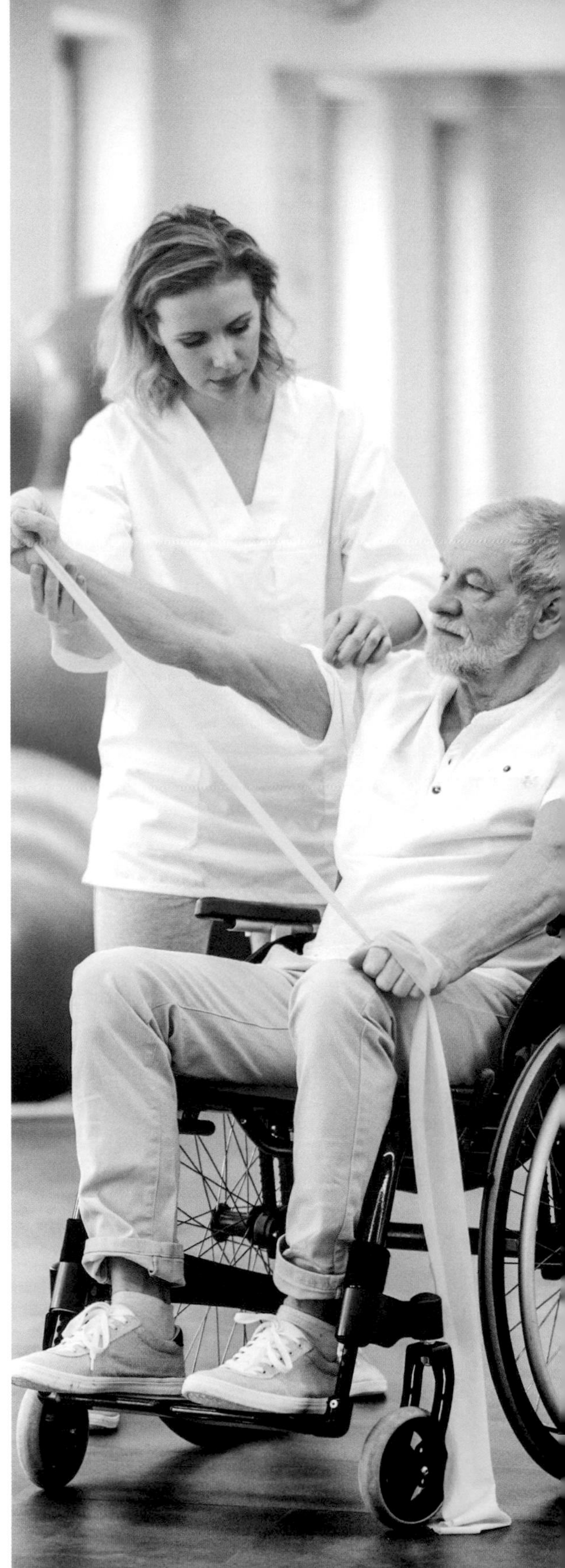

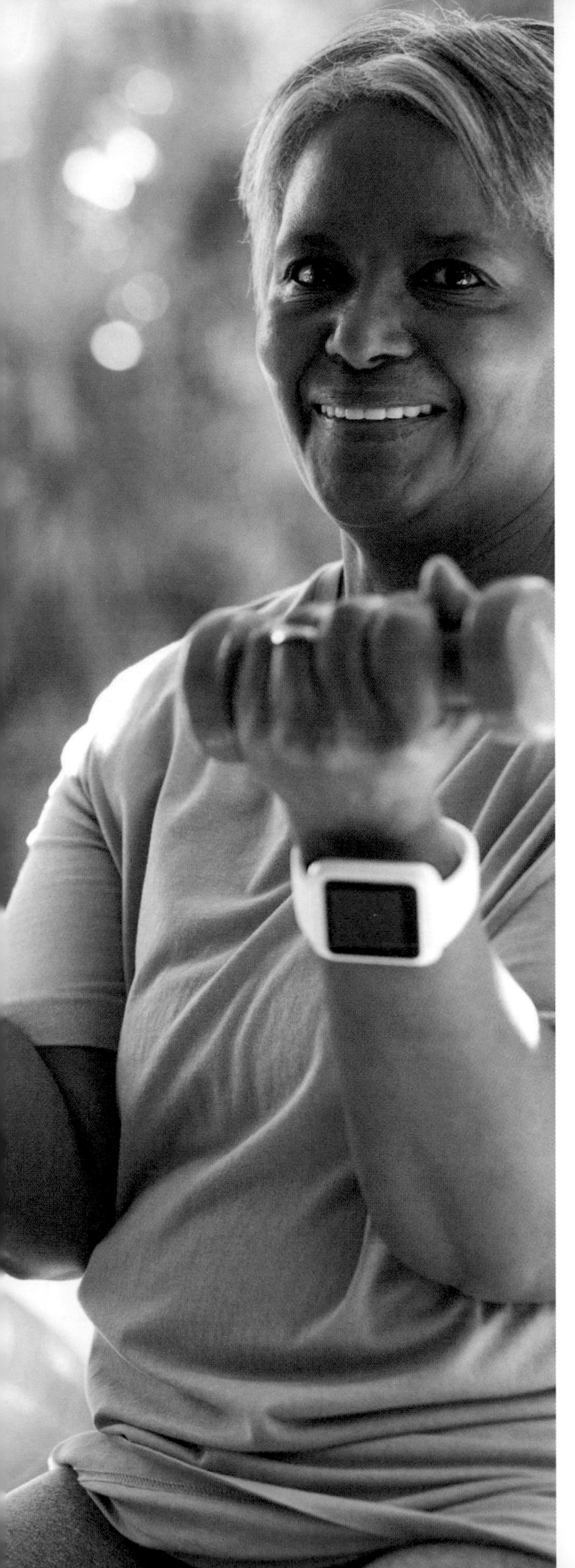

movement, as well as restoring function, preventing disability and enhancing overall wellness.

Many tenets of physical therapy have been shown to help people with Alzheimer's disease. For example, balance exercises and aerobic activity, including treadmill use and walking programs, seem to improve physical function as well as overall quality of life. Some research suggests that physical therapy may also help slow a decline in thinking skills.

Speech therapy

Language problems are the most common symptom of Alzheimer's disease dementia after memory loss. Early on, people with Alzheimer's may have trouble finding the words they want to say. When they have trouble naming an object, for example, they may use a generic term, like "thing," instead of calling the object by its name. As Alzheimer's progresses, language problems worsen to the point that the person may simply stop talking entirely.

Speech therapy can help people with Alzheimer's continue to use language well. In a small study of men, for example, speech therapy sessions improved how well they used words to identify pictures of objects. The men in the study were also better able to repeat words after hearing them.

Speech therapists use memory aids and other strategies to improve thinking and language skills. Speech therapy can be used as needed on an ongoing basis as Alzheimer's progresses.

Daily living strategies

In addition to occupational, physical and speech therapy, several lifestyle strategies can promote overall health and may help with maintaining thinking and memory skills.

Exercise The benefits of physical activity abound in all areas of health and well-being, including for those with Alzheimer's disease. For example, some research suggests that treadmill walking can improve quality of life and psychological well-being in Alzheimer's. Other researchers have found that home-based exercise may help support thinking and memory.

Put simply, physical activity is an important way to manage symptoms of Alzheimer's disease dementia. A daily walk can improve mood and keep the heart, muscles and joints healthy. Exercise is also helpful in promoting restful sleep, which can help improve behaviors. It also helps prevent constipation. If walking is difficult, doing household tasks like sweeping, riding a stationary bike, using stretching bands, and lifting weights or household items like soup cans are all options.

Nutrition People with Alzheimer's may forget to eat, lose interest in preparing meals or not eat a healthy combination of foods. They may also forget to drink enough, causing dehydration and constipation.

Care partners can help by offering healthy options that the person living with Alzheimer's likes and can eat. Encouraging water and other healthy beverages that don't contain caffeine is also helpful. Caffeine can increase restlessness, cause sleep problems and trigger a need to urinate more often. High-calorie, healthy meal replacement shakes and smoothies can be helpful when eating becomes more difficult.

Social engagement and activities People with Alzheimer's disease dementia can engage with others until later stages of the disease. Social engagement is an important way to manage symptoms and support quality of life.

Listening to music or dancing, attending social events in the community, and taking part in planned activities with children are all examples of social interactions that can bring meaning and enjoyment to someone living with Alzheimer's disease.

Adapting to cognitive losses Because Alzheimer's primarily affects thinking, it's helpful to compensate for those losses. Keeping a daily routine, using a calendar and allowing time for breaks between tasks are all examples.

Technology also can help. For example, a person with Alzheimer's dementia may feel less distracted and agitated when listening to a selection of favorite songs. Or a diffuser

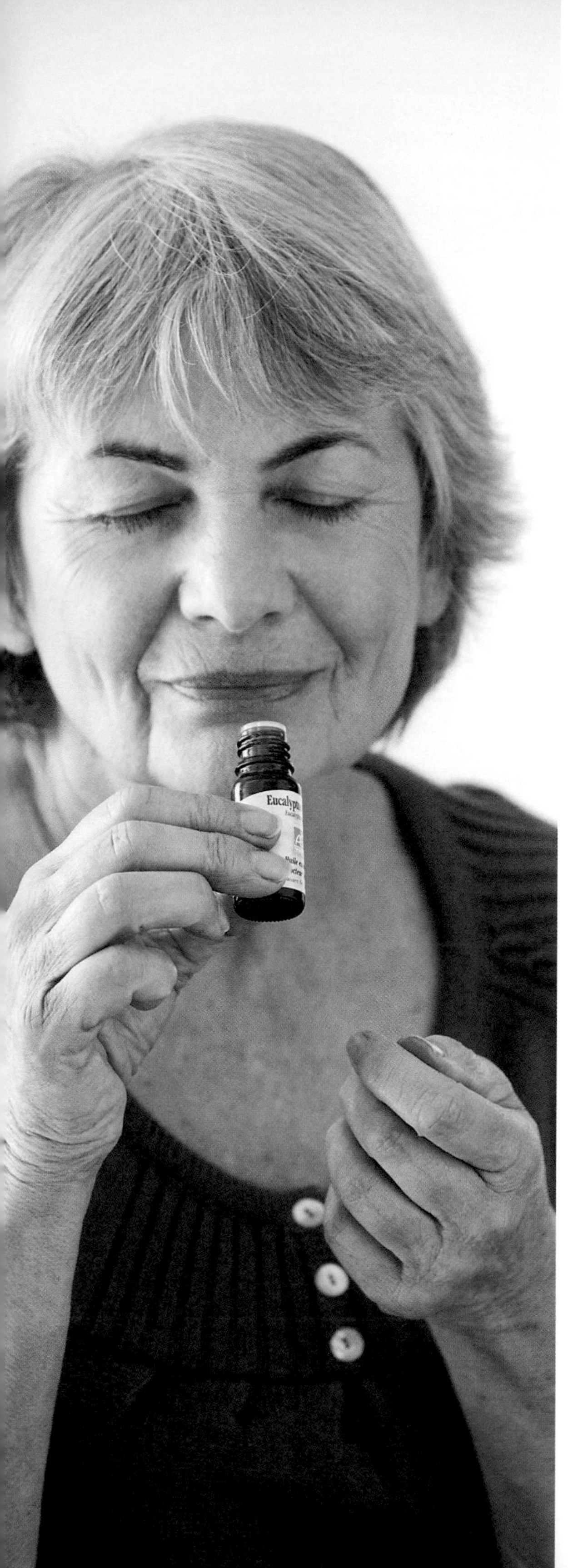

that disperses aromatherapy scents may offer a sense of calm.

Safety devices like medication organizers, wearable IDs, and door and window sensors can all help instill a sense of freedom for someone living with Alzheimer's, while also keeping the person safe. You'll learn more about how technology can improve quality of life for people living with dementia in Chapter 14.

Good sleep Dementia often causes sleep issues. Someone with Alzheimer's may wake up more often during the night, stay awake longer and feel sleepy during the day. Problems with sleep often increase as Alzheimer's progresses. In turn, sleep problems can increase confusion during the day and result in agitation or other behaviors.

Establishing a regular routine, treating underlying conditions like sleep apnea, and creating a comfortable sleeping environment with the right temperature and nightlights all help promote a restful night's sleep. Limiting screen time before bed, as well as alcohol, caffeine and nicotine, can also help. Getting regular physical activity, limiting daytime naps and managing the timing of medications that can interfere with sleep are other tips for making sure the person living with Alzheimer's sleeps well at night.

Managing stress Change can be stressful, especially for someone living with Alzheimer's disease. In turn, too much stress can affect well-being and the ability to function.

Managing stress offers many benefits, including better focus, decision-making and quality of life.

People living with Alzheimer's disease can reduce stress in a number of ways. Identifying sources of stress, getting help dealing with those situations and learning ways to relax are all helpful. Talking with a trusted friend also can help. Finding a place to relax and regroup can be useful during times of too much stimulation. Taking breaks and resting as needed are two ways to maintain energy levels.

Care partners can help with stress management by focusing on tasks that don't cause extra stress. For example, if grocery shopping is frustrating for the person living with Alzheimer's, a better option may be to make a grocery list together instead.

Music Listening to or singing songs can help people living with Alzheimer's disease dementia. That's due in part to the fact that areas of the brain linked to musical memory are relatively untouched in Alzheimer's. Music can relieve stress, reduce anxiety and depression, and lessen agitation. Music helps care partners, as well, by reducing their anxiety and distress and providing a way to connect with the person living with dementia.

The best choices are songs that the person with dementia enjoys or that remind the person with dementia of happy times in life. Clapping along or tapping one's feet to the music can enhance the experience.

Learn more about music and the brain in Chapter 17.

CREATING A PLAN FOR LIVING WELL

Living well means something different for every individual. But most often, it includes a balance of personal care, a sense of purpose and meaning, and a mix of activities that provide enjoyment and stimulation.

What living well means will also change over time, so what's helpful now may change in later stages of the disease. Keeping these main facets of well-being in mind throughout the process of Alzheimer's will help the person living with Alzheimer's and the care partner find a balance of wellness.

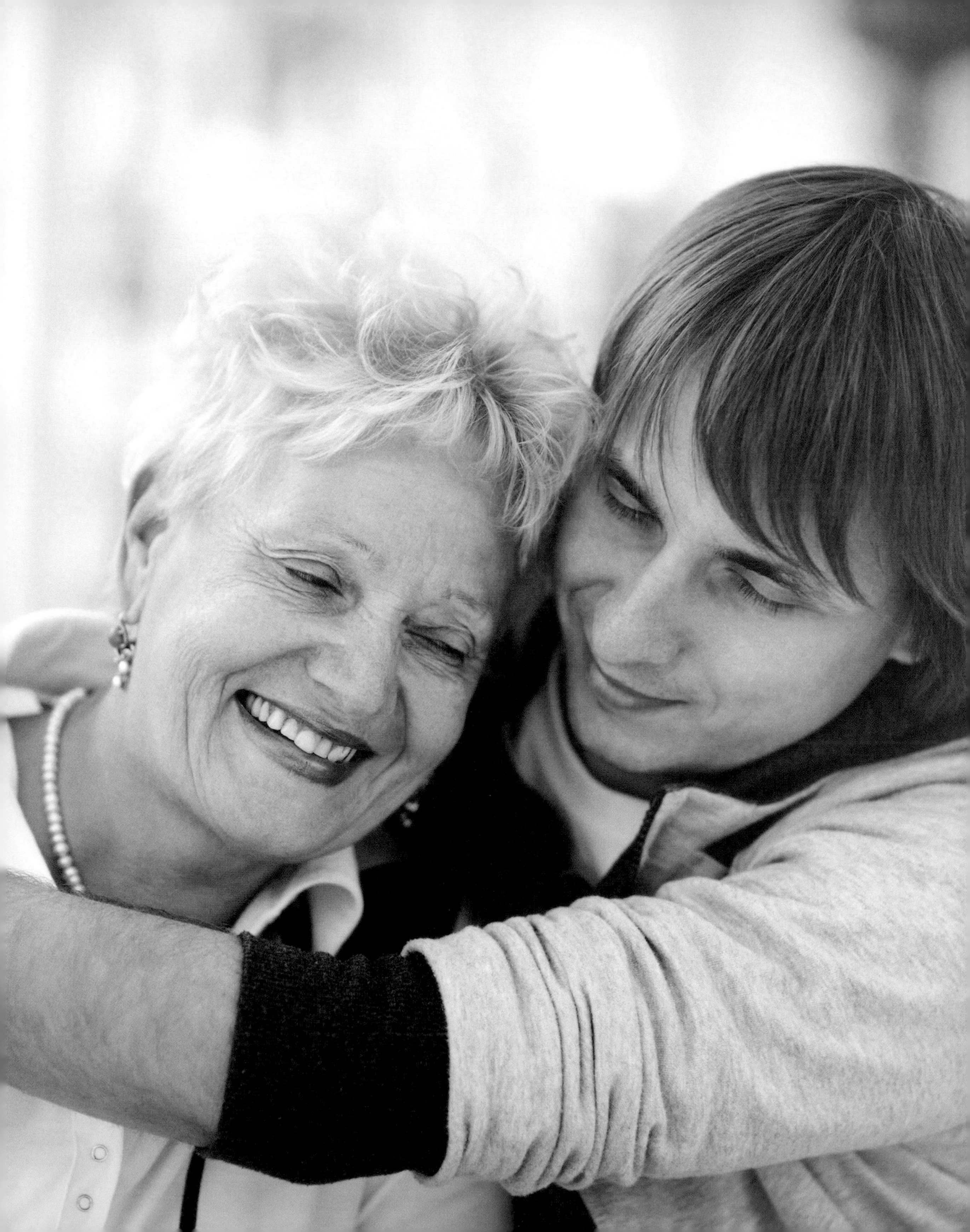

PART 3

Causes of dementia other than Alzheimer's

The terms *dementia* and *Alzheimer's disease* are often used interchangeably, as if they mean the same thing. However, these terms are different and have distinct meanings.

Dementia is a general term that refers to changes in thinking, remembering or reasoning that are severe enough to cause problems with day-to-day life.

Memory, language skills, problem-solving, and the ability to focus and pay attention are all affected by dementia. Dementia can also alter someone's personality and ability to regulate emotions.

Dementia is caused by physical changes in the brain. It's not a disease in itself; instead, it's a syndrome — a collection of signs and symptoms caused by a disease. Alzheimer's disease is the most common cause of dementia. But many other diseases can cause dementia, too. They include vascular cognitive impairment, Lewy body dementia and frontotemporal degeneration. You'll read about each of these disorders in the next few chapters of this book.

Each of these disorders can cause different symptoms. At the same time, someone can have more than one of these disorders, leading to an overlap in symptoms.

You'll get to know the signs and symptoms of each disorder, as well as changes that often happen over time and ways to adapt to these changes.

The first disorder you'll read about is frontotemporal degeneration.

“ALTHOUGH NO TREATMENT CAN CURE FRONTOTEMPORAL DEGENERATION OR SLOW ITS PROGRESS, MANY OPTIONS CAN HELP WITH SYMPTOMS.”

CHAPTER 9

Frontotemporal degeneration

Frontotemporal degeneration is the third most common neurodegenerative dementia. It refers to a group of disorders that mostly affect the frontal and temporal lobes of the brain. These parts of the brain are used for language. They're also linked to personality and behavior.

Major changes in personality and behavior are often seen in frontotemporal degeneration. Inappropriate actions, lack of empathy and lack of judgment are all examples. Frontotemporal degeneration can also cause problems with language use, as well as issues with movement, like tremors.

Symptoms worsen over time. People with frontotemporal degeneration may have just one symptom in the beginning, but have many symptoms in later stages as more parts of the brain are affected.

Frontotemporal degeneration often affects adults at a younger age than Alzheimer's disease does and can progress more quickly. It's also less common than Alzheimer's disease. As you'll learn in this chapter, these are just two of many differences between Alzheimer's disease and frontotemporal degeneration.

This type of dementia affects men as often as it does women, and nearly half of the people with it have a family history of some type of brain disease in a parent or sibling, including dementia, parkinsonism or amyotrophic lateral sclerosis (ALS), also known as Lou Gehrig's disease.

How quickly frontotemporal degeneration develops varies. Some people decline in two or three years, while others live with it for more than 20 years.

ALZHEIMER'S DISEASE VS. FRONTOTEMPORAL DEGENERATION

Alzheimer's disease	**Frontotemporal degeneration**
Mostly affects adults age 65 and older.	Usually affects adults between ages 40 and 65.
Time between the start of symptoms and a diagnosis is usually less than three years.	Time between the start of symptoms and a diagnosis is often more than is often more than three years.
Most common cause of dementia.	Accounts for 1 in 10 cases of dementia or fewer.
Memory loss is an early symptom.	Memory loss develops later on.
Behavior changes tend to happen later on.	Behavior changes are one of the first noticeable signs.
Getting lost in familiar places is a common symptom.	Getting lost in familiar places is not common.
Seeing or hearing things that aren't real is common as the disease progresses.	Seeing or hearing things that aren't real is not common.

TYPES OF FRONTOTEMPORAL DEGENERATION

Earlier, you learned that dementia is an umbrella term because it refers to several different disorders that affect the ability to think and remember. Like the term *dementia*, frontotemporal degeneration is also an umbrella term. Frontotemporal degeneration is broken down into different types of disorders, named based on the functions that are affected.

FRONTOTEMPORAL DEGENERATION

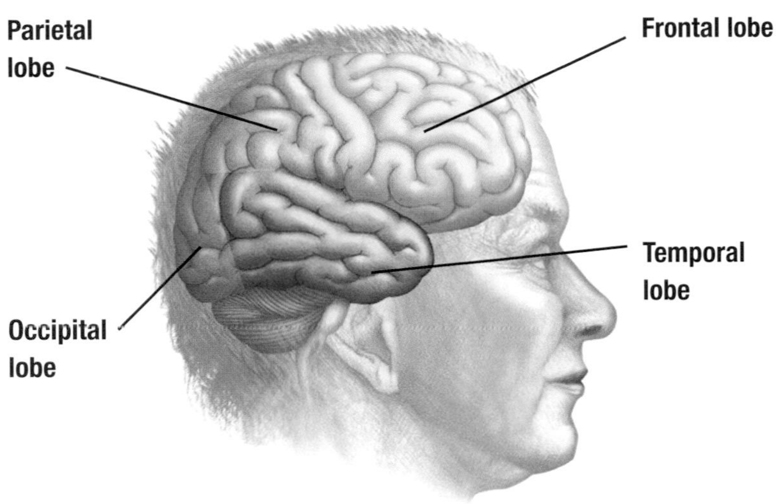

In frontotemporal degeneration, portions of the frontal and temporal lobes shrink (atrophy) and neurons die. This is different from Alzheimer's disease, which affects neurons in the hippocampus or medial portion of the temporal lobe of the brain and then spreads across most of the brain.

Signs and symptoms of these disorders vary widely. This can make it hard for a doctor to diagnose early on. Plus, signs and symptoms can be mistaken for other types of dementia or a mental health issue.

Later, you'll learn how frontotemporal degeneration is diagnosed. Find a full list of signs and symptoms for all of these disorders starting on page 192. For now, here's more on the disorders that fall under the frontotemporal degeneration umbrella.

Behavioral variant frontotemporal degeneration

The most common type of frontotemporal degeneration is behavioral variant frontotemporal degeneration (bvFTD). It affects

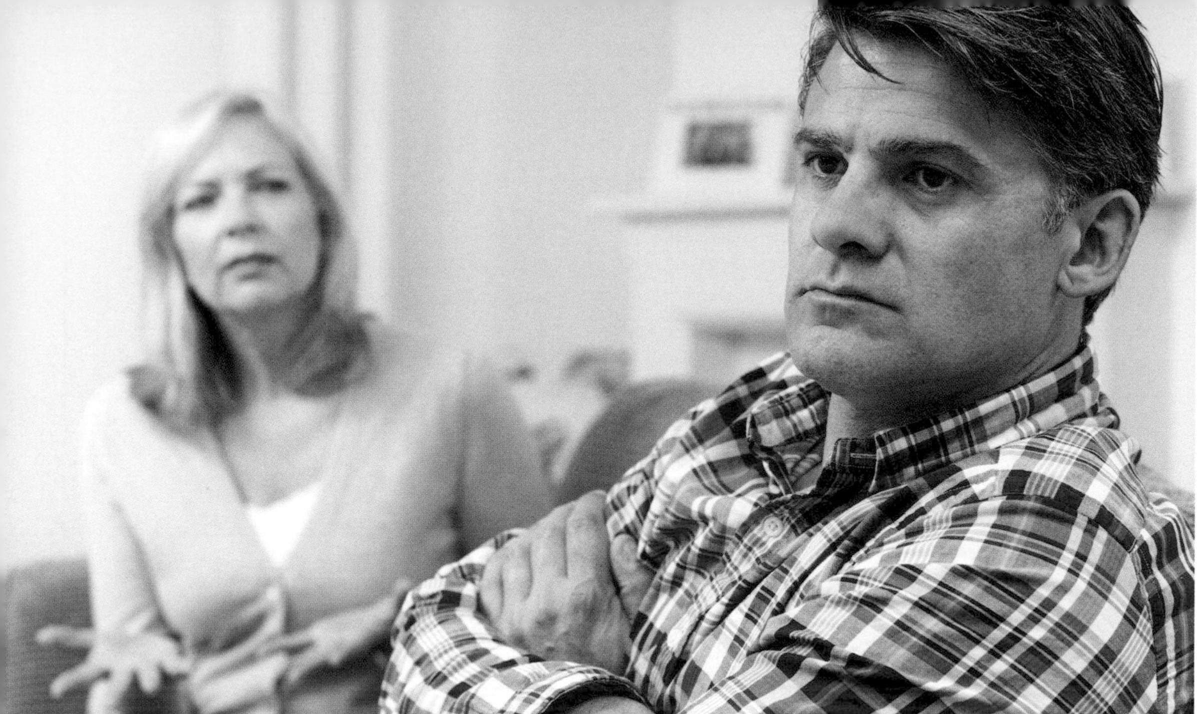

about half of the people with frontotemporal degeneration.

As its name suggests, behavioral variant frontotemporal degeneration is marked by changes in behavior and personality. Early on, this disorder may be mistaken for depression or another mental health condition because it can cause a loss of interest in things and activities that used to be important (apathy) and a loss of social graces, empathy and compassion.

Behavioral variant frontotemporal degeneration may cause someone to neglect family duties, ignore personal boundaries with strangers or say inappropriate things. Major events affecting a spouse or partner, like a death in the family, may get brushed off.

Speech and language disorders

The next most common types of frontotemporal degeneration make it hard to use language to speak, read, write or understand what other people are saying.

More than a third of people with frontotemporal degeneration have one of these types. With these disorders, problems with memory, reasoning and judgment don't happen at first but may develop over time. They may also cause changes in behavior.

The three main types of this kind of frontotemporal degeneration are all forms of primary progressive aphasia (PPA). Aphasia is trouble producing or understanding written or spoken language.

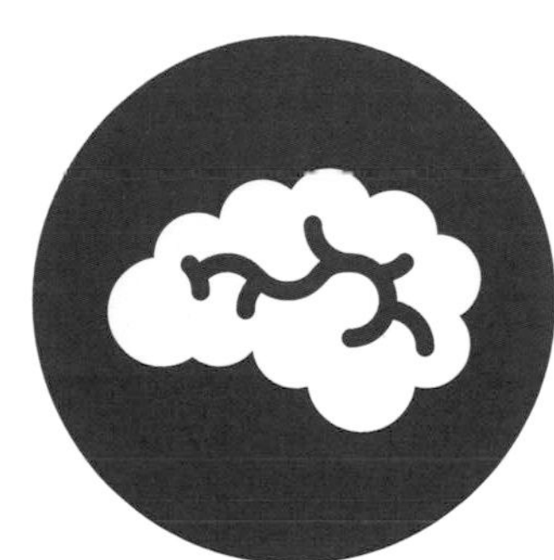
FTD
with motor
neuron disease/ALS
• Cognitive loss
• Behavior impairment
• Motor symptoms
Behavioral
variant FTD
• Cognitive loss
• Disinhibition
• Inflexibility
• Apathy
Semantic PPA
• Fluent speech
• Decreased word comprehension and recognition of objects and people
Agrammatic PPA
• Halting speech
• Short phrases
• Grammar errors
Logopenic PPA
• Spontaneous but slow speech output
• Word retrieval problems
Corticobasal
degeneration
• Asymmetric rigidity
• Apraxia
Progressive
supranuclear palsy
• Behavioral and cognitive loss
• Parkinsonism
• Eye movement disturbances

Semantic PPA First described more than 100 years ago, this type of frontotemporal degeneration is also known as semantic dementia. It causes a breakdown in the part of the memory you need to understand and describe everything you know about the world (semantic memory). Semantic memory is different from episodic memory, the part of the brain involved with recalling specific events or experiences.

Over time, people with semantic PPA are less able to recall knowledge about the world they're living in. Other types of memory — for example, past experiences — usually aren't as affected.

People with this disorder also have language issues. They usually have trouble naming an item when it's shown to them. They also tend to have problems remembering words or finding the right word when they're speaking.

In addition to these symptoms, people with semantic PPA lose knowledge about what an object is or how it's used. They may not realize, for example, that an elephant is large and a mouse is small. This kind of knowledge is needed for day-to-day function. For example, identifying a common kitchen utensil like a fork and how it's used for eating may be a challenge.

People with semantic PPA may also have problems reading or writing words that don't follow pronunciation or spelling rules; for example, using *no* instead of *know*.

Nouns are often the hardest words to use and remember; someone who can't think of the right word to say may use a more general word, like *thing*, in place of what they're trying to say. They may not even realize how often they're affected by these issues.

Not everything related to language use is affected by semantic PPA. People with this disorder can still use speech and proper grammar and repeat words they hear. They're often able to understand sentences better than they can understand single words that aren't used often.

During an exam, a doctor will likely use verbal tests to check word use. A person may be asked to identify an unnamed item that's shown to them by choosing a word from a small list. Someone with this disor-

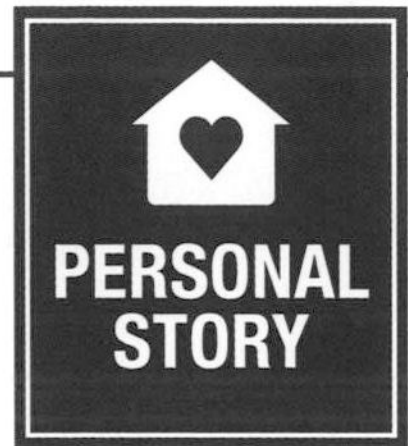

BEHAVIORAL VARIANT FRONTOTEMPORAL DEGENERATION: LINDA'S STORY

Linda was easygoing, generous and intelligent. But at age 51, Linda starting showing changes in her behavior and mood.

She spent days in bed watching television. She couldn't stop eating doughnuts by the package. When her husband tried to take away her doughnuts, she flew into a rage. Over time, she cared less about her appearance. When her best friend of 30 years told her that her mother had died, Linda showed no emotion.

Testing revealed some impairment in problem-solving and intellectual flexibility, but her general intelligence, memory and visuospatial skills were normal. An MRI of Linda's brain showed noticeable shrinkage of the frontal lobes.

Over the next few years, Linda became more and more apathetic. She also developed urinary incontinence. Linda's situation demonstrates many characteristics of behavioral variant frontotemporal degeneration.

der often has trouble choosing the correct word. A doctor may also ask family members about signs they've noticed. For example, a family member may recall a time when the person didn't know the name of a common fruit, like an orange.

People with semantic PPA almost always have degeneration affecting the left side of the brain; specifically, the front part of the left temporal lobe.

Agrammatic PPA A defining feature of agrammatic PPA is difficulty with grammar. Not using pronouns correctly and making mistakes in sentences are signs a doctor usually looks for during an exam. A person with agrammatic PPA may omit small words, use word endings and verb tenses incorrectly, and mix up the order of words in a sentence.

The second hallmark sign is difficulty producing words (apraxia of speech). People with agrammatic PPA have trouble making the right sounds to match the words they're trying to say. Apraxia of speech affects most people with the disorder at some point.

Speaking may take significant effort. This is caused by problems with the coordination of speech — issues with the parts of the brain that control the muscles that allow you to use your lips and tongue to form sounds. The muscles themselves aren't affected, but the ability to use them is. Over time, speech becomes slow and speaking becomes a struggle. Eventually, the person

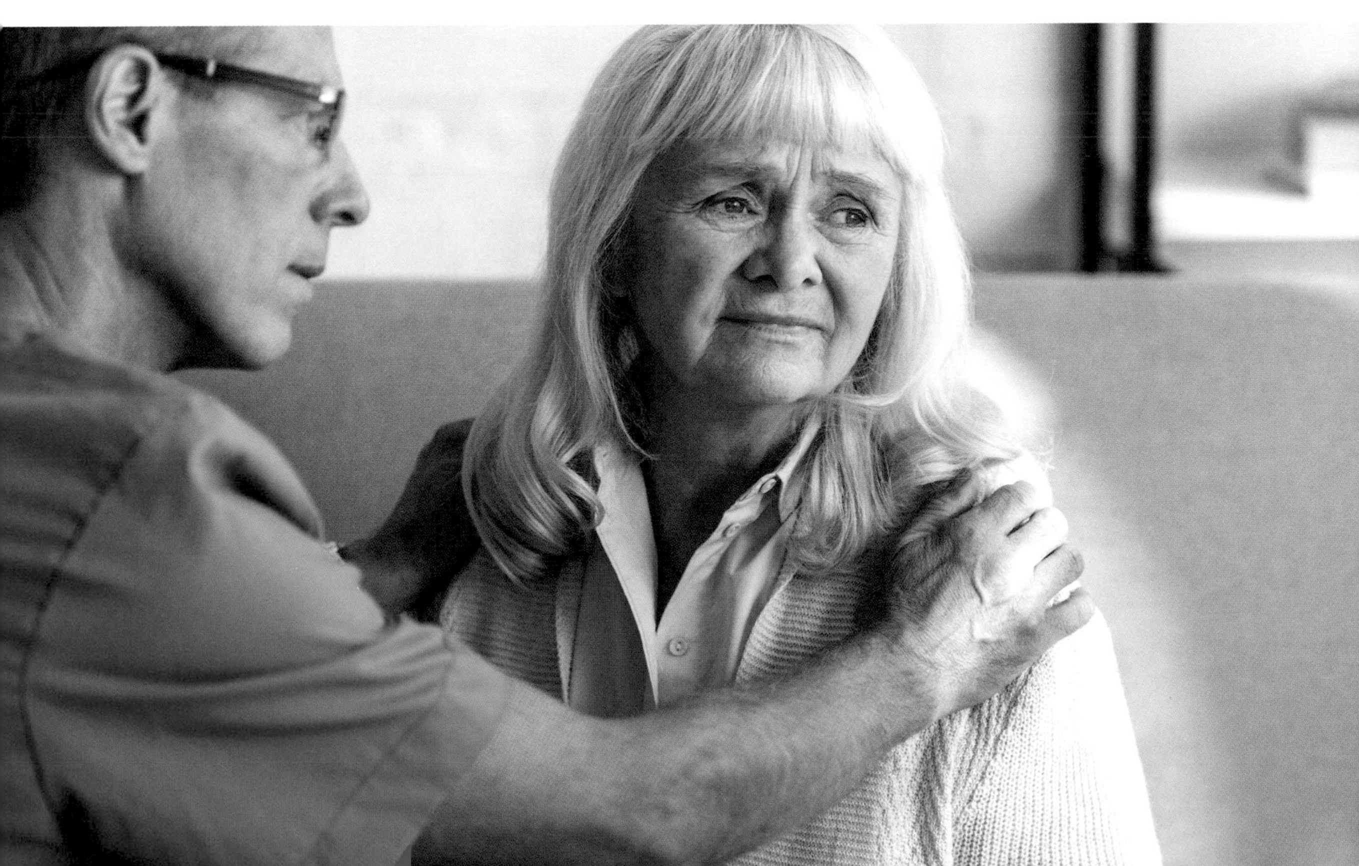

WHAT SEMANTIC PPA LOOKS LIKE

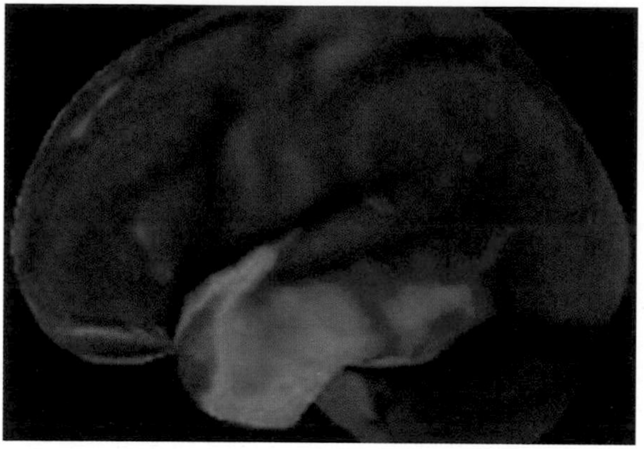

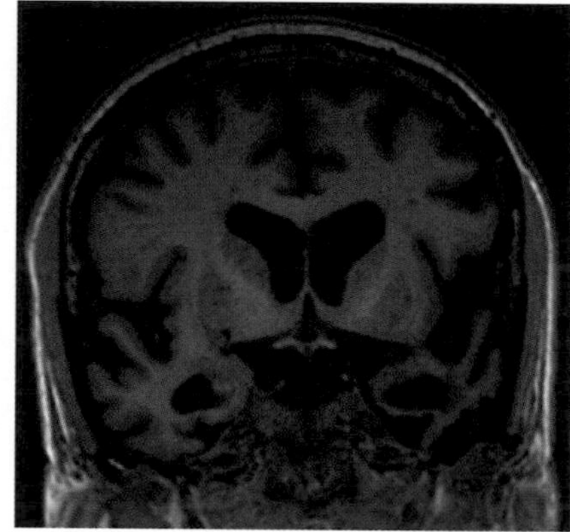

The left image is a PET scan showing semantic PPA. The colors in the image show areas of the brain that are affected by this disorder. Red shows the areas of the brain that are most affected, while dark blue areas are least affected. The area of the brain affected is the left temporal lobe, which is linked to word meaning and word association. The right image is an MRI of the same brain. Dark areas show damage to the left temporal lobe.

is unable to speak. Apraxia of speech that occurs without any language problems is called primary progressive apraxia of speech.

In addition to these signs and symptoms, a doctor may test how well a person can understand long and complex sentences. People with agrammatic PPA may have trouble in this area. A doctor may also test how well a person understands single words and what a person knows about specific objects. These areas usually aren't affected by agrammatic PPA.

Unlike people with semantic PPA, those with agrammatic PPA can usually recognize the name of an object if it's provided to them in a short list. They also don't usually have trouble repeating words, saying what a word means, matching a word with an object, or reading and writing single words. Because there's no standard way to test grammatical skills, a doctor or speech-language expert may rely on samples of a person's writing and conversations. A person may be asked to explain something familiar, like the rules of a favorite sport or something work related. A doctor may also review samples of written language, like emails.

People with agrammatic PPA almost always have degeneration affecting the left side of the brain. More specifically, it affects the language-producing structures in the middle parts of the frontal lobe.

Logopenic PPA This type of PPA is often caused by Alzheimer's disease, but it's also a type of frontotemporal degeneration.

This disorder causes people to have trouble finding the right words when they're speaking. However, they can understand words and sentences and use proper grammar. People with this disorder may speak slowly and hesitate often when they speak because they're trying to find the right word to say.

Unlike agrammatic PPA, people with logopenic PPA can speak fairly normally when making small talk with someone else. However, when they need to be specific or use words that aren't as familiar to them, they may hesitate.

An individual with logopenic PPA almost always has degeneration affecting the left side of the brain. More specifically, it affects the language-producing structures in the back part of the left temporal lobe and nearby regions.

Movement disorders

Some types of frontotemporal degeneration affect parts of the brain that control movement. These disorders may also affect thinking abilities. Here's more about the most common types of frontotemporal degeneration that affect movement.

Frontotemporal degeneration with motor neuron disease About 1 in 10 people with frontotemporal degeneration has a type that causes weakness and muscle wasting, as well as changes in behavior and language seen in other types of frontotemporal degeneration. Signs and symptoms are similar to those seen in amyotrophic lateral sclerosis (ALS), also known as Lou Gehrig's disease. Up to 1 in 5 people with ALS has the thinking and behavioral issues of this type of dementia.

Corticobasal degeneration Sometimes called corticobasal syndrome, corticobasal degeneration causes nerve cells (neurons) to waste away and die in the areas of the brain that control movement.

People with this disorder become unable to control movement little by little, usually starting in their 50s or 60s. It causes people to become unable to move their hands and arms, even though they have the muscle strength to do so.

Signs and symptoms first appear on one side of the body only, and then eventually affect both sides of the body. A person with this disorder may feel as if an arm or leg is no longer part of the body and that body part moves without the person consciously planning to move it (alien limb). Changes in balance and walking also can occur.

Not everyone with corticobasal degeneration will have the problems with memory, thinking, language or behavior seen in other types of frontotemporal degeneration.

Progressive supranuclear palsy Closely related to corticobasal degeneration, this disorder is also sometimes called Steele-Richardson-Olszewski syndrome, after one of the doctors who first described it.

As with corticobasal degeneration, progressive supranuclear palsy causes problems with balance and walking. That's because it,

WHAT AGRAMMATIC PPA LOOKS LIKE

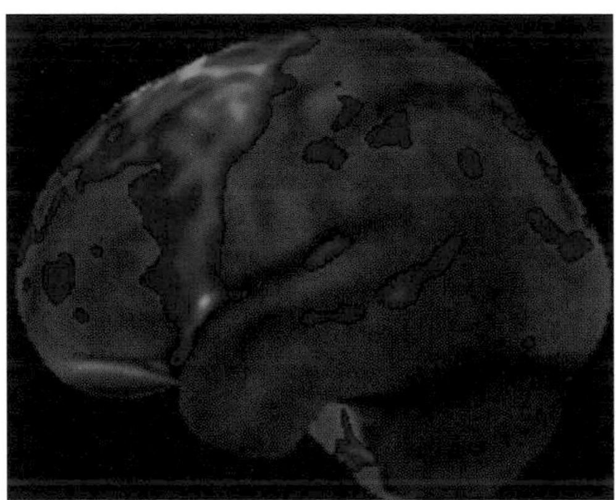

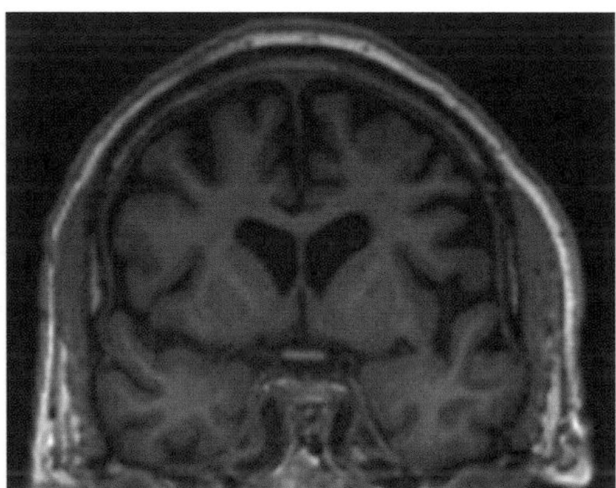

The left image is a PET scan showing agrammatic PPA. The colors show areas of the brain affected by this disorder. Green shows damage to the brain that's most severe, while dark blue areas of the brain are affected the least. In this image, the left frontal lobe of the brain is affected — this is the part of the brain that's typically associated with grammar and speech planning.

The right image is an MRI of the same brain. The dark areas show loss of volume in the same areas of the brain. This is another way to show damage to the part of the brain linked to grammar and speech planning.

too, affects the parts of the brain that control body movement.

People with this disorder are also affected by problems with eyesight. Vision may be blurry, and people with this disorder may have trouble looking down. Because of these issues, people with this disorder may seem uninterested in conversation.

Individuals with this disorder often have a fixed stare and can't make facial expressions. As with other frontotemporal disorders, progressive supranuclear palsy can cause problems with memory, reasoning, problem-solving and decision-making.

As with corticobasal degeneration, progressive supranuclear palsy is linked to the tau

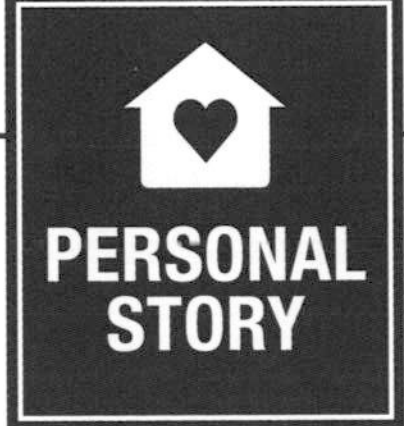

SEMANTIC PPA: JOHN'S STORY

For two years, John, age 53, had struggled to find the words for ideas he wanted to express. He decided to seek help from his doctor. John and his wife felt that all of his other intellectual functions were intact, including memory and language comprehension. His personality remained unchanged. His wife even noted John's continued ability to tinker in the workshop and fix small engines — a task requiring considerable skill and patience.

John was fully aware (and frustrated by) his difficulties with language, sometimes making self-deprecating remarks about the problem. A mental status examination showed some difficulty with abstract thinking, general knowledge awareness and verbal recall. Though he couldn't remember the specific words for various items on a naming test, he could describe details about them. He also had trouble understanding spoken words such as *pyramid* and *compass*.

An MRI of John's brain showed prominent shrinkage in the left temporal lobe, while the hippocampus appeared relatively normal. This is fairly typical of a person with semantic PPA.

protein, but it's different from the tau protein seen in Alzheimer's disease.

SIGNS AND SYMPTOMS

Signs and symptoms of frontotemporal degeneration affect people in different ways from those of other types of dementia. First, they tend to change a person's personality or language abilities. Second, these signs and symptoms often affect adults in the most active time of life, when they're working and raising families.

Not everyone has all the signs and symptoms of frontotemporal degeneration or has them in the same way. In addition, the combinations of signs and symptoms in frontotemporal degeneration are many. However, there's enough in common to allow for a general picture of what frontotemporal degeneration looks like. Changes usually occur a little at a time, although some forms progress more quickly.

Early symptoms generally develop in one of three areas: personality and behavior, language and communication, or movement and motor skills. Behavioral and emotional changes usually take place before thinking skills decline.

Memory may not be affected for a long time. The same can be said for visuospatial skills, like moving about or judging the height of a step or navigating familiar places.

Language issues can happen with any type of frontotemporal degeneration, but they tend to be a main symptom in primary progressive aphasia types of the disorder.

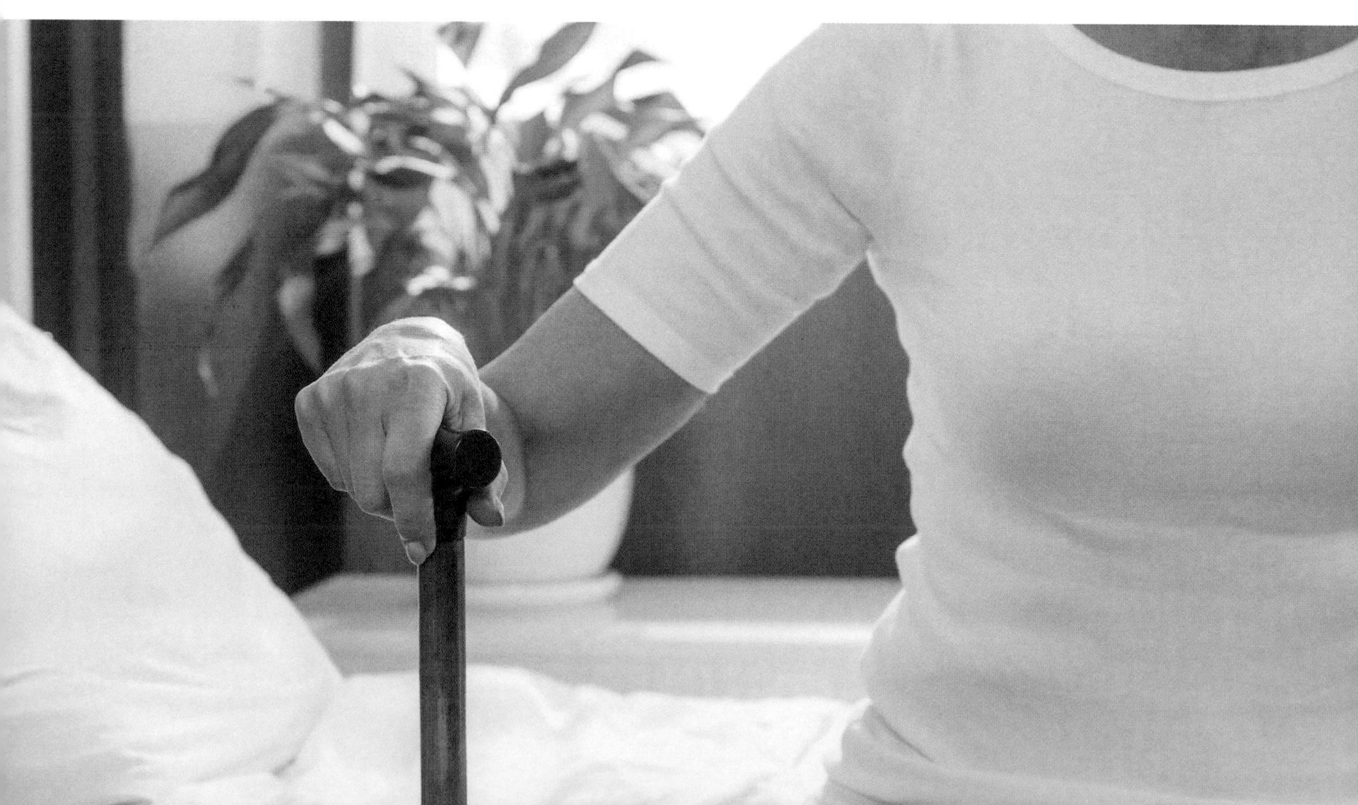

WHAT CAUSES FRONTOTEMPORAL DEGENERATION?

In most cases, what causes frontotemporal degeneration isn't known. But as with Alzheimer's, it's linked to abnormal protein deposits in the brain. Instead of the amyloid protein, as in Alzheimer's, many cases of frontotemporal degeneration show changes in the tau protein, which causes nerve cells to collapse and die. The type of tau associated with frontotemporal degeneration is different from tau seen in Alzheimer's disease.

Researchers have found that a protein called TDP-43 is also linked to frontotemporal degeneration. About half of the cases of behavioral variant frontotemporal degeneration are caused by TDP-43, and half are caused by tau. In rare cases, it's caused by a protein known as fused in sarcoma. Similar to the tau protein in Alzheimer's disease, TDP-43 proteins cause nerve cells in the brain to stop communicating with each other and die.

At this point, there's no way of testing someone who's living with frontotemporal degeneration to find which protein is causing it. This is a very active area of research.

DIAGNOSIS

It can be hard for a doctor to tell if someone has frontotemporal degeneration.

In part, no single test can identify it. Plus, signs and symptoms of this disorder can overlap with those of other conditions. A doctor may also diagnose frontotemporal degeneration as something else. It may look like another type of dementia, or like schizophrenia, bipolar disorder or depression.

The fact that frontotemporal degeneration isn't just one disorder adds another challenge to the mix. Symptoms can vary, and as the disease progresses, the symptoms of different types of frontotemporal degeneration can overlap. For example, someone with the behavioral variant form will likely show early signs of thinking problems and apathy. Later on, the person may develop trouble producing or understanding written or spoken language (aphasia). The longer it takes to diagnose, the more delayed treatment becomes.

The process of diagnosing frontotemporal degeneration usually starts with tests to help show — and rule out — possible causes for the symptoms. First, a doctor will get a person's medical history and perform a physical exam that includes testing thinking abilities. Blood tests may be used spot thyroid disease or a vitamin deficiency.

An MRI may be used to look for strokes or tumors that can mimic symptoms of frontotemporal degeneration. If a doctor isn't sure whether a person has Alzheimer's disease or frontotemporal degeneration after a routine exam, a fluorodeoxyglucose (FDG) PET scan may be used to tell the difference between the two. This type of PET scan shows areas of the brain where there's decreased glucose metabolism, meaning that fewer nutrients are broken down.

CATEGORIES OF SYMPTOMS IN FRONTOTEMPORAL DEGENERATION

Emotions	Behaviors	Speech and language	Thinking skills	Movement
Apathy toward people, surroundings and events	Loss of social skills, like tactfulness and manners	Not speaking as much or speaking very softly	Unable to focus on a task or being easily distracted	Less facial expressions
Loss of emotional warmth, sympathy and empathy toward others, including loved ones	Lack of hygiene	Muscle coordination problems that make it hard to talk	Getting stuck in familiar patterns and having trouble adapting to new circumstances	Slow movements
Abrupt mood changes	Overeating, excessive drinking and smoking	Not using proper grammar	Trouble planning daily tasks or appointments	Rigid muscles
	Repetitive behavior	Being unable to name familiar people or objects	Poor financial judgment	Weak muscles
	Hypersexual behavior — loss of inhibition, explicit sexual comments, obsession with pornography	Not understanding words as well when reading or being spoken to	Trouble detecting sarcasm or irony	Poor arm or leg coordination
	Impulsive behavior	Repeating words and phrases		Poor balance
	Hyperactivity, including agitation, pacing, vocal outbursts, aggression	Gradual loss of all speech		

HOW PET SCANS WORK

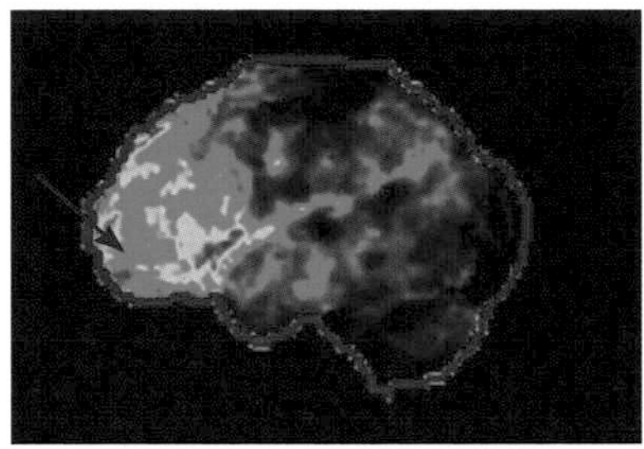

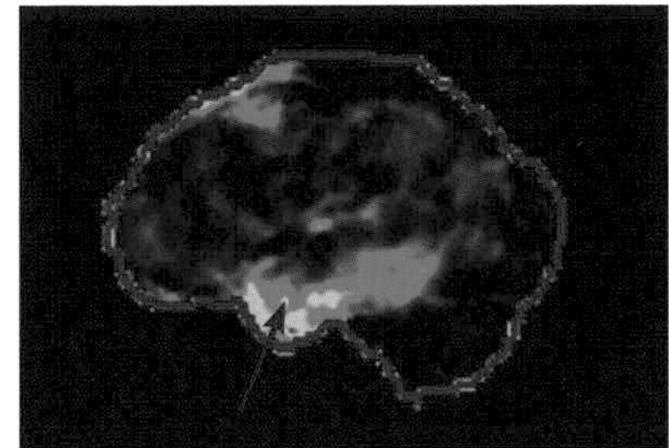

PET scans use a radiotracer to detect different levels of activity in the brain. Blue is normal, while green, yellow, orange and red show less activity in the brain.

The PET scan on the left is of a brain affected by behavioral variant frontotemporal degeneration. You'll see less activity in the frontal lobes of the brain. The frontal lobes control thinking, planning, organizing, problem-solving, short-term memory and movement.

The PET scan on the right is of someone with semantic PPA. It shows less activity in the left temporal lobe of the brain. The temporal lobes process information from your senses, especially sound. They also play a role in memory storage.

Early on, it can be hard to spot the exact type of frontotemporal disorder. Symptoms can vary, as can the order in which symptoms appear. For example, language problems may come on first in some disorders; in others, they may appear later on.

Each type of frontotemporal degeneration is linked to damage in a different area of the brain. To help tell which disorder someone has, MRI and other imaging tests can help. Imaging tests give doctors a picture of the brain that can show which areas are being affected. Researchers are also looking into biomarkers in the brain that may someday help tell one type of frontotemporal degeneration from another.

See how MRI scans can help identify frontotemporal degeneration on page 194.

COMMON SIGNS AND SYMPTOMS, BY DISORDER

Here are some of the most common signs and symptoms of the different forms of frontotemporal degeneration.

Personality and behavior disorder	
Name	Symptoms
Behavioral variant frontotemporal degeneration	• Increasingly inappropriate actions • Lack of judgment and inhibition • Apathy • Lack of empathy • Repetitive, compulsive behavior • Decline in personal hygiene • Changes in eating habits, especially overeating • Being unaware of changes in thinking and behavior • Eating nonfood objects
Speech and language disorders	
Name	Symptoms
Semantic PPA	• Trouble understanding words and recognizing names of people and objects • Difficulty with nouns
Name	Symptoms
Agrammatic PPA	• Halting speech that sounds telegraphic • Short phrases • Grammar errors, misusing pronouns and making errors in sentences
Name	Symptoms
Logopenic PPA	• Speech is spontaneous but slow, often due to trouble finding words • Trouble following long directions • Problems finding words

Name	Symptoms
Primary progressive apraxia of speech	• Speech becomes slow • Longer than expected pauses between words or within multiple syllable words • Knowing what you want to say, but unable to say it correctly • Sounds that don't come out right • Difficulty saying longer or harder words
Movement disorders	
Name	Symptoms
Frontotemporal degeneration with motor neuron disease	• Changes in behavior and language • Muscle weakness and cramping • Difficulty making fine movements
Name	Symptoms
Corticobasal degeneration	• Difficulty moving on one or both sides of the body • Movement gets more difficult over time • Stiffness • Poor coordination • Trouble with thinking, speech and language
Name	Symptoms
Progressive supranuclear palsy	• Losing balance, falling backward • Stiffness • Trouble looking down; blurry or double vision • Unable to make facial expressions • Fixed stare • Laughing or crying for no reason • Problems with speech and swallowing • Sensitivity to light • Problems with memory, reasoning, problem-solving, decision-making

WHAT AN MRI SHOWS

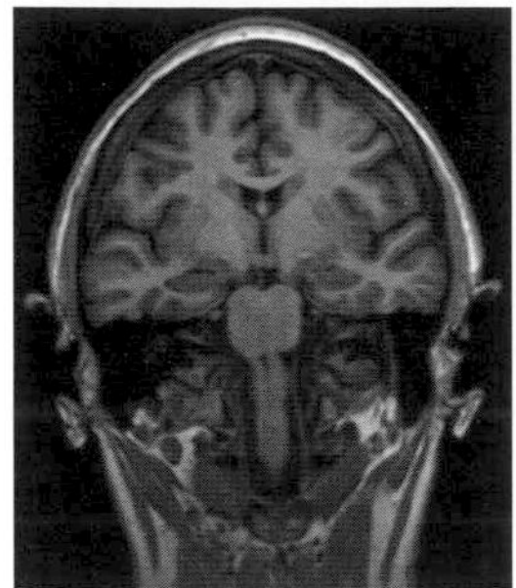
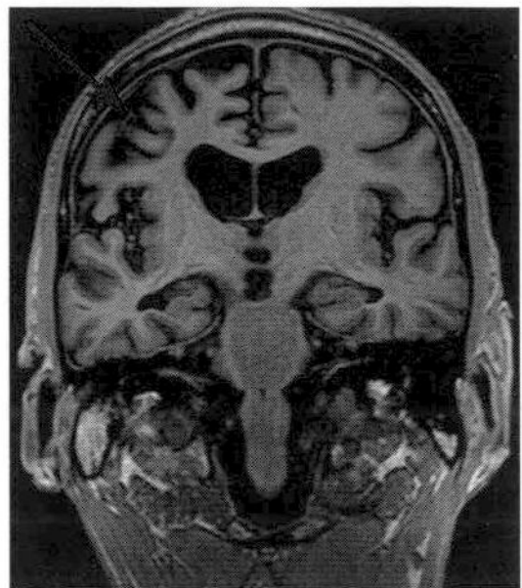
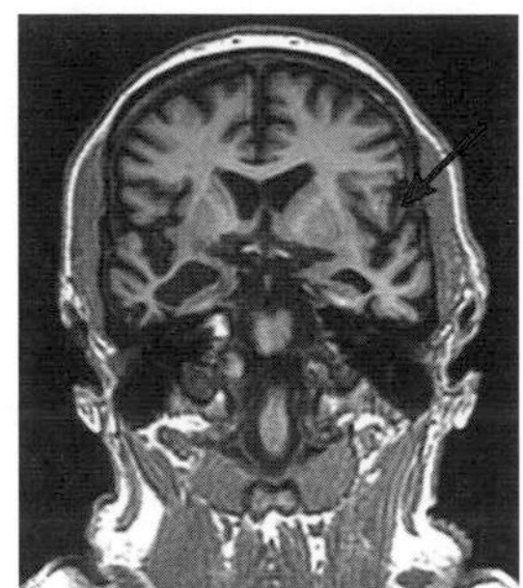

MRI scans can help a doctor identify a type of frontotemporal degeneration. That's because many types follow certain patterns of brain shrinkage as nerve cells become damaged and die.

The MRI on the left is of a normal brain. The image in the middle shows shrinkage in the right frontal lobe (red arrow). This pattern is typical of behavioral variant frontotemporal degeneration, which causes changes in behavior and personality.

The image on the right shows shrinkage in both temporal lobes (red arrow). This pattern shows semantic PPA. This type of frontotemporal degeneration makes it hard for someone to understand words or name objects or people.

Receiving a diagnosis

While receiving a diagnosis of frontotemporal degeneration is critical, understanding what it means takes time — both for the people affected by it and for others who interact with and care for them. A diagnosis will explain troubling changes in language or behavior, but it also poses many unanswered questions. Signs and symptoms of frontotemporal degeneration vary, and it's impossible to know how quickly the disease will progress or what symptoms someone will have now, as well as later on.

What experts do know is that someone with frontotemporal degeneration will need more help as the disease progresses —

BIOMARKERS: DIAGNOSIS OF THE FUTURE

You learned earlier that biomarkers are under study to help diagnose Alzheimer's disease long before symptoms have a chance to develop. Scientists are looking into biomarkers specific to frontotemporal degeneration for the same purpose.

Studies involving imaging and blood and spinal fluid tests are helping researchers see what's possible in terms of diagnosing frontotemporal degeneration before changes take hold in the brain. These tests aren't in widespread use by doctors yet; at this point, they're available only in specialty clinics or as part of research studies.

Clear guidelines around frontotemporal degeneration biomarkers don't exist yet, but researchers think that work being done on a blood test to detect Alzheimer's disease biomarkers may be helpful in developing tests for frontotemporal degeneration, too.

which means care partners' needs will increase with time, too.

People diagnosed with frontotemporal degeneration may:

- Be aware or unaware of the changes happening to them. Some people may feel losses related to these changes deeply.
- Feel isolated and scared if they don't have opportunities to meet others with the disorder.
- Need to find ways to feel productive.
- Want to take part in a support group.

The spouse or partner of someone with frontotemporal degeneration may:

- Face difficult emotions, like guilt, anger, loneliness, disappointment and grief. Learn ways to cope in Chapter 18.
- Feel overwhelmed without help.
- Feel loss in companionship and intimacy because of changes in behavior, personality and language.
- Need to take on more responsibility for household duties and decision-making.
- Become a single parent to a child and a care partner at the same time.

An adult child may:

- React differently to a parent's needs than his or her siblings do. Each adult child has a different relationship with a parent.

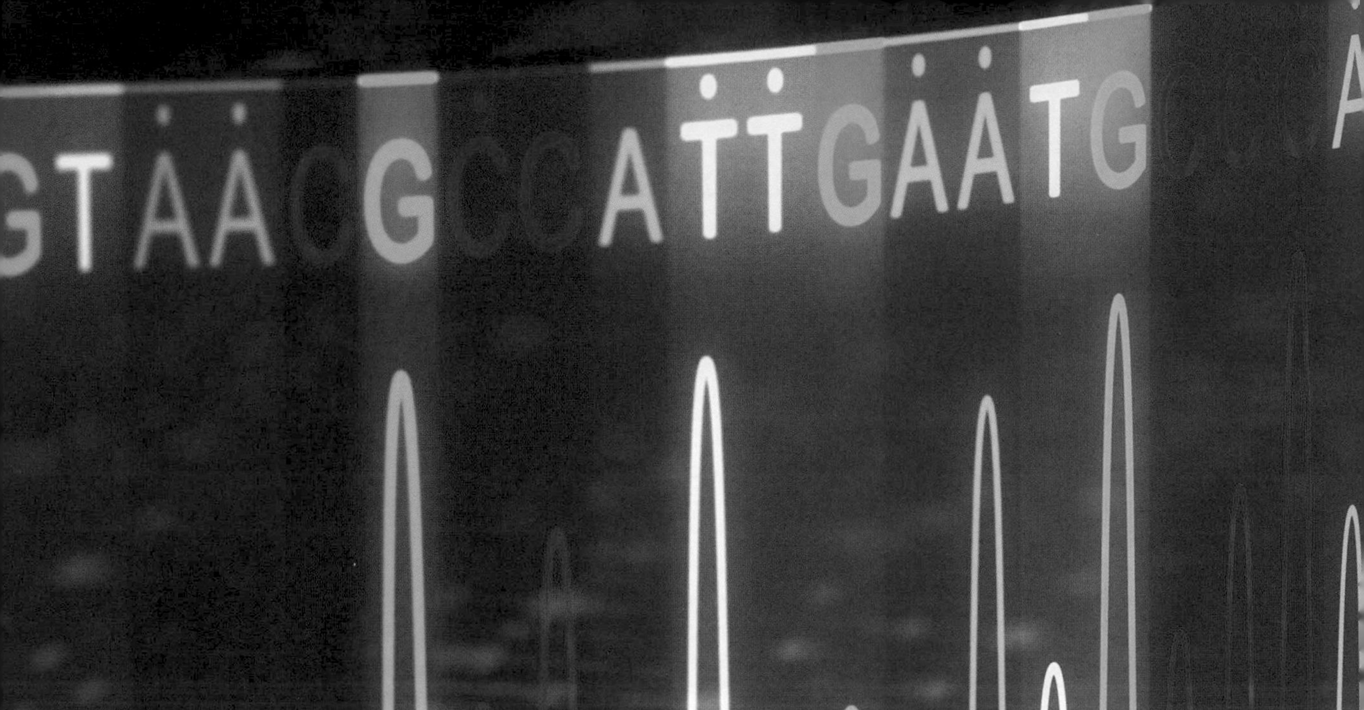

WHAT ROLE DOES GENETICS PLAY?

Although what causes frontotemporal degeneration is unknown in most cases, researchers have learned that genetics plays a strong role. In fact, as many as half of the people with frontotemporal degeneration have a family history of a brain disorder like dementia, parkinsonism or ALS.

Genes tell the cells in the body how to make the proteins it needs to function. Even a small change can cause the body to make abnormal forms of proteins that lead to changes in the brain — and, in time, disease. This is what happens in forms of frontotemporal degeneration that run in families.

The study of genetics in frontotemporal degeneration began more than 20 years ago when researchers found that people with frontotemporal degeneration and parkinsonism had changes to a gene known as the microtubule associated protein tau (MAPT). This gene makes the tau protein. Since then, researchers have discovered that many more gene changes are linked to frontotemporal degeneration.

Here's what's known about the three most common genetic causes of frontotemporal degeneration.

The MAPT gene — also called the tau gene — was the first gene linked to frontotemporal degeneration. Problems with this gene cause tangles to form in the brain's nerve cells (neurons). Eventually, these tangles brain cells to

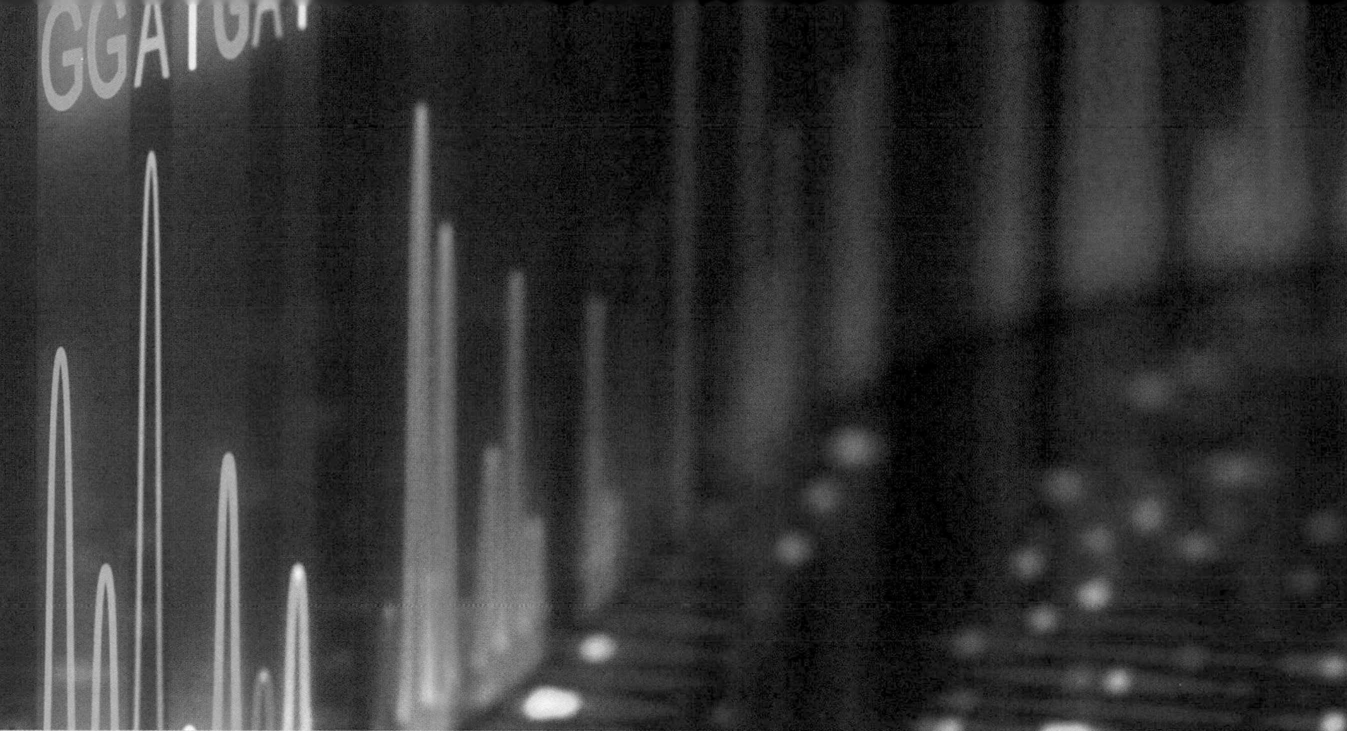

become damaged and die. Researchers are developing therapies aimed at treating this genetic mutation.

Progranulin, also called granulin, is another gene that's linked to frontotemporal degeneration. It's expressed by many cells in the body, including neurons in the brain. Mutations in the progranulin gene cause much less progranulin to be made in the brain. As many as 1 in 5 people with frontotemporal degeneration that runs in families has low levels of progranulin. Researchers think that boosting low levels of progranulin may treat or even delay this type of dementia.

A mutation to the C9orf72 gene is the most common hereditary cause of frontotemporal degeneration, particularly behavioral variant frontotemporal degeneration, as well as ALS.

This mutation leads to a buildup of certain forms of RNA in the brain and spinal cord. RNA is a chemical that carries instructions from DNA and helps cells throughout the body do their jobs. Researchers are developing ways to spot this mutation and use drugs to prevent it from causing frontotemporal degeneration.

Knowing what happens at the molecular level in almost every case of frontotemporal degeneration that runs in families will ideally lead to better care and, one day, ways to detect this type of dementia before it takes shape in the brain.

- Need to make difficult choices or changes in order to care for a parent.
- Face difficult emotions like guilt or anger, concern, disappointment and grief.
- Feel isolated and poorly understood.

Extended family and friends may:
- Have trouble appreciating the impact of the disease on the person living with it and his or her care partner if they don't stay in touch regularly.
- Not know what to do when their relationships with the person living with dementia and his or her care partner change.

It's important to know that you're not alone. The number of people and support groups focused on this type of dementia is growing. Find organizations dedicated to these disorders in the Additional resources section.

TREATING THE DISORDER

No treatment can cure frontotemporal degeneration or keep it from progressing. Therapies for these disorders are focused on symptoms and quality of life.

As with other types of dementia, researchers continue to study frontotemporal disorders to find medications that may help treat or prevent them in the future.

In particular, researchers are looking into how the disease develops so that when treatments are available, they can be directed to people when they can be most helpful. What's known about the genes and proteins involved in frontotemporal degeneration is evolving rapidly. This is leading to the development of new therapies. Most of these therapies are still in the early stages of development, which means it will take time before they can be tested in humans. But some are being tested in humans at specialized research centers.

Visit *www.clinicaltrials.gov* to learn more about what clinical trials are underway in frontotemporal degeneration.

MANAGING SYMPTOMS

Although no treatment can cure frontotemporal degeneration or slow its progress, many options can help with symptoms. This is especially important for two reasons: Symptoms can change over time, and people can live for many years with frontotemporal degeneration.

A team of specialists familiar with these disorders, including doctors, nurses, and speech, physical and occupational therapists, can help guide therapies that can help most with specific symptoms. The following therapies are among the most common used to manage symptoms of frontotemporal degeneration.

Medications

Current guidelines focus on using therapies other than medications to treat symptoms of frontotemporal disorders. In part, this is because not enough research proves that certain drugs are helpful and safe. With this said, some medications are used to treat symptoms. Medications for symptoms of frontotemporal disorders include:

Antidepressants Some types of antidepressants may reduce behavioral symptoms. Trazodone is an example. Selective serotonin reuptake inhibitors (SSRIs) like sertraline (Zoloft) have been suggested for treating impulsive behavior, irritability, apathy and unusual eating behaviors in some people. However, most research hasn't been definitive. More study is needed.

Antipsychotics These medications are also sometimes used to help with behavioral problems. Quetiapine (Seroquel) is an example. Some experts believe that low doses can help with aggression and seeing or hearing things that aren't real (hallucinations). However, these drugs can cause side effects, some of which are serious.

The decision to use an antipsychotic drug must be considered carefully. Older adults with dementia who take these drugs have a higher risk of stroke and death. The Food and Drug Administration requires these medications to carry a black box warning label about these risks, as well as a reminder that while they may be used, they're not approved for treating dementia symptoms.

Other medications Behavior problems like aggression and socially inappropriate behavior can be hard to manage. To treat these

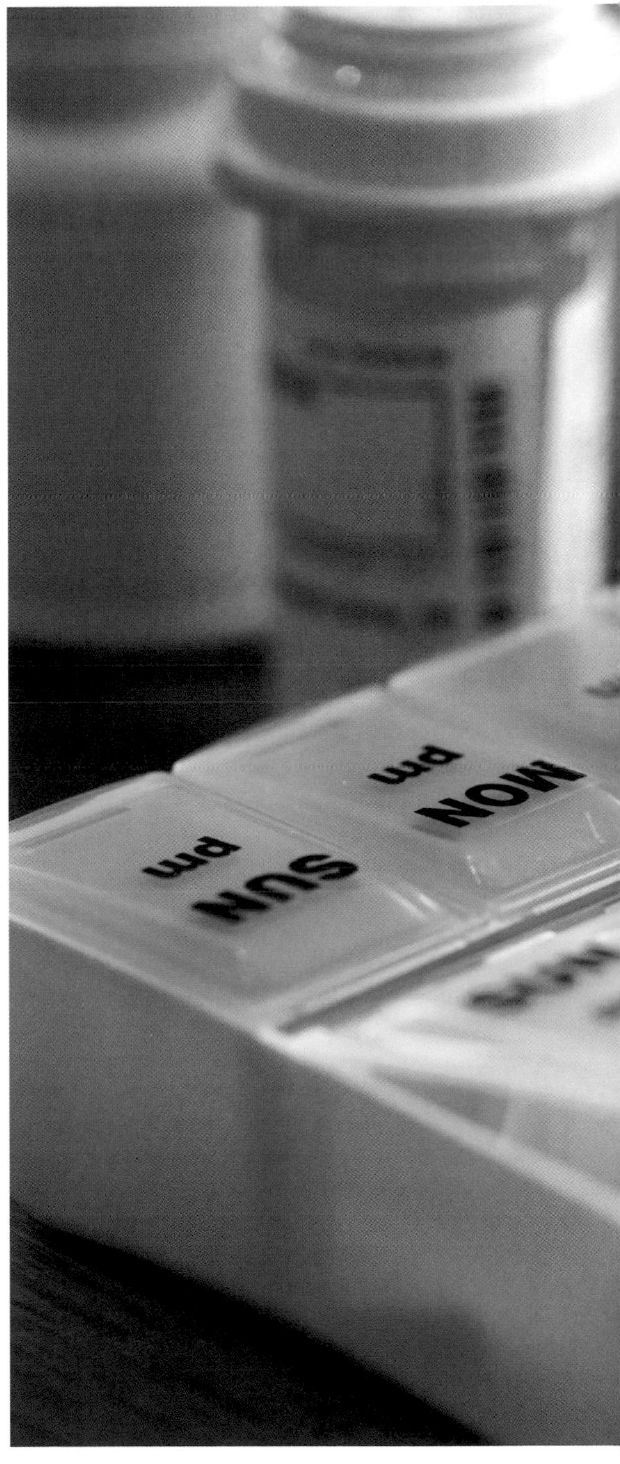

CHALLENGES FOR CARE PARTNERS AND FAMILIES

Frontotemporal degeneration, as you've learned, tends to strike adults earlier than other types of dementia do. Someone with frontotemporal degeneration may be enjoying a successful career, raising a family and planning for the future. A diagnosis of behavioral variant frontotemporal degeneration is likely to cause a significant shift in future plans, which can take time to accept and adapt to.

Relationships may change and stress may increase for care partners and families, especially as symptoms progress. A care partner may have to take on more of the household duties and child rearing or take a second job or quit working altogether to provide care. Children may feel that they're losing a parent at a critical time in their lives.

Behavioral signs, like public outbursts, may embarrass friends and loved ones and cause additional challenges. Frontotemporal degeneration affects the areas of the brain that tell someone the appropriate ways to interact with other people in social situations. Someone with behavioral variant frontotemporal degeneration may be hurtfully honest or not be able to suppress impulses, like hugging a stranger on the street. It can be hard to remember to not hold the person with this disorder completely responsible for actions like this. These actions are a sign of the disease. At the same time, it's important to find ways to help the person with frontotemporal degeneration act appropriately, while also keeping in mind that this disease affects a person's ability to make the right decisions in social situations.

symptoms, the antidepressant Trazadone may be prescribed.

This medication may cause mild side effects, including fatigue, dizziness and low blood pressure.

Therapies outside of medication

Approaches outside of medication can also help relieve symptoms. As with medication, these approaches can't cure frontotemporal degeneration or stop it from progressing.

Frontotemporal degeneration can be stressful. If you're caring for someone with frontotemporal degeneration, keeping these thoughts in mind can help:

- *Maintain perspective.* Remember that some types of frontotemporal degeneration affect a person's social behavior, self-regulation and emotion. This means someone may say or do things that are hurtful. These are not deliberate actions or personal attacks — they are symptoms of the disease.
- *Accept your feelings as normal.* It's hard to feel compassion for someone who no longer senses your emotional needs, as is common in behavioral variant frontotemporal degeneration.
- *Reach out for help.* When possible, ask for help with child care, errands and other tasks.
- *Join a support group.* Talking with others in the same position can help you share your feelings and find effective ways to cope. Find a list of support groups in the Additional resources section of this book.
- *Take time to do things you find enjoyable.* This may involve enlisting care services or enrolling the person with dementia in an adult day program for people with dementia or other disabilities.
- *Trust yourself.* Keep in mind that you're caring for someone you know better than anyone else; someone who deserves respect, as well as the right care.

The Association for Frontotemporal Degeneration offers awareness cards, one for people with frontotemporal degeneration and one for care partners. They let people know that language ability and behavior may be altered due to disease. Find contact information for this organization in the Additional resources section.

Occupational therapy and physical therapy These therapies are used for managing the movement-related symptoms of frontotemporal degeneration. They're especially helpful later on when movement becomes more difficult. Physical therapy, for example, can help with balance and help keep an individual with frontotemporal degeneration active. Physical therapy can also help with the muscle symptoms of some types of frontotemporal degeneration.

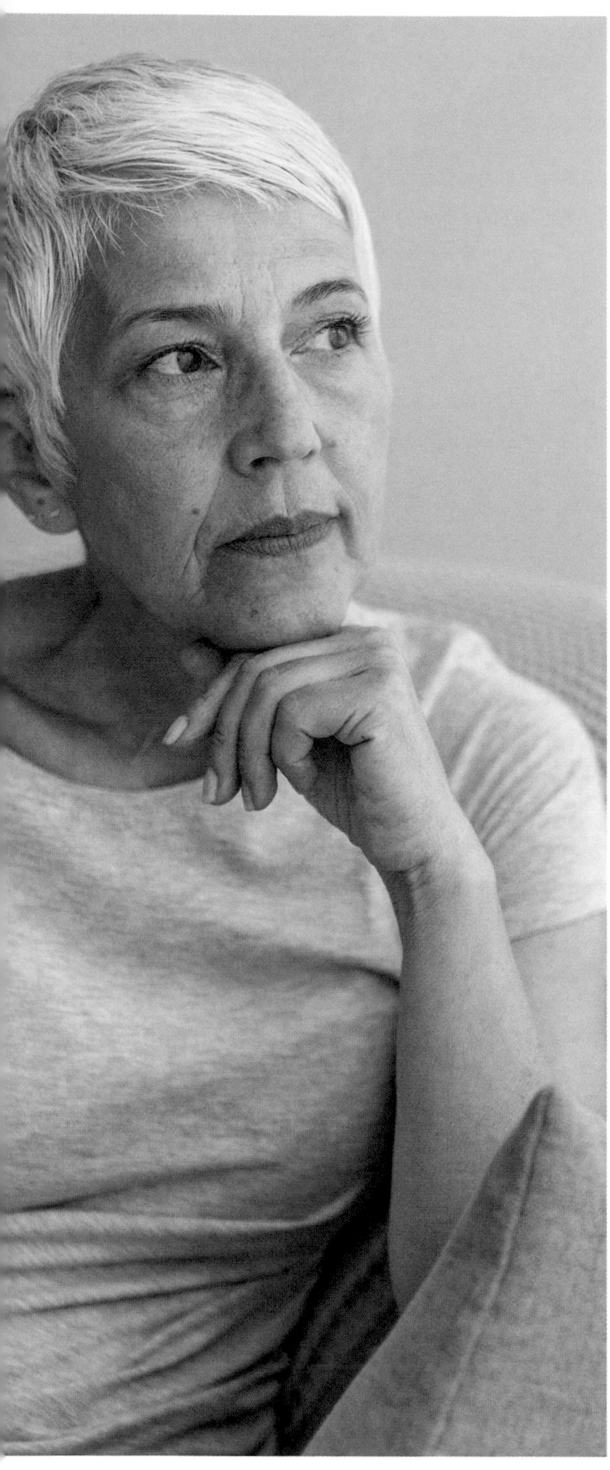

Despite the changes that take place in the brain during frontotemporal degeneration, someone with this disorder can learn new ways of taking part in daily activities. This is where occupational therapy can help.

Occupational therapists learn about a person's interests and routines, as well as what the person can still do. From there, an occupational therapist assesses the skills a person needs for a specific task and breaks them into smaller steps, tailored to the person's abilities.

Occupational therapists also look for possible hazards in a person's environment and makes suggestions geared toward safety. They also teach care partners strategies they can use to help the person with frontotemporal degeneration stay as engaged as possible in the activities of daily living and have a good quality of life.

Speech therapy Speech therapy can be helpful in both early and late stages of frontotemporal degeneration, especially the primary progressive aphasia variants. Early on, speech therapy can help someone living with frontotemporal degeneration speak more clearly.

Therapists can work with people with frontotemporal degeneration and their care partners to troubleshoot communication challenges. For example, if a person has trouble understanding a question like, "Do you want oatmeal or scrambled eggs for breakfast?" a speech therapist can help train care partners to simplify their language. In this situation and for some types of this dementia, it might be better to ask a yes-no question rather than offer a choice or ask a question with longer words or phrases.

Speech therapy is tailored to the challenges each person has and focuses on communication challenges in everyday life. For example, if the person with dementia is still working, it may be helpful to focus on how to complete tasks in a work setting.

Speech therapy may also help people with dementia maintain their level of functioning. In later stages of frontotemporal degeneration, speech therapy can help people find new ways to communicate when they can no longer speak. Writing and using apps on a smartphone or tablet are examples.

Integrative medicine The practice of using conventional medicine alongside evidence-based complementary treatments is known as integrative medicine.

Several integrative therapies can help by promoting relaxation. They include music therapy, which involves listening to music, as well as playing music and singing. Art therapy, shown to reduce anxiety and improve well-being, offers opportunities for creativity using many different mediums. Interacting with pets can also bring comfort and joy.

Changes to the environment People living with frontotemporal degeneration can feel overwhelmed when there's too much going on around them. This can lead to irritability, anxiety and aggression because overstimulation makes it hard to process information from the world around them.

Certain adjustments can help. An environment that offers consistency, routine and structure is most helpful. For those with behavioral variant frontotemporal degeneration, a safe environment that provides both novel and interesting activities may prevent undesirable outcomes like agitation or the desire to go somewhere else.

Additional considerations include reducing noise and limiting interaction to just a few people at a time. For some people, individual, rather than group, activities work best.

Nutritional support Proper nutrition helps brain function and reduces the risk of heart disease, which in turn, helps the brain. A brain-healthy diet is low in fat and cholesterol, and high in fruits and vegetables. Good nutrition can help the parts of the brain that aren't damaged work as well as possible.

People with behavioral variant frontotemporal degeneration face different challenges in terms of nutrition. They may feel an overwhelming urge to eat certain foods and may seem to not be able to eat enough of them, like sweet-tasting foods and carbohydrates. They may eat quickly, want to eat all the time, and get angry if they can't eat what they want, when they want, in the amounts that they crave.

This can be challenging for care partners. Restricting foods can cause aggression and tension, and mealtimes may require extra supervision.

To address these challenges, experts advise:

- Locking cupboards and refrigerators
- Reducing access to large amounts of food
- Avoiding restaurant buffets
- Setting out portions at mealtimes, offering only small amounts of food at a time
- Making healthy options more available than sweets are
- Keeping food that could be unsafe out of reach; uncooked meat and inedible items that might look like food are examples

In later stages, swallowing may become difficult. Mild problems with swallowing have been seen in more than half the people with frontotemporal degeneration. Coupled with the tendency to eat quickly and eat large amounts of food at one time, this can pose a safety risk.

These behaviors can cause coughing and choking and lead to pneumonia, a common cause of death for people with frontotemporal degeneration. A dietitian can recommend foods that are healthy but easy to swallow. Sometimes a feeding tube inserted into the stomach is needed.

Interventions for behavioral variant frontotemporal degeneration People with behavioral variant frontotemporal degeneration have increasing trouble controlling their behavior.

They commonly show apathy or lack of interest, loss of sympathy or empathy for others, disinhibition, difficulty resisting impulses, and overeating. Repetitive or compulsive behaviors, like hoarding and doing the same thing over and over, are also possible. People with behavioral variant frontotemporal degeneration may also develop excessive or inappropriate elation (euphoria).

Care partners and families may find these strategies helpful as they care for and support a person with behavioral variant frontotemporal degeneration:

- Try not argue and never point out a problem or try to reason. Reasoning won't make a person with frontotemporal degeneration see things differently.
- Don't feel you need to explain why.
- Encourage and praise often. People with frontotemporal degeneration often understand positive emotional expressions better than they do negative ones.
- Communicate in ways that are firm, with clear limits that are enforced.
- Incorporate daily activities that have value to the person even if they seem odd. For example, someone with frontotemporal degeneration may want to spend hours swinging in the backyard, playing video games or counting the cars that go by. It's best to accommodate and accept the behavior as long as it's not harmful to the person or others.
- Communicate in a way that offers a sense of control. (Learn more in Chapter 17.)
- Limit and offer specific choices. For example, ask, "Do you want to walk to the park or walk to the river?" instead of, "What do you want to do today?"

- Try not to take the person's behavior personally.

Safety is also important. Removing guns, weapons, power tools and other potentially dangerous items is often necessary.

Palliative care This type of therapy focuses on relief from pain and other symptoms of a serious illness. It's different from hospice care, which is used at the end of life and doesn't use medications meant to prolong life. Palliative care can be used at any time during the course of dementia. It centers around relieving symptoms, offering support and advice for care partners, and teaching techniques that help provide comfort.

OPTIMIZING WELL-BEING

It's important to tell family and friends about a frontotemporal degeneration diagnosis so they're prepared and less likely to avoid the person with the disorder or drift away.

Many people have never heard of frontotemporal degeneration and may feel uncomfortable by what they see if they're not informed. They will need to learn what frontotemporal degeneration is, what to expect, and the best ways to connect with and support the person with frontotemporal degeneration and the person's care partner.

At the same time, it's important for people with frontotemporal degeneration to stay engaged with others and in life, doing the things they enjoy. Staying active and engaged is important and can make a significant difference in overall well-being and quality of life.

"THIS TYPE OF DEMENTIA AFFECTS MORE THAN A MILLION PEOPLE IN THE UNITED STATES ALONE."

CHAPTER 10

Lewy body dementia

Earlier, you learned that an abnormal buildup of protein in the brain is a key feature of many diseases that cause dementia. In Alzheimer's disease, for example, fragments of the protein beta-amyloid clump together *outside* of brain cells, causing plaques. Fragments of the protein tau stick together *inside* brain cells, causing tangles. Plaques and tangles disrupt communication within and between nerve cells (neurons) in the brain. In time, nerve cells stop working and die.

In this chapter, you'll read about a brain disorder called Lewy body dementia. It involves the buildup of a different protein, called alpha-synuclein.

Normally, alpha-synuclein helps nerve cells in the brain send and receive messages. But in Lewy body dementia, too much of this protein is produced, causing clumps of it to form. These clumps keep brain cells from working properly, make it harder for them to talk to each other and cause them to die.

Lewy body dementia is an umbrella term that refers to both dementia with Lewy bodies and Parkinson's disease dementia, which you'll learn about in this chapter.

Both dementia with Lewy bodies and Parkinson's disease dementia are caused by abnormal deposits of alpha-synuclein. Lewy body dementia is the second most common form of degenerative dementia, behind only Alzheimer's disease.

DEPOSITS IN THE BRAINSTEM

In the early 1900s, Friedrich H. Lewy, a German neurologist, was working in Dr. Alois

Alzheimer's lab when he came across abnormal protein deposits in the brains of people who died of Parkinson's disease. Lewy saw rounded deposits in brain cells in the brainstem and in the area right above the brainstem. These deposits were later named after him, called Lewy bodies.

Then in the 1990s, scientists discovered that alpha-synuclein is the main protein in Lewy bodies. In Lewy body disorders, alpha-synuclein was also found in the branches of the brain cells that receive information from other cells. These deposits are called Lewy neurites.

Lewy bodies and Lewy neurites interrupt the normal functioning of the brain. Together, they represent Lewy body disease. The areas of the brain most sensitive to Lewy body disease are the parts that produce two brain chemicals, dopamine and acetylcholine. These brain chemicals and the brain pathways that use them are important for attention, visual perception, thinking, movement, motivation and emotion.

Studies of Lewy body disease show that deposits of alpha-synuclein start in the olfactory brain region and the lower part of the brainstem. For some, the progression stops there. But for others, the deposits spread to the upper brainstem. For some people, the progression stops there. But again, for others, the deposits go on to spread to the middle (subcortical) part of the brain. Again, for some people, the progression stops there. But for others, it spreads to the outer (cortical) part of the brain.

When Lewy body disease is confined to the brainstem, a person may only develop parkinsonism or sleep issues, and be diagnosed with Parkinson's disease at some point. When Lewy body disease spreads to other parts of the brain and dementia and other symptoms develop, a person is more likely to be diagnosed with Parkinson's disease dementia or dementia with Lewy bodies.

That's because different brain regions are responsible for different functions. The olfactory region is important for the sense of smell. The lower brainstem is important for regulation of blood pressure and sleep. The upper brainstem is important for motor function. The middle (subcortical) region is connected to parts of the brain involved in movement, attention, alertness, visual perception, motivation and emotion.

Because of its array of symptoms, Lewy body dementia can be difficult to diagnose. To complicate things, some people with Lewy body disease also have Alzheimer's disease. Scientists are working to understand what causes the spread of Lewy body disease, why it's more widespread in some people and not others, and why some people also have plaques and tangles. A great deal of work is focused on ways to try to stop its progression.

WHAT HAPPENS IN LEWY BODY DEMENTIA?

Lewy body dementia usually progresses little by little over several years, but how it

FOUR BASIC TERMS

The terms Lewy body disease, Lewy body dementia, dementia with Lewy bodies and Parkinson's disease dementia are related — but distinct — terms. Here's what each of them means and how they're related.

Lewy body disease refers to the abnormal buildup of alpha-synuclein. Lewy bodies result from a buildup of this protein inside cell bodies. A buildup of this protein in cell branches causes Lewy neurites to form.

Lewy body disease that's seen only in the brainstem tends to lead to Parkinson's disease. Lewy body disease that spreads to other areas of the brain causes people to develop Lewy body dementia, which results in either dementia with Lewy bodies or Parkinson's disease dementia.

Lewy body dementia refers to either dementia with Lewy bodies or Parkinson's disease dementia.

Dementia with Lewy bodies causes problems with thinking and daily activities that a person has always been able to do.

Dementia with Lewy bodies is characterized by the presence of at least two of these symptoms: acting out dreams during sleep (REM sleep behavior disorder); motor symptoms that may include stiffness, slowness, stooped posture, masked face, tremor, imbalance (parkinsonism); times when attention, alertness and abilities are impaired and then improve (fluctuations); and seeing images of objects, animals or people that aren't really there (visual hallucinations). Symptoms of parkinsonism (motor stiffness, slowness, stooped posture, masked face, tremor, imbalance) typically come on less than a year before symptoms of dementia do.

Parkinson's disease dementia, as you may expect by its name, is dementia that affects someone with Parkinson's disease. It refers to parkinsonism that's followed by the development of dementia. Parkinson's disease dementia often progresses more slowly than dementia with Lewy bodies does.

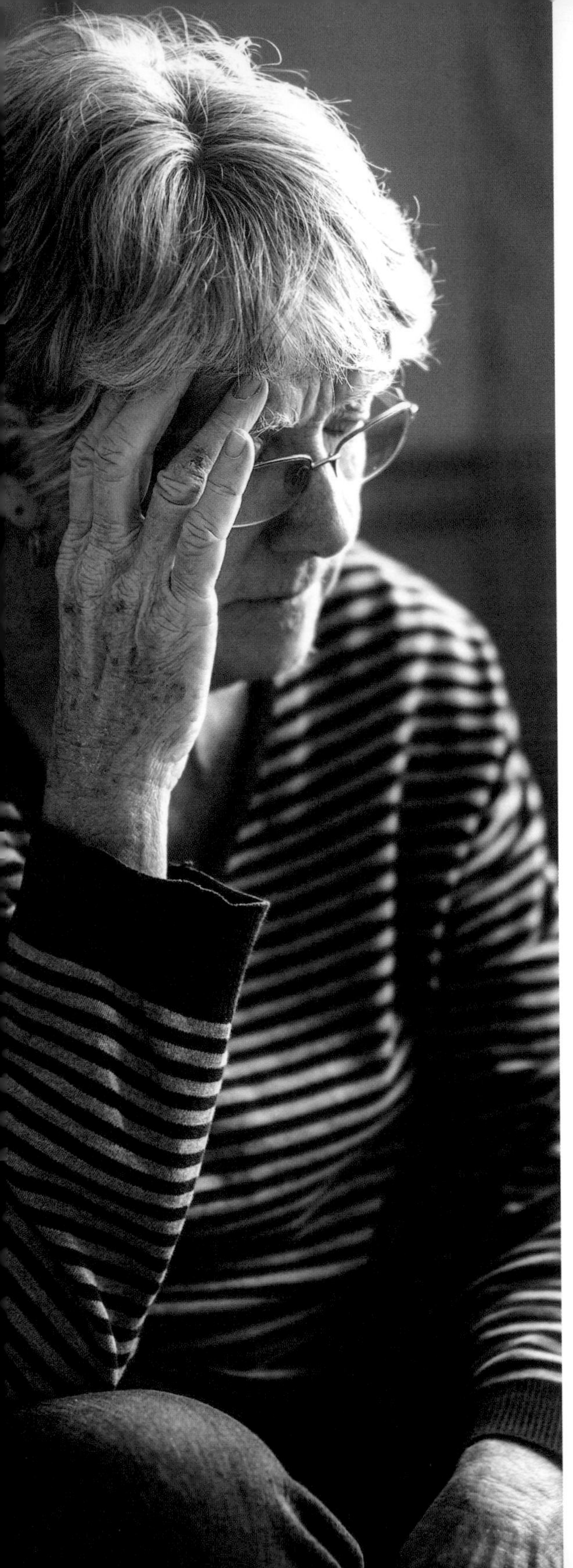

progresses varies. Acting out dreams while asleep is often one of the first symptoms. This symptom may occur years or even decades before other symptoms appear.

In dementia with Lewy bodies, thinking tends to be affected before movement problems like stiffness, slowness, imbalance and tremor (parkinsonism) appear. In Parkinson's disease dementia, problems with movement start before thinking abilities are affected. Varying levels of attention, alertness and abilities that come and go (cognitive fluctuations) are also seen in Lewy body dementia. Seeing things that aren't actually there (visual hallucinations) also may occur.

On average, people live five to 10 years with Lewy body dementia after it's been diagnosed. Some people decline quickly, while in others, the disease progresses slowly. Some people live for well over 10 years, while others live only a few years after they're diagnosed. Lewy body dementia tends to progress more quickly in people who also have Alzheimer's disease.

Many factors are involved in how quickly Lewy body disease progresses. Medications that lower dopamine or acetylcholine in the brain may make symptoms worse and cause the disease to progress more rapidly, for example. You'll learn more in this chapter.

Who's at risk?

Lewy body dementia is more common in people older than 60, and men are more likely to have it than are women. Women who have one or both ovaries removed early, before age 45, seem to have a somewhat higher risk of this type of dementia.

This type of dementia affects more than a million people in the United States alone. Lewy body dementia usually affects adults between ages 50 and 85. In people with dementia, as many as 2 in 10 people have Lewy body dementia on its own, but many also have some degree of Alzheimer's disease changes in the brain.

Family history may play a role in a person's risk of Lewy body dementia, but usually this is only the case when several family members have a history of dementia or parkinsonism. When only one family member has it, the risk of others developing it is only a little bit higher. Rare, inherited forms of the disease can be passed down through generations. These forms usually affect people in their 20s, 30s or 40s. Even if a family has a known genetic form of the disease, there's still a chance that individual family members won't get it.

A lot of research has been done to improve how well Lewy body dementia is identified. A person's medical history, neurologic exam, imaging, and certain markers in the blood and fluid around the brain and spinal cord (cerebrospinal fluid) all play a role in diagnosis, as you'll learn later on.

In this chapter, you'll learn that medications and other therapies may help with symptoms. However, common over-the-counter and prescription drugs may make symptoms worse. In addition, people with Lewy body dementia tend to respond better to certain medications than people with Alzheimer's do. This is one reason why an early and proper diagnosis is important. Given early, the proper treatment can promote a longer and higher quality of life.

SIGNS AND SYMPTOMS

As you've learned, in Lewy body dementia, changes may be limited to certain parts of the brain, or they may spread to other areas of the brain. Because of these differences, not everyone gets the same combination of symptoms or has the same amount of cognitive change over time.

Here's more on each of the core signs and symptoms of Lewy body dementia.

Cognitive changes and dementia

Problems with attention, visual perception and spatial processing are often among the first challenges of Lewy body dementia. This is different from Alzheimer's disease, in which these symptoms don't develop until later on. Like in Alzheimer's disease, some people with Lewy body dementia may also have trouble keeping track of details of conversations or recalling recent events.

These changes commonly make it harder to think quickly and pay attention to more than one thing at a time. A person with Lewy body dementia may take longer to process what someone says, may not catch all of the details of information that's given quickly, and may take longer to respond or express thoughts or ideas. Problems with attention also make it more likely for a person to get distracted.

Here are examples of how these changes may take shape.

Lapses in attention are common for everyone, but a person with Lewy body dementia may be more likely to say things like, "I lost my train of thought," or "I forgot what I was going to say" or ask, "What did I come in here for?" Distracted thinking like this can make it harder to plan, prioritize, do math in one's head, or understand lengthy explanations, text or story plots. Sometimes, these issues interfere with memory.

Visual perception and spatial processing problems may make it hard to recognize an object from an unusual angle or in dim light. For example, someone may think crumbs are bugs or a lamp is a person. These difficulties can make it harder to find an object that's among several other objects. It may also be harder to judge distance. It may be more difficult to figure out how to fit an object into a certain space.

These issues aren't always noticeable, but sometimes they can affect how well a person can do certain things. Making repairs, using carpentry skills, sewing, crafting or packing a suitcase are all examples.

People with Lewy body dementia are usually able to recognize faces and emotions, but some may misidentify people as the disease progresses. Although the visual problems in Lewy body dementia aren't caused by poor vision, regular eye exams are a good idea.

REM sleep behavior disorder

Rapid eye movement sleep behavior disorder affects more than half of people with Lewy body dementia. It causes people to physically act out their dreams while they're sleeping.

Movements during sleep match the dream the person is having. They may be subtle or vigorous and may result in injuries to the person with dementia or a bed partner. Common themes include fighting, defending oneself or others, playing sports, or running. Women tend to dream less vigorously than men do.

Rapid eye movement sleep behavior disorder is linked to disrupted function in the lower brainstem and a loss of the normal paralysis of dream sleep. Unless it causes someone to wake up, rapid eye movement sleep behavior disorder doesn't usually interfere with a person's sleep.

There's usually no need to wake a person who's acting out a dream unless there's a safety concern. Moving sharp objects away from the bed, lowering the bed and having bed partners move to another room can help with safety.

This sleep disorder may occur years and even decades before other symptoms of Lewy body dementia appear. One study shows that nearly two-thirds of people diagnosed with this sleep disorder go on to develop either parkinsonism or dementia. Rapid eye movement sleep behavior disorder often lessens as other symptoms of Lewy body dementia emerge.

Symptoms of other sleep disorders, like severe sleep apnea, sleepwalking and nighttime confusion, can look like rapid eye movement sleep behavior disorder, so a proper diagnosis is important. Treatment for rapid eye movement sleep behavior disorder varies from that of other sleep disorders. An overnight sleep study (polysomnogram) may be needed.

Fluctuating attention, alertness and thinking abilities

In Lewy body dementia, the word *fluctuations* describes episodes when attention and alertness worsen and then improve to a normal or near-normal level. Then they worsen again, and then improve, and so on.

This leads to situations in which a person can carry out a task, then can't, and then later on can do it again. Care partners often describe these episodes as "good times and bad times" that come and go.

During "bad" episodes, a person with Lewy body dementia may:

- Be less able to follow what's being said

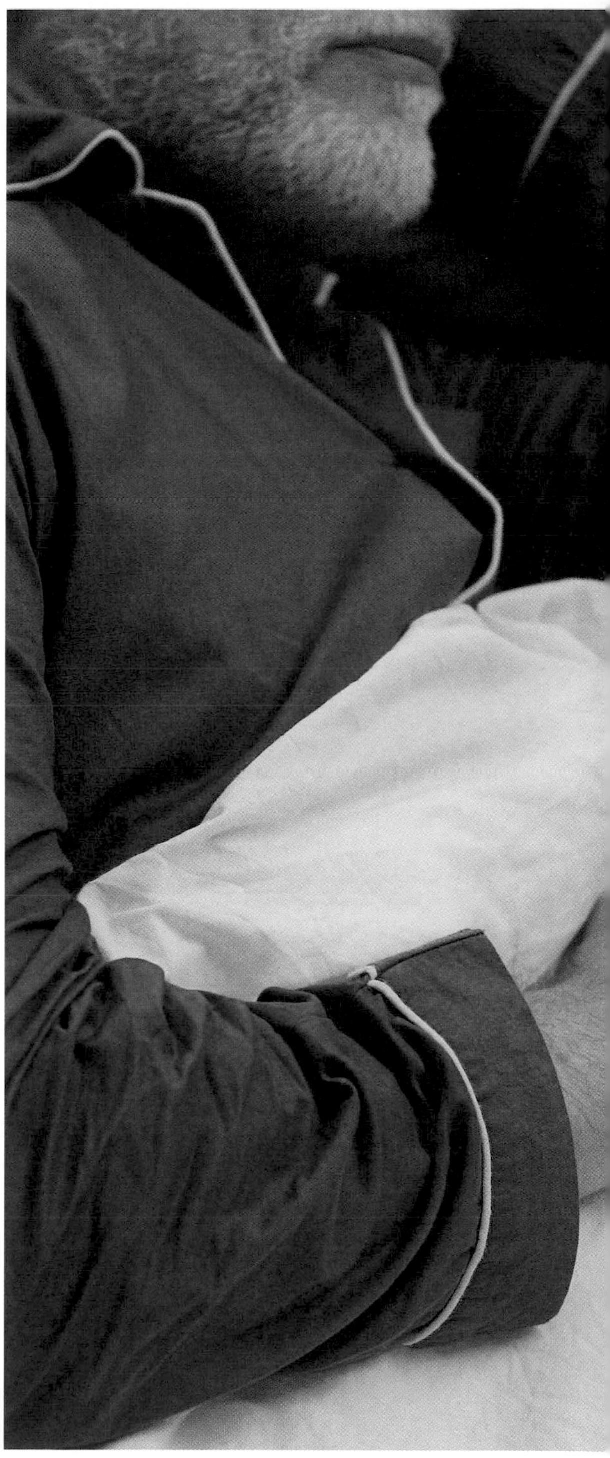

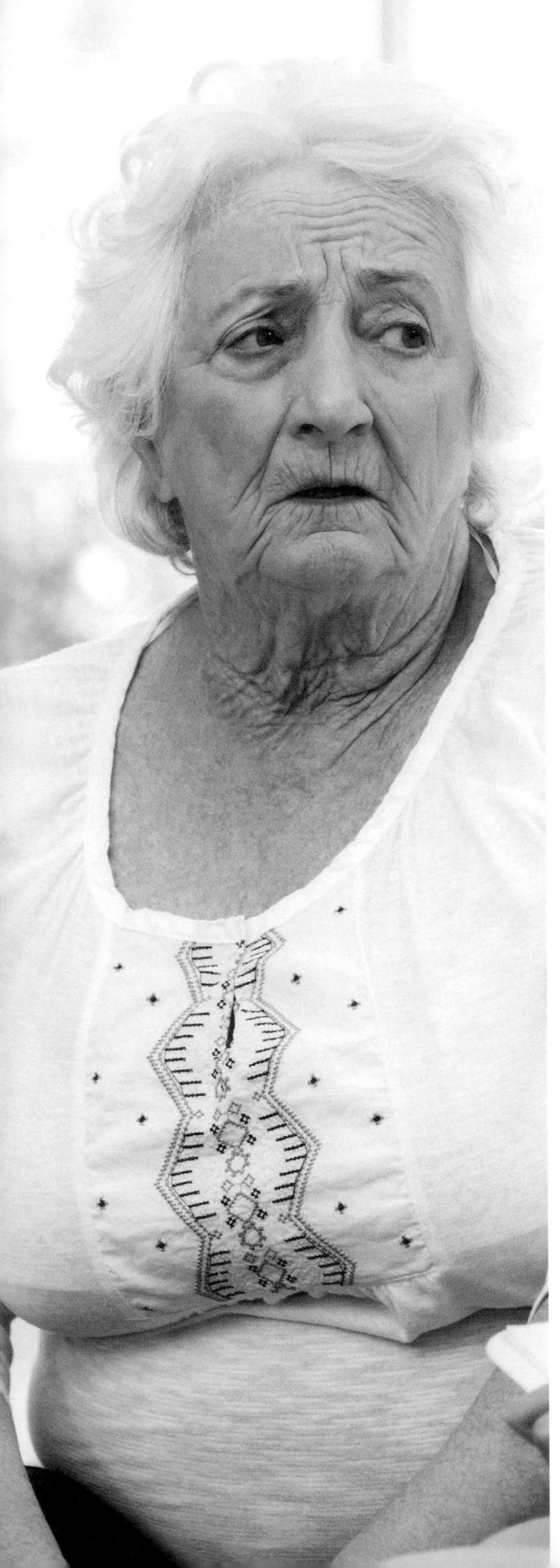

- Process information more slowly than usual
- Stare off into space (but respond when spoken to)
- Seem zoned out, glazed over, drowsy or more distracted than usual
- Speak out of context or off topic
- Speak in ways that are disorganized, disjointed or that don't make sense
- Be unable to figure something out or carry out a task, but be able to do it later on

"Bad" episodes are followed by "good" episodes when a person appears much more alert, lucid, attentive, logical, able to understand and communicate, and able to carry out tasks they couldn't manage before.

Fluctuations between "bad" and "good" episodes may alternate back and forth within minutes, hours or days. Each episode may even last weeks at a time. Fluctuations can occur at any time of the day. They're not restricted to the late afternoon or evening hours. As dementia progresses and cognitive abilities worsen, fluctuations may become less extreme.

Fluctuations occur in about 3 out of 4 people with Lewy body dementia. They're one of the biggest sources of care partner stress and can be costly in terms of emergency room visits and testing needed to rule out other causes, like seizures or strokes. Alcohol, medication side effects, infections, pain, stress, and other causes of drowsiness or confusion also need to be ruled out. These can all cause or worsen changes in mental status and functioning.

Parkinsonism

Lewy body dementia can cause some or all of these movement-related symptoms:

- Slowed movement
- Rigid muscles, including stiffness in the throat that makes swallowing more difficult and drooling more common
- Stooped posture
- Reduced facial expression (like a masked look on a person's face)
- Reduced blinking
- A tendency not to swing the arms when walking
- Short, shuffling steps
- Hand tremor
- Balance issues

Movement-related symptoms are like those in Parkinson's disease, which is why they're referred to as parkinsonism.

While parkinsonism affects many people who have dementia with Lewy bodies, some never develop it. Sometimes parkinsonism and cognitive changes happen at the same time; for other people, parkinsonism develops shortly after or several years after cognitive changes start.

Parkinsonism in Lewy body dementia and Parkinson's disease are both caused by Lewy body disease and cell loss in the dopamine-producing area in the brainstem.

The motor symptoms in Lewy body dementia and Parkinson's disease are the same, but in Lewy body dementia, they tend to be milder, the stiffness usually occurs on both sides of the body and hand tremors are less common.

Visual hallucinations

Visual hallucinations involve seeing fully formed images that aren't actually present. They're usually images of people, children or animals, but may also be images of objects or insects. The images often look quite solid. They may or may not move, and they can sometimes can be quite detailed.

Visual hallucinations may occur occasionally, once a month, once a week or daily. The person experiencing the images may not know if they're real or not, but the images often aren't frightening or distressing.

In Lewy body dementia, visual hallucinations can develop in the mild or early stages of the disease. In Alzheimer's disease, on the other hand, visual hallucinations tend to occur in the advanced stages.

More than two-thirds of people with Lewy body dementia have visual hallucinations within five years after problems with thinking appear.

Visual hallucinations seem to be related to having very low levels of the brain chemical acetylcholine. This chemical is associated with confusion and hallucinations. Visual hallucinations may also be caused by problems with the areas of the brain responsible for visual processing or dreams that cross over into wakefulness.

Visual misperceptions

Since it causes issues with visual processing, Lewy body dementia commonly causes someone to see an object and mistake it for something else.

A person with Lewy body dementia may think a lamp is a person, mistake a fire hydrant for a child, think that specks of dirt are bugs, or mistake a pattern in carpeting or a bedspread for bugs, snakes or animals. Sometimes, the objects may appear to move.

These errors in vision are called misperceptions and not hallucinations because they involve actual objects. Moving an object, replacing it or increasing the lighting may help. People with Lewy body dementia who have visual misperceptions are more likely to also see things that aren't actually there (visual hallucinations).

Delusions or false beliefs

False beliefs or delusional thinking may occur in Lewy body dementia. When someone with Lewy body dementia can't grasp the reality of the images that they're seeing, this can lead to false beliefs. For example, if a person with Lewy body dementia sees someone in a room but there's no one there, the person with dementia may think there's a stranger in the house even when no one is there.

A second common type of false belief in Lewy body dementia is known as Capgras syndrome. Capgras syndrome is the false belief that a loved one, almost always a spouse but sometimes an adult child, is an exact duplicate or an imposter.

In this situation, the person with Capgras syndrome may believe an individual looks, sounds and acts just like their loved one, but it's not. Sometimes people with Lewy body dementia believe there's more than one version of their loved one, like "the good Louise" and "the bad Louise." While Capgras syndrome can be seen in other types of dementia, it's more common in dementia with Lewy bodies.

Other types of delusions or false beliefs may occur, like feeling paranoid or suspicious or falsely believing that a spouse has been unfaithful. These delusions are often related to longstanding worries or fears, to current fears or discomfort of being left alone, or to worry about being unable to manage alone. These delusions may also occur in someone who has problems with intense emotions (fear, anxiety, anger), impaired reasoning skills, and limited or no awareness of one's cognitive difficulties.

Misinterpreting social cues is another symptom of Lewy body dementia. Someone with Lewy body dementia may believe people are laughing at or talking about them when they see people laugh or talk. Including the person with Lewy body dementia in the conversation by looking at the person's eyes or smiling and explaining things briefly and in a way he or she can understand can help relieve these misunderstandings.

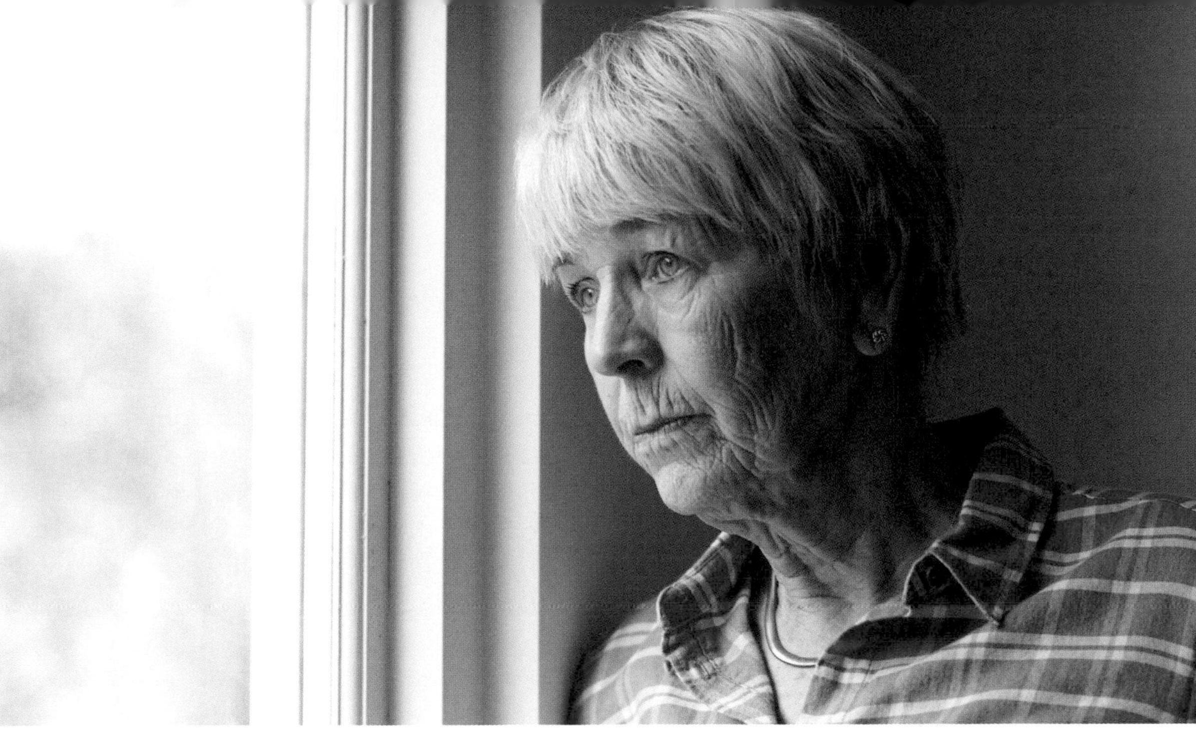

Poor body function regulation (autonomic dysfunction)

Lewy body dementia affects the autonomic nervous system, which is the part of the brain involved in processes that the body regulates without any effort on your part. Blood pressure, heart rate, sweating, digestion and bladder function are all examples. Autonomic dysfunction describes issues with these processes.

Problems with blood pressure may cause feelings of lightheadedness upon standing, when climbing stairs or after standing for a period of time. A drop in blood pressure may also cause someone to fall or faint. Or, urine may not flow or the bladder may not empty completely. This can lead to problems with urinary retention and bladder infections. These are just some examples of autonomic dysfunction.

Daytime sleepiness

Daytime drowsiness involves feeling so tired that you're ready to fall asleep. Excessive daytime sleepiness, on the other hand, is when someone sleeps a lot during the day, even after a good night's sleep. Both are common in Lewy body dementia. It's important to rule out other causes of these issues first, like not getting enough sleep at night, snoring, too much alcohol, medication side effects, infection, a recent injury or other medical reasons for drowsiness.

What's considered excessive depends on how much daytime sleepiness disrupts a person's daily life and how it compares to a person's previous levels of daytime wakefulness. Two or more hours of daytime sleep is usually considered more than expected.

Whether to address daytime drowsiness and excessive daytime sleepiness depends on how disruptive it is. Sometimes doing more during the day and building in periods of rest is helpful. For others, short naps help promote better daytime functioning. Improving nighttime sleep, reducing snoring and considering medication to increase daytime alertness are other options.

Apathy

In Lewy body dementia, apathy can be related to moving more slowly and taking longer to find words, come up with ideas, or complete a task. Apathy is also often related to cognitive issues, like knowing what needs to be done first (prioritizing).

Lack of interest or emotion also are features of apathy. A person may seem indifferent, not express emotion, not appear to care, and may have less or no interest in activities or people. Emotional features like these may be related to lower levels of dopamine in the brain caused by Lewy body dementia.

Apathy may also be a symptom of depression, and it may be associated with feelings of sadness, a sense of loss and feeling overwhelmed. One of the best ways to tell the difference between apathy or depression may be to ask the person directly about mood and feelings. People who are experiencing apathy usually don't describe themselves as feeling emotionally distressed.

Depression

In Lewy body dementia, depression may be a reaction to the losses and physical limitations associated with having dementia. This is commonly seen in people who are aware of their difficulties and feel saddened and frustrated by their inability to do the things they used to enjoy.

Depression may also be related to chemical changes in the brain, and to changes in the emotion areas of the brain affected by Lewy body disease. Sometimes depression looks like sadness. In others, depression is expressed as anxiety or fear. Still others express depression in terms of irritability or agitation.

Anxiety, fear, agitation

Lewy body dementia can cause emotional outbursts or emotional responses that are inappropriate or out of proportion to the situation. They may involve anger, panic attacks, combativeness, or any type of intense or extreme expression of emotion. Common triggers include frustration, feeling that one's needs or wishes are being blocked, a feeling of being in danger, a feeling of not being heard or taken seriously, or a belief that a person is against them or keeping them from getting what they need.

It's important to recognize that agitation and other signs of distress in a person with Lewy body dementia are often reasonable reactions to the environment and situation. For example, losing independence, feeling left out of decisions, or having someone who's nearly a stranger help with bathing can make anyone — with or without dementia — respond with agitation or anger. In these circumstances, addressing the root cause of the distress is critical.

In addition, remaining calm and warm and using a patient and agreeable tone of voice is important. It's best not to argue, raise your voice, talk the person out of his or her concern, or provide lengthy explanations. Instead, speak slowly and use short sentences. Tell the person that you understand and hear the concern. Reassure the person, validate the person's feelings and make it known that you're on the person's side. This is known as the "go along to get along" approach. You'll learn more about approaches like this in Chapter 17.

Sometimes, medication is used to help calm a person in the short run. An antidepressant may be prescribed to help with intense reactions related to Lewy body dementia.

DIAGNOSIS

No single test can positively identify Lewy body dementia. It can only be confirmed when the brain is examined after a person has died. During a person's life, doctors diagnose Lewy body dementia based on the presence of the signs and symptoms you're reading about in this chapter.

In general, a person diagnosed with Lewy body dementia is experiencing a change in thinking skills. Thinking skills have become impaired, and this makes it hard for a person to handle daily activities that he or she used to be able to manage independently.

A person who's diagnosed with dementia with Lewy bodies also has two or more of these signs and symptoms:

- Fluctuations in attention and alertness
- Acting out dreams during sleep (rapid eye movement sleep behavior disorder)
- Movement symptoms (parkinsonism) like motor stiffness, slowness and imbalance that aren't caused by medications, stroke or another known brain injury
- Seeing things that aren't real (visual hallucinations), including people, animals or objects

Other signs and symptoms that can suggest someone has Lewy body dementia include:

- Problems with processes the body regulates (autonomic dysfunction), like blood pressure, temperature and sweating, digestion, and bowel and bladder function
- False beliefs or delusions
- Hearing things that aren't real (auditory hallucinations), like buzzing, a doorbell, music, a car door or muffled voices
- Apathy, depression, anxiety or agitation
- Sensitivity to neuroleptics or other medicines that block dopamine and cause or worsen parkinsonism (see page 233)
- Loss of sense of smell

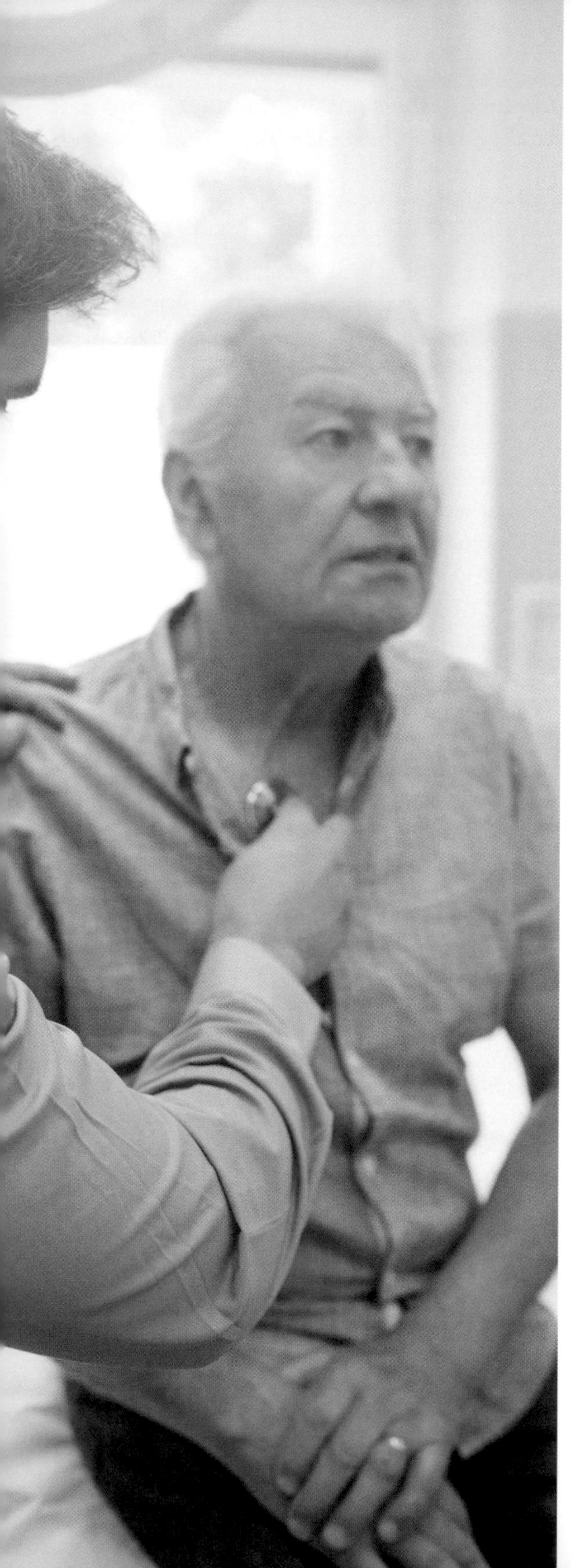

- Sensitivity to anticholinergic medicines that block acetylcholine, causing or worsening cognitive impairment, fluctuations, and hallucinations (see page 233)

Tests you may have

After considering symptoms and medical history, a doctor may suggest additional tests to confirm or rule out Lewy body dementia. You'll read about them next. These tests are similar to those used to diagnose other forms of dementia. You can revisit these tests and read about them in more detail in Chapter 4.

Neurological and physical exam A doctor may look for signs of parkinsonism or other medical conditions that may explain signs and symptoms. A doctor may also test reflexes, strength and muscle tone. A sense of touch and smell and how well a person walks and maintains balance also may be tested.

Mental abilities tests A doctor may use a brief screening test to look for general changes in thinking. This test can't tell the difference between Lewy body dementia and Alzheimer's disease dementia, but it can show if more tests are needed.

From there, neuropsychological tests offer a more detailed look at a person's thinking skills (attention, memory, language, visual processing and reasoning), as well as emotional function. The scores on these tests are compared with those taken by people who are the same age and have completed the same level of education.

Neuropsychological tests help show if problems with cognitive function are greater than what's expected with normal aging. They show patterns of strengths and difficulties and help to determine if a person has normal cognition, mild cognitive impairment or dementia. They can also show how severe dementia is. Neuropsychological testing may be repeated over time to help monitor the disease's progression.

Blood tests Blood tests may be used to show if a metabolic problem, like a low level of vitamin B-12 or an underactive thyroid, may be causing dementia-like signs and symptoms. Although no blood test can detect Lewy body dementia currently, researchers are studying people with Lewy body dementia in an effort to develop markers that can one day be tested in the blood to help diagnose this type of dementia.

Brain scans An MRI or a CT scan may be used to see if a structural problem like a stroke, bleeding, tumor or fluid on the brain from normal-pressure hydrocephalus is causing symptoms.

Imaging tests can also show differences between types of dementia. An MRI, for example, may help tell the difference between Alzheimer's disease dementia and dementia with Lewy bodies. In Alzheimer's, an MRI or CT scan is likely to show shrinking in the hippocampus, part of the brain that's linked to memory. A hippocampus that doesn't appear to be shrinking may mean a person has dementia with Lewy bodies.

A diagnosis of dementia with Lewy bodies can most often be made after a routine clinical evaluation and an MRI or CT scan, but additional imaging tests may be done if the diagnosis isn't clear after a routine exam. For example, one additional imaging test that can be used is a PET scan that looks at brain function (fluorodeoxyglucose). A certain pattern of changes on this scan can show if someone has dementia with Lewy bodies. See examples on page 223.

An imaging test known as ioflupane SPECT (also called a DaTscan) also may be used. It measures the level of the dopamine transporters in the brain. Lewy bodies in the brainstem are associated with lower levels of dopamine transporter. As you learned earlier, a drop in dopamine causes problems with motor skills and other brain functions. See examples of a DaTscan on page 224.

Cardiac metaiodobenzylguanidine (MIBG) is one more imaging test that may be used. It shows changes in the heart's function that are linked to dementia with Lewy bodies. This test can help tell the difference between dementia with Lewy bodies and Alzheimer's disease. Commonly used in Japan, this test is rarely used in the United States to diagnose dementia with Lewy bodies.

Other tests An overnight sleep study (polysomnogram) may be used to check for rapid eye movement sleep behavior disorder or find other causes of daytime sleepiness.

For this test, electrodes are placed on the head and legs, and soft sensor bands are placed around the chest and on the finger. This test shows if someone twitches and jerks during sleep, has restless legs or stops breathing during sleep (sleep apnea). Any of these can cause a poor night's sleep and daytime sleepiness. A sleep study also checks for muscle tone. Muscle tone that's present during sleep may be a sign of rapid eye movement sleep behavior disorder. Autonomic function tests also may be used.

RECEIVING A DIAGNOSIS

Even though there's no cure for Lewy body dementia, a diagnosis is important because it can help guide treatment and inform a person with dementia about what to expect.

The MRIs below illustrate one of the key differences between Alzheimer's disease and Lewy body dementia: how much memory is affected. The image on the right is of the brain of someone with Alzheimer's disease. The arrow points to the hippocampus, which is smaller than normal. (You'll recall that the hippocampus is the central switchboard for the brain's memory system.)

Compare that to the left image, a brain affected by Lewy body dementia. The hippocampus is roughly the same size as that in a normal brain. The smaller hippocampus in the Alzheimer's image shows why memory problems are one of the first symptoms of Alzheimer's disease, but not of Lewy body dementia.

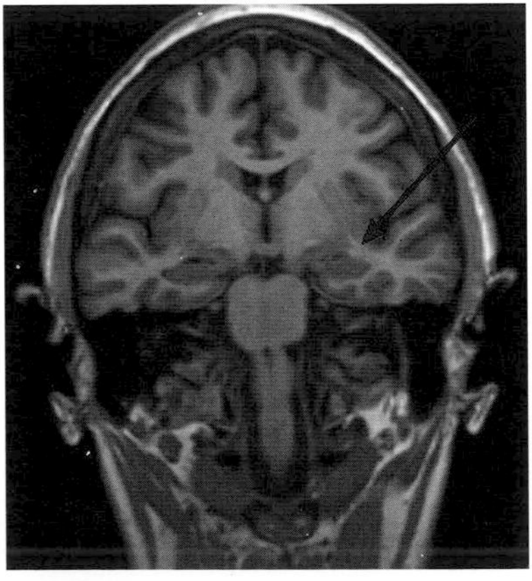

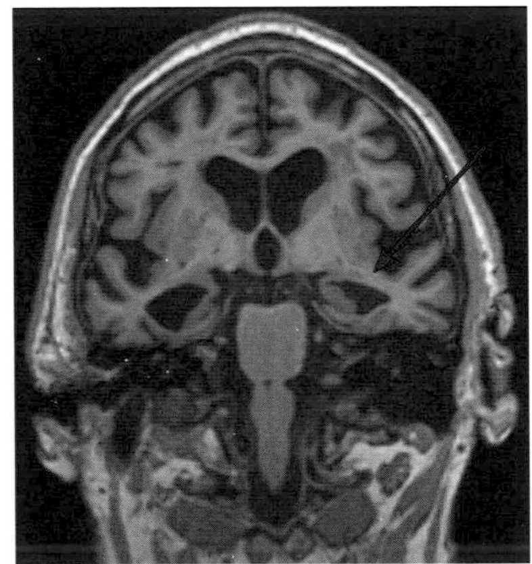

DEMENTIA WITH LEWY BODIES VS. ALZHEIMER'S DEMENTIA

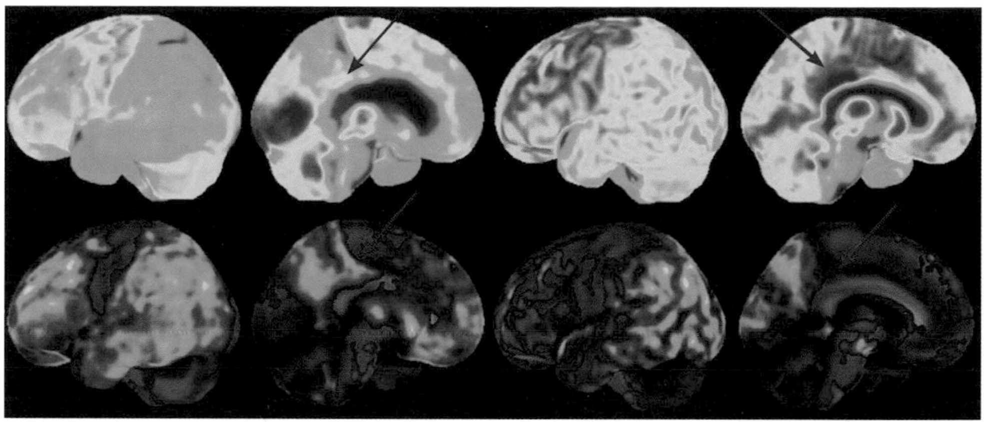

These fluorodeoxyglucose (FDG) PET scans help show the difference between dementia with Lewy bodies and Alzheimer's disease dementia. The left two columns show the brain of someone with Alzheimer's disease dementia. The right two columns show the brain of someone with Lewy body dementia. Dark blue areas are less affected, while green areas are the most affected. You'll see that Alzheimer's disease dementia and dementia with Lewy bodies both cause changes to the brain. But in Lewy body disease, the area of the brain known as the posterior cingulate (see arrow) is spared. The posterior cingulate plays a role in many processes, including memory, attention, emotional responses, and processing things you see and hear. In addition, the back of the brain is more involved in dementia with Lewy bodies than it is with Alzheimer's dementia.

These days, doctors are more able to tell the difference between Lewy body dementia and other types of dementia. This means that someone with this disorder is may get treatment for symptoms sooner — and avoid treatments that may make symptoms worse. A diagnosis also offers answers for troubling symptoms, many of which are related to behavior and emotions.

Talking about the diagnosis offers people living with dementia and their care partners an opportunity to maximize quality of life. This includes gathering support from family, friends and health care professionals, creating a safe environment and planning for the future. Learn more in Chapter 13.

It can be helpful to share this diagnosis to help others understand the changes they may see as the disorder progresses. Although Lewy body dementia was discovered in the early 1900s, the first case wasn't

On a DaTscan, cool colors (blues and greens) show low levels of dopamine transporter. Warm colors (oranges, reds and whites) show high levels. The brain scan of a person with Alzheimer's disease (right), shows a dopamine transporter level in the brain that's close to normal (a normal scan is on the left). The brain of someone with Lewy body dementia (center) shows much lower dopamine transporter level in the brain.

A reduced dopamine transporter level is a biological sign of disease (biomarker) that can show if someone has dementia with Lewy bodies. A person who has one of the core symptoms you read about earlier and a reduced dopamine transporter level, shown by this imaging test, helps show the difference between dementia with Lewy bodies and Alzheimer's disease. While a reduced dopamine transporter level can help diagnose dementia with Lewy bodies, it may also have other causes, so a doctor will need to rule out other causes first. It's also important to note that a scan that comes back normal doesn't necessarily rule out dementia with Lewy bodies.

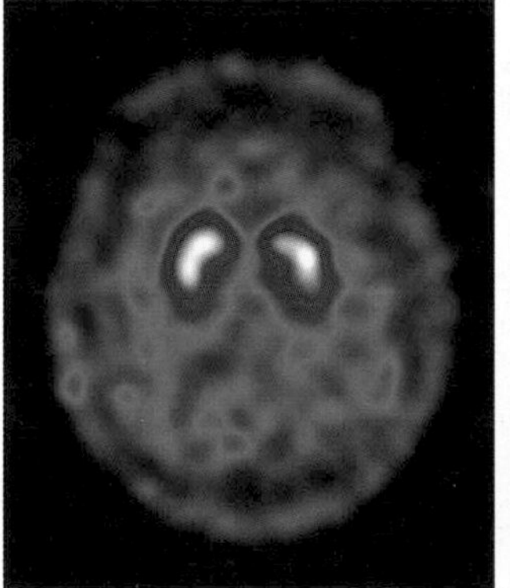

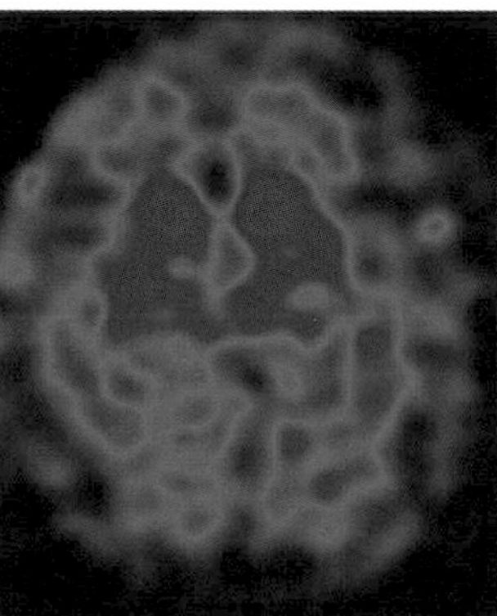

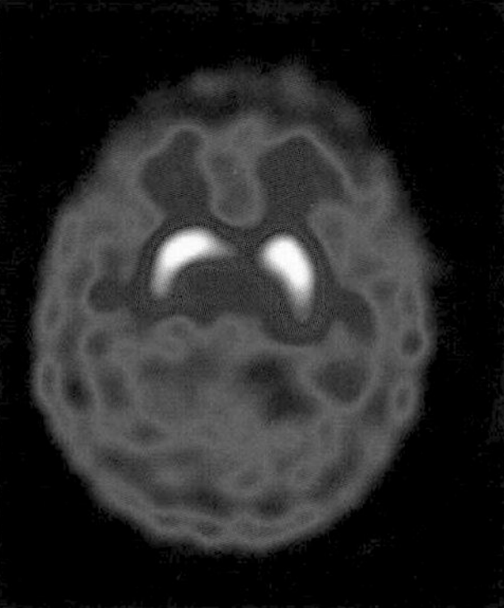

described until 1961, and the first set of criteria used to diagnose it wasn't available until 1996. So in many ways, people are still in the early stages of recognizing and learning about this type of dementia.

Above all else, after receiving a diagnosis, it's important to focus on strengths, enjoy each day and make the most of your time. This goes for people living with Lewy body dementia as well as their care partners.

Parts 4 and 5 of this book are dedicated to strategies for coping with a dementia diagnosis and living a full life with dementia. There, you'll find strategies for people with dementia and for care partners.

TREATING THE DISEASE

Because there's no cure for Lewy body dementia, treatment is aimed at lessening the impact of symptoms on quality of life. This typically involves a combination of several therapies.

People with Lewy body dementia and their care partners play important roles in identifying the symptoms that need the most attention as they change over time.

MANAGING SYMPTOMS

Some symptoms of Lewy body dementia respond well to treatment for a period of time.

Medications, physical and other types of therapy, and counseling can all help. Changes made at home also can lessen symptoms and make everyday living a little easier. Because Lewy body dementia can cause a vast range of symptoms, a team of care providers is generally needed. Learn about managing symptoms starting on page 228.

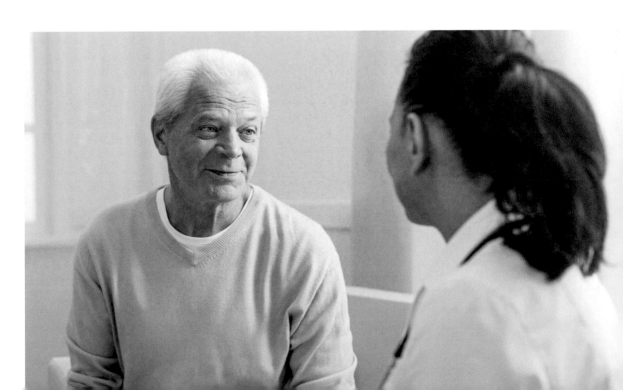

LEWY BODY DEMENTIA VS. ALZHEIMER'S DISEASE DEMENTIA

People with Lewy body dementia may have a decline in thinking skills that looks like Alzheimer's disease. In fact, it can be hard to tell the difference between Lewy body dementia and other dementias at first. Here are some of the key differences between Lewy body dementia and Alzheimer's disease dementia.

Alzheimer's disease dementia	Lewy body dementia
Mostly affects adults age 65 and older	Usually affects adults between ages 50 and 85
May live for more than 10 years after diagnosis	Most live for 5 to 10 years after diagnosis
Most common cause of dementia	Second most common cause of degenerative dementia
Memory loss is common early on	Memory problems may happen in later stages
Seeing and hearing things that aren't real may not happen; when it does, it occurs later in the disease	Causes someone to see things that aren't real early on
Thinking skills get worse and worse over time	Thinking skills and attention fluctuate; they're better some days, worse on other days, and they can get better or worse throughout the day
Don't tend to have daytime sleepiness	More likely to have daytime sleepiness

While Lewy body dementia and Alzheimer's disease dementia are different in many ways, they do have features in common. For example, autopsies show that some people with Lewy body dementia can have the same hallmark plaques and tangles seen in Alzheimer's disease. On the flip side, it's possible for someone with Alzheimer's disease to have Lewy bodies in the brain but not have any symptoms of Lewy body dementia.

About half of people with Lewy body dementia also have Alzheimer's disease. In people who have both, those with fewer tangles in the brain tend to mostly have symptoms of Lewy body dementia. Those with more tangles have symptoms closer to those of Alzheimer's disease.

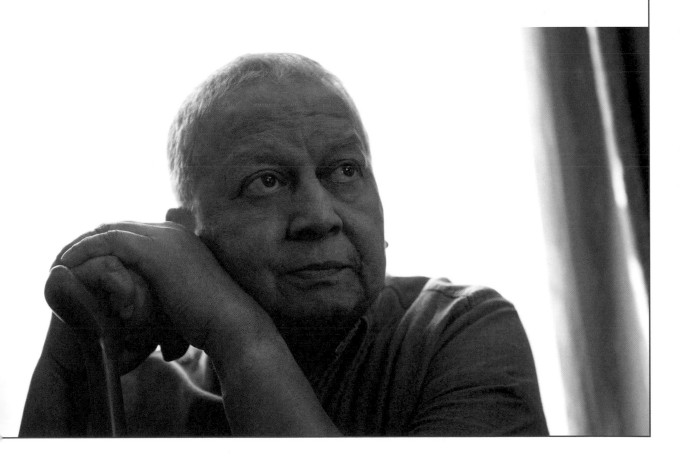

Medications

Before reading on, it's worth repeating that an accurate Lewy body dementia diagnosis is needed, ideally from a doctor experienced in treating this type of dementia. It's important, in part, because some dementia medications can make Lewy body dementia symptoms worse. Plus, with some drugs, dosages must be adjusted and side effects balanced often for optimal benefit.

With this said, medications are often needed to manage symptoms. Although no medications are approved by the Food and Drug Administration specifically for Lewy body dementia, medications can help manage the symptoms it often causes, like sleep disorders and low blood pressure. In this way, medications can improve quality of life.

The following is a review of the most troubling symptoms of Lewy body dementia and the medications used to relieve them.

Thinking issues (cognitive impairment)
In Lewy body dementia, cognitive impairment can cause:

- Slowed thinking, including taking longer to come up with words or ideas
- Feelings of getting distracted easily or losing a train of thought
- Trouble with visual tasks like putting things together, matching or lining things up, or organizing things visually
- Issues with planning and managing time

The first step in managing these symptoms is to stop taking medications that may be causing them or making them worse. Medications with anticholinergic side effects are one example. These drugs can make cognitive impairment, confusion and hallucinations worse.

As you learned earlier, Lewy body dementia causes a sharp drop in the level of acetylcholine, a brain chemical that's important for attention and concentration, judgment, thinking, and memory. Taking drugs with anticholinergic side effects lowers the level of acetylcholine even further, making symptoms of cognitive impairment much worse.

You'll find drugs with anticholinergic side effects available over-the-counter and by prescription. They're used for allergies, ulcers, muscle spasms, asthma, incontinence and tremors.

Cholinesterase inhibitors, on the other hand, *boost* the level of acetylcholine in the brain. Although cholinesterase inhibitors were originally developed for Alzheimer's disease, some research suggests that they're far more helpful for Lewy body dementia, and the improvements they offer can be dramatic.

Cholinesterase inhibitors can help improve alertness and thinking and may make hallucinations and other behavioral issues like apathy less severe and less frequent.

Sometimes people who take cholinesterase inhibitors have temporary side effects, including nausea, diarrhea, urinating more often and vivid dreams when they're taken

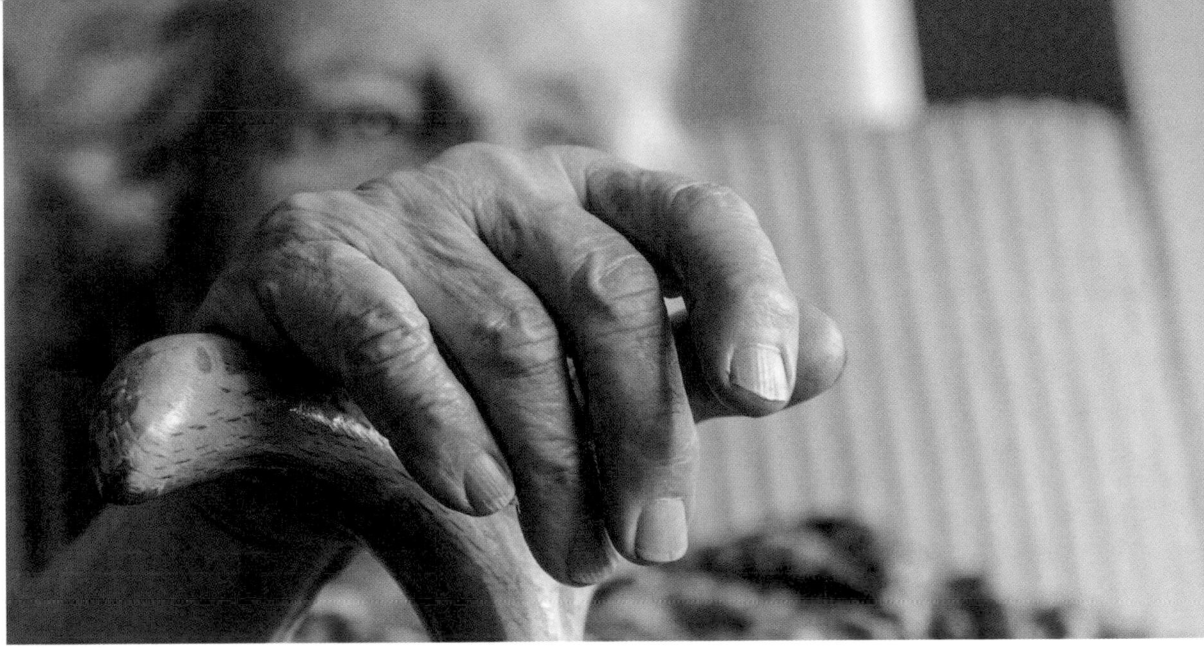

at night. Some people with certain heart issues shouldn't take these drugs because they can cause a heart rhythm problem.

Another medication sometimes used for thinking issues is memantine (Namenda), an N-methyl-d-aspartate (NMDA)-receptor antagonist. It's thought to help protect brain cells and keep them working longer.

Motor symptoms Lewy body dementia can cause parkinsonism. Symptoms of parkinsonism include slow movements, rigid muscles, a shuffling gait, stooped posture, reduced facial expression, trouble speaking loudly and trouble with fine motor skills. Tremors are also sometimes a symptom.

Often, parkinsonism is so mild that there's no need to treat it with medication. Instead, exercise and activity may be enough to keep the muscles strong and limber. But if symptoms interfere with daily activities, medication may help. When medications are used to treat these symptoms in Lewy body dementia, their use must be monitored closely.

The first medication used to treat parkinsonism is carbidopa-levodopa. It helps with rigid muscles and slow movement, sometimes helps tremors, and can make it easier to walk, get out of bed and move around.

Many people with Lewy body dementia have found carbidopa-levodopa helpful. It doesn't cause side effects for most people, but it's important to start with a low dose first and then increase the dose gradually over time. Side effects may include lightheadedness, low blood pressure and nausea, and it may turn urine a dark color.

In some individuals, this medicine may cause or worsen hallucinations, though this usually happens when high doses are taken. To reduce the risk of making hallucinations worse, doctors often prescribe cholinesterase inhibitors first.

Dopamine agonists should not be used in dementia with Lewy bodies. They can make thinking problems worse and are more likely than carbidopa-levodopa to cause hallucinations and delusions.

Another medicine used to treat tremors is amantadine. An anticholinergic medication, this drug can worsen cognitive impairment and cause confusion, hallucinations and delusions in Lewy body dementia.

Neuropsychiatric symptoms False beliefs that a person thinks are real (delusions), seeing things that aren't real (visual hallucinations), agitation, aggression, and Capgras syndrome, which causes a person to believe that someone has been replaced by an imposter, are all neuropsychiatric symptoms of Lewy body dementia. Depression and anxiety also fall in this category.

Sometimes, visual hallucinations don't need to be treated with medication — especially when they don't cause distress. It's not necessary to convince the person that what he or she is seeing isn't there. Instead, acknowledging the image, validating the person's feelings, expressing understanding, asking about the image and providing a response that makes sense to the person ("He'll be gone soon") is often all that's needed.

Keep in mind that your response to the images — and your efforts to convince your loved one that the images aren't real — may cause the person distress.

The main reason to treat visual hallucinations is when the images cause the person experiencing them tremendous distress. If hallucinations interfere with daily living, for example, medication may be helpful.

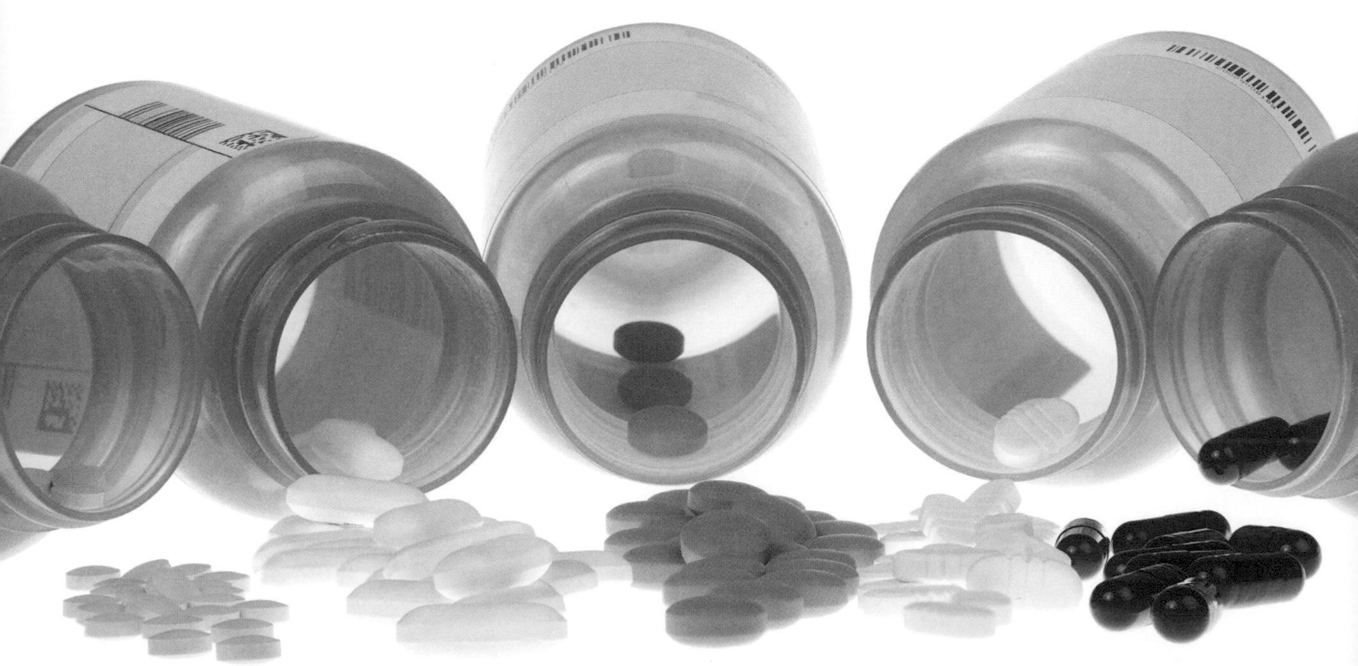

Cholinesterase inhibitors are the first choice for managing hallucinations and delusions. These drugs can make hallucinations less frequent and less intense.

Atypical antipsychotic drugs are rarely prescribed and only when they're absolutely needed. In these cases, a low dose of quetiapine (Seroquel) may be an option. As doses of this medication increase, it can cause tiredness, confusion and falls. Higher doses may also worsen the symptoms it's being used to treat. If this drug is used after a careful discussion of its risks, benefits and alternatives, it should be used at the lowest dose necessary, for the shortest time possible.

Pimavanserin, an antipsychotic drug that's FDA-approved to treat Parkinson's disease psychosis, is being researched as a treatment for dementia-related psychosis. It may be an option in the future.

These drugs must be used with extreme caution; they can cause serious side effects in as many as half of the people who take them for this type of dementia. Older adults with dementia who take these drugs have a higher risk of strokes and death. The Food and Drug Administration requires these medications to carry a black box warning label about these risks, as well as a reminder that they're not approved for treating dementia symptoms.

Atypical antipsychotic drugs like haloperidol (Haldol) and thioridazine and newer dopamine-blocking drugs can cause severe reactions that can lead to severe parkinsonism, involuntary movements, a permanent loss of some motor skills and even death. The risk of death is higher with these medications; they should never be used in dementia with Lewy bodies.

Bottom line: older antipsychotics and dopamine-blocking agents should never be used to treat symptoms of Lewy body dementia.

Side effects may include sudden changes in consciousness, trouble swallowing, confusion that comes on quickly, paranoia, seeing things that aren't real, extreme sleepiness, fainting caused by low blood pressure, new or worsening parkinsonism, and involuntary movements of the hands, feet and mouth.

Depression and anxiety can be treated with selective serotonin reuptake inhibitors, the most commonly prescribed antidepressants, or bupropion (Wellbutrin SR, Wellbutrin XL, others).

SSRIs are more helpful than tricyclic antidepressants. Acetylcholine, you'll recall, is a chemical that's important for judgment, thinking and memory, and it's already lower in people with dementia. Tricyclic antidepressants reduce the level of this chemical even more, which can make cognitive issues worse and may cause confusion, hallucinations and delusions.

Sleep issues Rapid eye movement sleep behavior disorder, which causes people to physically act out dreams while they're sleeping, is a common sleep issue in Lewy

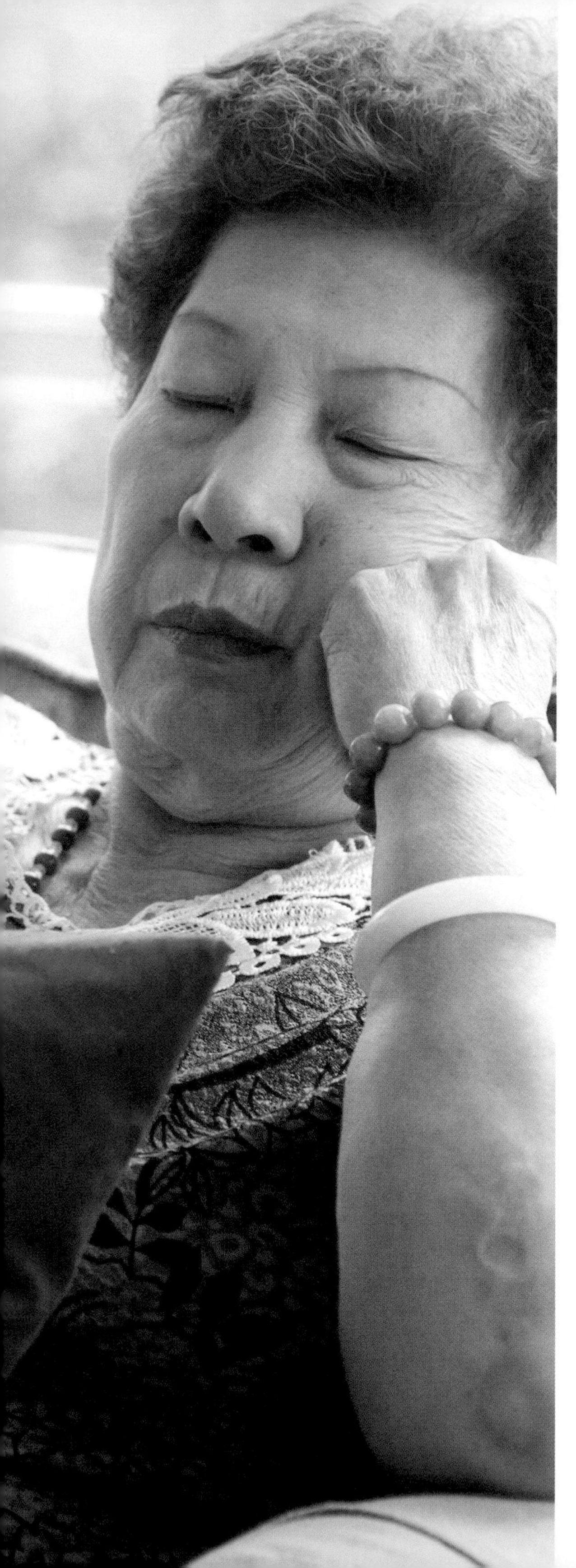

body dementia. Excessive daytime sleepiness and obstructive sleep apnea are also common sleep-related symptoms.

Because obstructive sleep apnea is common in Lewy body dementia, it's usually treated first. From there, several medications can treat other sleep-related symptoms.

Melatonin is usually the first medical treatment used for rapid eye movement sleep behavior disorder if nonmedication treatments don't help.

If melatonin doesn't help, a low dose of clonazepam (Klonopin) may be prescribed. This drug is commonly used for anxiety, panic attacks and seizures. Clonazepam is the only prescription drug known to improve symptoms of rapid eye movement sleep behavior disorder. A very low dose can help reduce vigorous movements. This drug is also sometimes used to treat restless legs syndrome. Clonazepam can cause daytime sleepiness, either on its own or because it worsens sleep apnea at night. For some, it may also increase the risk of falls, so it should be used with caution.

After other causes for excessive daytime sleepiness are ruled out, drugs that promote wakefulness may be used. Modafinil (Provigil) or armodafinil (Nuvigil) are usually used first. Unlike older stimulants, they don't produce extreme highs and lows, and they don't cause problems with insomnia or appetite. Side effects are uncommon but may include headaches, nausea or anxiety. Some people use stimulants like methyl-

MEDICATIONS TO AVOID

Before starting any medication, it's important to talk with a doctor about possible side effects.

These drugs, for example, can cause extreme sleepiness, problems with motor skills and confusion:

- Benzodiazepines, like diazepam (Valium) and lorazepam (Ativan), which are used to relax muscles.
- Anticholinergics, which include anti-nausea drugs like cimetidine (Tagamet HB), drugs used to treat ulcers (antispasmodics), some types of bladder medications like oxybutynin (Ditropan XL, Oxytrol), tricyclic antidepressants, heartburn medications like metoclopramide, drugs like benztropine (Cogentin) and amantadine that are used to treat tremors, and glycopyrrolate (Cuvposa, others), which is used to treat ulcers and drooling.
- Certain over-the-counter drugs with anticholinergic effects, like the antihistamine diphenhydramine (Benadryl) and dimenhydrinate (Dramamine), used for motion sickness.
- Atypical antipsychotic drugs like haloperidol (Haldol) and thioridazine and newer dopamine-blocking drugs. As you learned earlier, these drugs can cause severe side effects, including worsening thinking problems, confusion, and an increase in parkinsonism symptoms that may be irreversible, and may even cause death.

It's always best to keep a doctor informed about medications being taken, both over-the-counter and prescription, as well as supplements. Keeping an eye on side effects is also important. All of this information helps ensure that the best combination of drugs is being used at the appropriate doses.

phenidate (Aptensio XR, Concerta, Ritalin, others) to help with daytime alertness. Side effects include reduced appetite, insomnia, and a fluttering or rapid heart rate.

Autonomic dysfunction Lewy body dementia can cause problems with processes that the body regulates on its own (autonomic dysfunction), including sweating, heart rate, blood pressure and body temperature. Symptoms may include low blood pressure, urinary incontinence and constipation. Drugs aren't often used to treat these symptoms, but they can be managed with several strategies.

Some people experience a drop in blood pressure upon standing after sitting or lying down (orthostatic hypotension). It can make a person feel dizzy or lightheaded or even faint. Lifestyle changes like drinking enough water, not drinking alcohol, elevating the head of the bed and standing up slowly can all help. A doctor may also suggest taking in more salt if a person doesn't have high blood pressure. Compression stockings and garments and binders worn over the stomach also may help.

A dysfunction in the part of the brain that controls the muscles involved in urination can lead to urinary incontinence. This is the inability to hold urine. Avoiding medications that block acetylcholine can help improve this symptom. Constipation, a related symptom, can be addressed by increasing fiber intake. Fiber supplements like psyllium (Metamucil, Konsyl, others) can also help. Polyethylene glycol also can be effective. Sometimes stronger forms of therapy are needed to reduce constipation.

If nondrug options aren't helpful, medications may be used.

Future drug therapies Many drugs are in development. Learn more by visiting *www.clinicaltrials.gov.* Use search terms like *Lewy, Lewy body dementia* and *alpha-synuclein*.

Options outside of medication

Many strategies that don't involve medication can improve quality of life for someone living with Lewy body dementia. They include various types of therapy and changes

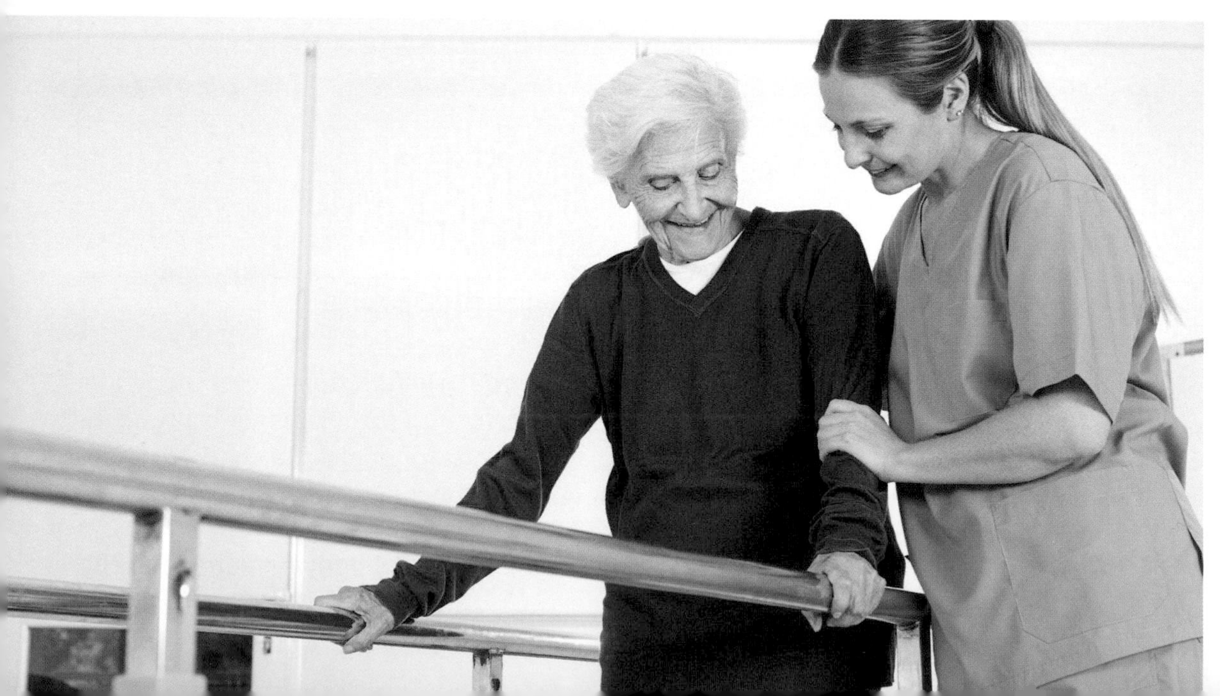

that can be made at home, both in the physical environment and in terms of lifestyle approaches.

Occupational therapy Occupational therapy helps improve quality of life by helping with daily skills and promoting function and independence. Occupational therapy teaches easier ways to carry out everyday activities, like eating, dressing, using the bathroom and walking safely. People living with dementia, as well as their care partners, are encouraged to take part in occupational therapy sessions.

Physical therapy A physical therapist can help address movement issues through exercise and training. Aerobic physical activity, strength training and water exercise may all be included in a general fitness program as part of physical therapy.

Speech therapy Someone who speaks softly or has trouble saying words may benefit from speech therapy. It can also help with swallowing difficulties.

Integrative medicine The practice of using conventional medicine alongside evidence-based complementary treatments is known as integrative medicine. Many integrative therapies have been shown to help with symptoms of Lewy body dementia.

For example, frustration and anxiety can worsen dementia symptoms. Several therapies have been shown to help by promoting relaxation. They include music therapy, which involves listening to music, as well as playing music and singing. Art therapy, shown to reduce anxiety and improve well-being, offers opportunities for creativity using many different mediums. Interacting with animals through pet therapy can improve mood and behavior in people living with dementia. And aromatherapy, which uses scents from fragrant plant oils, can lessen anxiety and improve mood.

Counseling Licensed mental health professionals can help people living with Lewy body dementia and their care partners work through challenging emotions and address changes and behaviors. They can also help with planning for the future.

Palliative care This type of therapy focuses on relief from pain and other symptoms of a serious illness. It's different from hospice care, which is used at the end of life and doesn't use medications meant to prolong life.

Palliative care can be used at any time during the course of dementia. It can also be given alongside other treatments and can improve quality of life for people living with dementia and their care partners. Using a whole-person approach, palliative care centers around relieving symptoms, offering support and advice for care partners, and teaching techniques that help provide comfort.

Changing the environment Hallucinations, stress, anxiety, fear and frustration can cause someone with Lewy body dementia to lash out verbally or physically.

Making changes to the living environment can help with these feelings and the behavior issues they may cause. Simple tasks, a regular routine and lighting that's not overly stimulating can all help. Reducing clutter, avoiding large crowds and keeping noise levels low are also helpful strategies.

Lifestyle interventions In addition to making changes to the environment, care partners can help someone living with Lewy body dementia by:

Offering reassurance. Correcting and quizzing someone with dementia may make behaviors worse.

Speaking clearly and simply. Maintain eye contact and speak slowly. Speak in simple sentences, and don't rush a response. Offer just one idea or instruction at a time. Gestures and cues, like pointing to objects, can also help.

Encouraging exercise. Exercise can help improve physical function, as well as behavior and depression symptoms.

Stimulating the mind. Games, staying engaged socially and activities that encourage thinking may help slow mental decline.

Establishing a nighttime ritual. A calming bedtime ritual can help with behavior issues, which may worsen at night.

Eliminate the distraction of television, meal cleanup and active family members. Leave nightlights on to help someone with dementia feel less disoriented. Limit caffeine during the day and discourage daytime naps to help with nighttime restlessness.

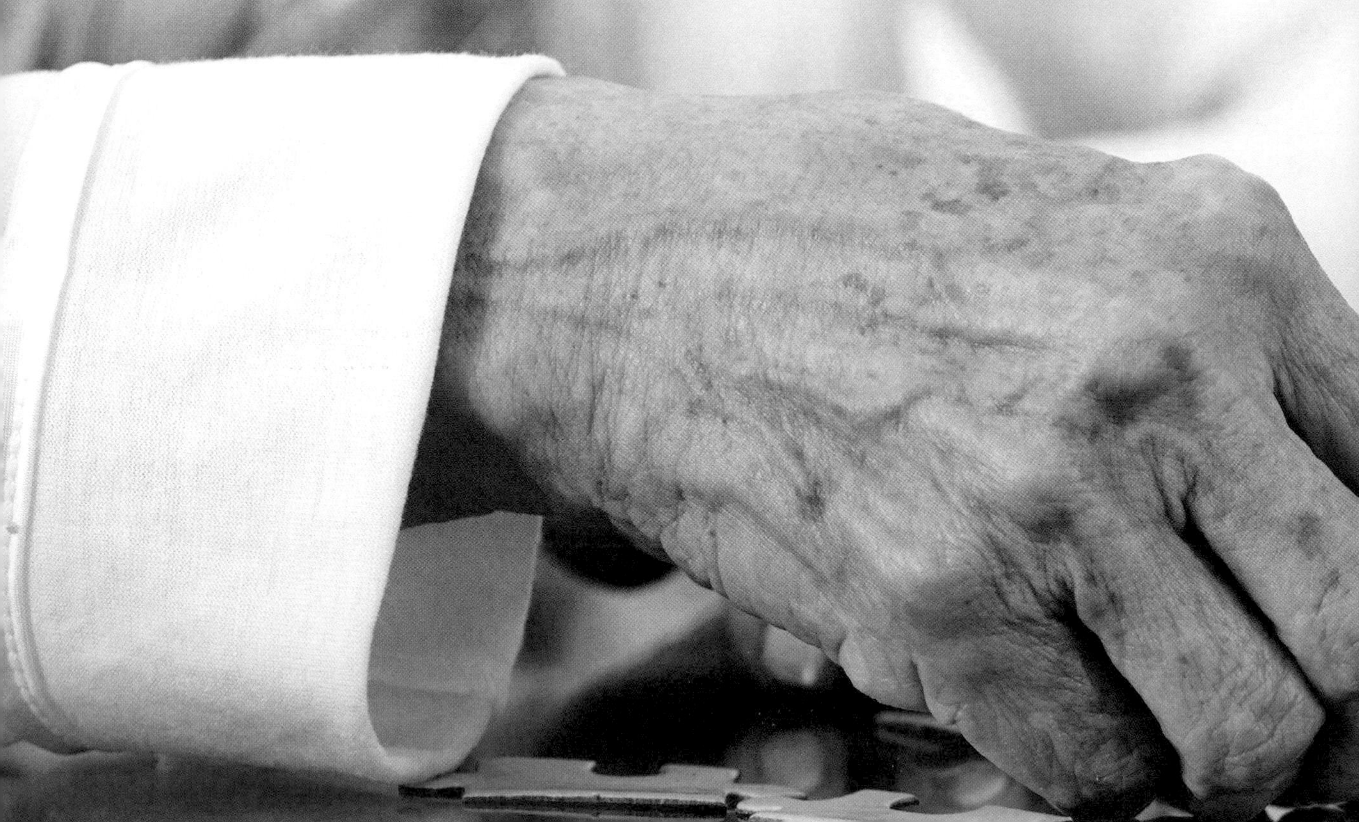

There are ways to address some of the more specific issues that come up with Lewy body dementia, too. For example, to decrease risk of injury from nighttime concerns, such as rapid eye movement sleep behavior disorder, consider moving lamps, nightstands and other furniture away from the bed and placing padding or cushions on the floor beside the bed, in case of a fall. If a bed partner is at risk, sleeping in separate beds should be considered.

Rearranging the dosing periods of drugs known to cause insomnia, like cholinesterase inhibitors, also may help improve sleep.

OPTIMIZING WELL-BEING

Although well-being means something different for every individual, people with Lewy body dementia may experience some of the same struggles — and likewise, have similar opportunities — for well-being.

But people living with Lewy body dementia can't achieve well-being on their own. Support from family, friends, health care professionals and society in general all play a role. While people with Lewy body dementia recognize that there will be a time when they'll need more help and support from others, surveys of people with this type of dementia emphasize the need for support that's given respectfully and at a level that helps them maintain their highest level of functioning and sense of self.

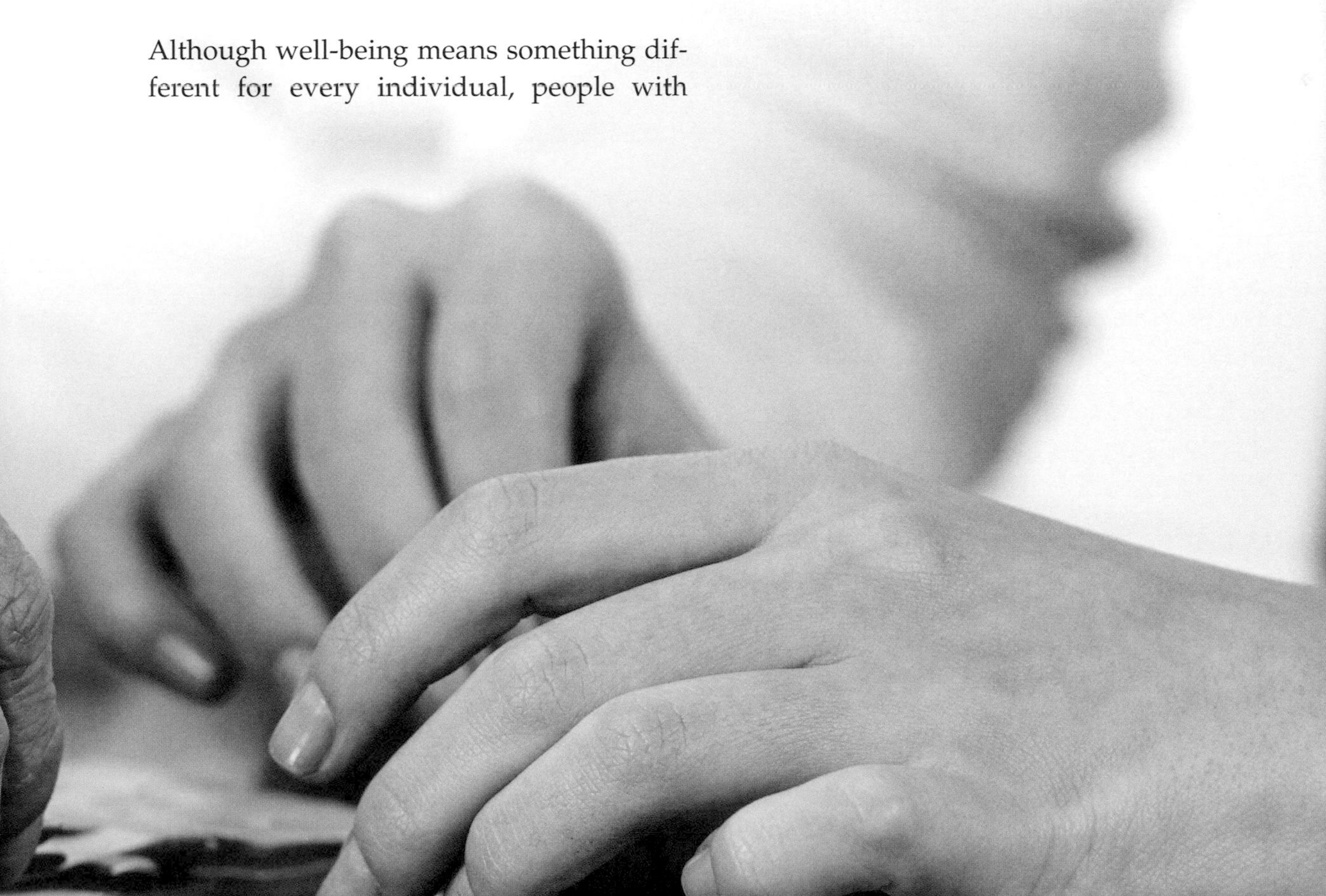

"MUCH CAN BE DONE TO NOT JUST KEEP VASCULAR COGNITIVE IMPAIRMENT FROM PROGRESSING BUT ALSO PREVENT IT FROM HAPPENING AT ALL."

CHAPTER 11

Vascular cognitive impairment

Vascular cognitive impairment stands out from many other conditions associated with dementia, including Alzheimer's disease, because its cause is relatively well understood. The condition stems from chronic damage to the complex network of blood vessels that supply the brain with the nutrients it needs to function.

When blood flow in the brain is disrupted or blocked, not enough nutrients, like oxygen and glucose, reach brain cells. In turn, the cells in the brain get damaged or die.

From there, areas of damaged or dead cells called infarcts form permanent scar tissue and aren't replaced by new cells. Infarcts can cause problems with reason, judgment, memory, personality, emotions and other cognitive functions, depending on the location and extent of the damage in the brain.

Vascular cognitive impairment used to be called vascular dementia. The name change reflects the fact that vascular disease can cause milder forms of cognitive impairment that don't necessarily meet the strict criteria for dementia.

Your risk of vascular cognitive impairment is linked to the health of your blood vessels. Conditions like high blood pressure and changes to the blood vessels, like atherosclerosis, increase your risk. Factors that increase your risk of heart disease and stroke — including diabetes mellitus and cigarette smoking — also raise your risk of vascular cognitive impairment.

The good news is that you can take steps to reduce all of these risks and prevent further damage if symptoms of vascular cognitive impairment start to appear.

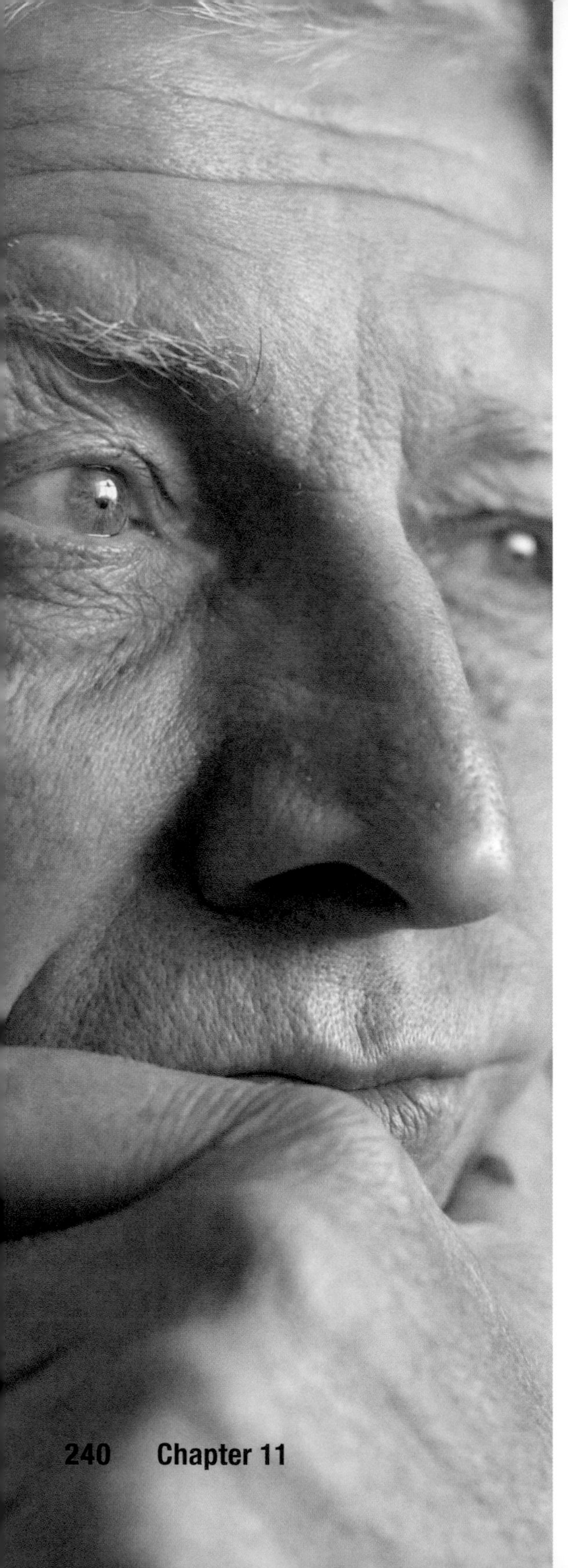

YOUR BRAIN'S VASCULAR SYSTEM

As the operational control center for your entire body, your brain requires a lot of blood — almost a quarter of the blood your heart pumps out. Two main arteries (carotid arteries) and two smaller arteries that run along the vertebrae of your neck (vertebral arteries) meet up at the base of your brain. From there, a network of smaller blood vessels reaches deep inside brain tissue. Any interruption in the blood supply deprives brain cells of essential nutrients, like oxygen and glucose. Without these nutrients, the cells get damaged quickly or die.

When the blood supply to the brain is blocked or reduced, a stroke is a common result. Stroke may occur if a blood clot keeps blood from flowing through an artery or if an artery leaks or ruptures, bleeding into surrounding tissue. This disruption of normal blood flow — even for a few seconds — can dramatically affect brain function.

Most people think of stroke as a major event that instantly causes severe problems with movement and speech. A stroke like this is a medical emergency. It can permanently damage structures in the brain needed for thinking and other functions, and it can lead to vascular cognitive impairment. In cases like these, the right treatment can only be given within a narrow time frame.

But strokes may also occur on a milder or silent level. In these cases, a stroke may cause minimal symptoms — or no symptoms at all. A series of these minor strokes

STROKE AND VASCULAR COGNITIVE IMPAIRMENT

Vascular cognitive impairment commonly occurs in people who've had a major stroke. According to some estimates, between 20% and 30% of people who've had a stroke go on to develop cognitive impairment, usually within several months of the event. One study found that having a stroke doubles a person's risk of dementia.

At the same time, not all strokes lead to vascular cognitive impairment. Although stroke can cause confusion, memory loss, and trouble with language and perception, these effects are typically severe immediately after a stroke but then gradually improve with time. This temporary impairment isn't the same thing as having vascular cognitive impairment — in which the signs and symptoms of dementia get worse over time, never better.

may damage enough brain cells over time to cause cognitive impairment.

In addition, if vascular disease causes the small blood vessels throughout the brain to weaken and narrow, it may reduce blood supply. Reduced blood supply may damage or destroy tissue, even if the blood vessels aren't completely blocked or ruptured.

Years ago, doctors believed that most often dementia was caused by diseased arteries in the brain. However, researchers now see it differently. Research now suggests that neurodegenerative conditions like Alzheimer's are the primary causes of dementia, and they're a result of many factors, not just problems with blood vessels.

For a number of reasons, it's hard to say how many people vascular cognitive impairment affects. For one, the term *vascular cognitive impairment* includes vascular dementia as well as milder forms of cognitive impairment. In addition, symptoms of vascular cognitive impairment often overlap with other causes of dementia, especially Alzheimer's disease. Plus, vascular cognitive impairment and Alzheimer's disease often occur together, so diagnosing one may not rule out the other.

For all of these reasons, it's hard to say how many people are affected by vascular cognitive impairment. Estimates show that vascular cognitive impairment affects at least 1 in 5 people with dementia.

HIGH BLOOD PRESSURE AND DEMENTIA: THE SPRINT STUDIES

High blood pressure increases the risk of stroke, and a stroke increases the risk of dementia. This makes lowering blood pressure and then controlling it an important part of treating — and preventing — vascular dementia. The key question is this: What blood pressure target should you aim for?

In 2010, researchers set out to answer this question when they launched the Systolic Blood Pressure Intervention Trial (SPRINT) study. The goal was to see how well lowering systolic blood pressure to 120 millimeters of mercury (mm Hg) could prevent heart and kidney disease as well as a decline in thinking skills. Systolic pressure is the top number in your blood pressure reading.

More than 9,000 adults age 50 or older took part in the trial; participants had a systolic blood pressure of 130 mm Hg or higher and at least one other risk factor for heart disease when they entered the trial. Participants took medication to lower blood pressure to one of two targets, based on the flip of a coin. Researchers found that reaching the lower blood pressure target reduced the risk of heart disease — including stroke — by nearly a third. It also reduced the risk of death from heart disease by nearly 25%. In short, this research showed that a lower blood pressure can save lives.

An offshoot of this study, known as SPRINT MIND, focused on how well this lower blood pressure target could reduce the risk of mild cognitive impairment and dementia. The results of this study showed that reducing blood pressure to the lower target was helpful; there were fewer cases of mild cognitive impairment among participants who reached the lower target.

When these studies were done, a systolic blood pressure of less than 140 mm Hg was considered acceptable. Since then, guidelines have been revised, and national recommendations are now in line with what researchers learned in these two studies. Now, a systolic blood pressure of 140 mm Hg or higher is described as stage 2 high blood pressure, and a systolic blood pressure of 120 mm Hg or lower is the desired target.

CAUSES

Vascular cognitive impairment can have several causes. Here's more on each one.

A single stroke

When a stroke blocks a brain artery, it can cause a number of symptoms, including dementia. Dementia can come on suddenly if a key part of the brain important for cognition, like a memory hub, is affected by a stroke.

For example, a small stroke that affects the thalamus — a relay station of the brain — can interrupt the brain's memory network and lead to sudden memory problems. Many studies show a link between stroke and the development of dementia. Dementia is nine times more likely after a stroke than it is in those who haven't had a stroke.

Silent strokes and ministrokes

Some strokes don't cause any noticeable symptoms. These so-called silent strokes (silent infarcts), seen in brain imaging, also increase the risk of dementia. They contribute to cognitive issues before dementia can be diagnosed.

A so-called ministroke, known as a transient ischemic attack (TIA), also can increase the risk of vascular dementia. This type of stroke resolves on its own without any noticeable symptoms or issues. About a third of people who have a TIA go on to have a full-blown stroke at some point. The risk of stroke is especially high within 48 hours after a TIA. This is why TIAs must be treated like a stroke, as a medical emergency.

Multiple strokes

The risk of vascular dementia increases with the number of strokes that occur over time. One type of vascular cognitive impairment that involves several strokes is called multi-infarct dementia. You'll recall from earlier in this chapter that an infarct is an area of damaged or dead cells. This area isn't filled in with new cell growth. Infarcts can cause a variety of problems depending on where they're located in the brain.

Having several minor strokes can affect smaller blood vessels. In turn, these minor strokes cause thinking problems that start out mild but worsen as more strokes and other conditions cause damage to the blood vessels in the brain.

Narrowed or damaged blood vessels

Damage to the brain's blood vessels can lead to vascular dementia. Widespread damage from narrowed vessels and reduced blood flow leads to a slow, subtle onset of cognitive impairment.

This damage increases with age and is made worse by conditions like high blood pressure and diabetes.

Combined Alzheimer's disease and vascular cognitive impairment

Many people with Alzheimer's disease dementia also have a disease that affects the blood vessels in the brain (cerebrovascular disease). In fact, researchers have learned that most people with dementia have more than one cause of the disease, and Alzheimer's disease with vascular disease seems to be the most common combination. One study of autopsies in those with dementia found that more than a third had Alzheimer's disease *and* vascular disease.

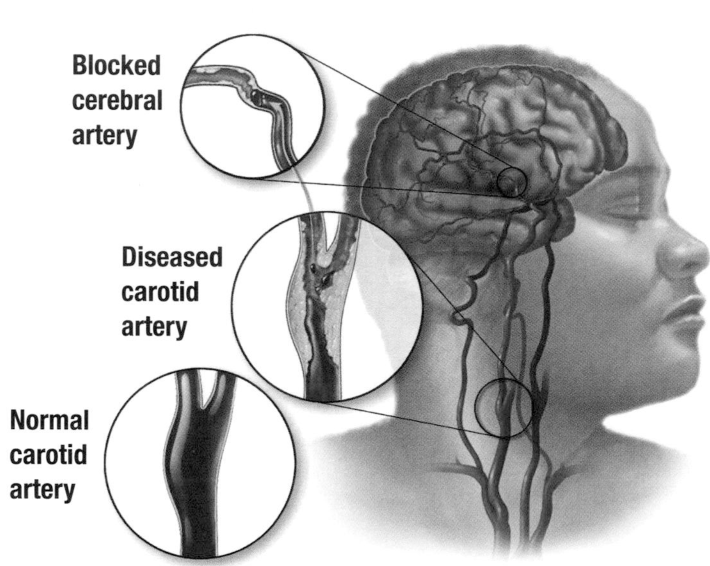

HOW A BLOOD CLOT CAN LEAD TO A STROKE

The formation of a blood clot in one of the carotid arteries of the neck may set the stage for a stroke. If the blood clot breaks free, it will travel through the vascular system and may become lodged in an artery of the cerebrum, blocking blood flow and causing a stroke.

Bleeding in the brain (hemorrhagic stroke) also can cause dementia. This type of stroke is caused by the rupture of a blood vessel in or on the brain's surface, causing bleeding into the surrounding tissue.

CAN LIFESTYLE HABITS HELP?

You're already learning how lifestyle choices and healthy habits can help with managing symptoms of dementia. But these habits can do even more. Later on, you'll learn how they can help your brain age well — and maybe even prevent dementia altogether. For now, here's a sneak peek at what's known about lifestyle habits and their potential to prevent cognitive decline, especially as it relates to the risk factors that can lead to vascular dementia.

For two years, researchers followed more than 600 people between ages 60 and 77 with a high risk of dementia as part of the Finnish Geriatric Intervention Study to Prevent Cognitive Impairment and Disability (FINGER). Participants were randomly put into one of two groups. The first group received general health advice, while the second group followed a program of diet, exercise, cognitive training, and monitoring of blood pressure and other heart disease risk factors. People in the second group also had about 200 meetings with health professionals and trainers during the two years of the study.

People in the second group improved in how quickly they processed information. They also improved their executive function — how well they could organize tasks, think abstractly, manage time and solve problems. People in the first group who only received general health advice didn't show the same improvements.

Researchers think that when they're used together, these habits have the potential to enhance thinking ability in people who are at risk of dementia, keeping these skills sharp and possibly preventing dementia from developing.

More research is underway to determine how well lifestyle habits can protect against dementia. One example is the U.S. Study to Protect Brain Health Through Lifestyle Intervention to Reduce Risk (U.S. POINTER). This research is focused on how well lifestyle changes like exercise, diet and cognitively stimulating activities can protect memory and thinking in adults between ages 60 and 79 who have a higher risk of significant memory loss. Another initiative known as World Wide FINGERS (WW-FINGERS) is aligning these efforts around the world.

SIGNS AND SYMPTOMS

Symptoms of vascular cognitive impairment can vary widely. What causes it, how severe it is and what parts of the brain are affected all play a role in what symptoms it may cause.

Common signs and symptoms include:

- Confusion
- Trouble paying attention and concentrating
- Reduced ability to organize thoughts or actions
- Decline in ability to analyze a situation, develop an effective plan and communicate that plan to others
- Difficulty deciding what to do next
- Problems with memory
- Restlessness and agitation
- Unsteady gait
- Sudden or frequent urge to urinate or inability to control passing urine
- Depression or apathy

It may be easiest to spot vascular cognitive impairment right after a stroke. Changes in thinking and reasoning that seem to be linked to a stroke and are severe enough to result in dementia are sometimes described as post-stroke dementia.

Sometimes a pattern of decline follows a series of strokes or ministrokes. After one stroke occurs, thinking skills decline and then stay steady for a while until another stroke happens. Then thinking skills decline again. This is different from the steady decline seen in Alzheimer's disease.

Because the symptoms that appear and how severe they are depend on the parts of the brain that are affected, some thinking abilities may become impaired while others stay the same. For example, you may have trouble following instructions or calculating numbers and know that this is a challenge for you. Being aware of an impairment like this can be frustrating and lead to depression — a condition that often accompanies vascular cognitive impairment. In turn, depression can make vascular cognitive impairment worse.

Compared with those in the early stages of Alzheimer's disease, people in the early stages of vascular cognitive impairment may experience greater physical disability and problems with movement. In general, people with Alzheimer's live longer than do those with vascular cognitive impairment, who are more likely to die of heart disease or stroke.

Sometimes, vascular cognitive impairment progresses in a fashion similar to that of Alzheimer's disease, with a slow but steady rather than a steplike decline in cognitive and, eventually, physical functions.

DIAGNOSIS

Vascular cognitive impairment is diagnosed in much the same way other forms of dementia are. A doctor will likely:

- Review your medical history, especially as it relates to any history of stroke or problems with the heart or blood vessels

PERSONAL STORY

JEAN'S STORY

Jean, an independent-minded, 80-year-old woman living on her own, had a stroke. Based on the location of the damage from the stroke, which could be seen on a CT scan, the stroke appeared to have affected the occipital lobe of her brain, which is mostly responsible for vision. Although Jean's symptoms improved right after the stroke, her son noticed that she wasn't as able to think clearly or take care of herself.

A year after her stroke, Jean could dress and feed herself but needed help with most other activities of daily living, including bathing. She could no longer drive, pay bills or do household chores. She also became increasingly quiet and withdrawn. Although she could write and name a few simple items, she lost the ability to read.

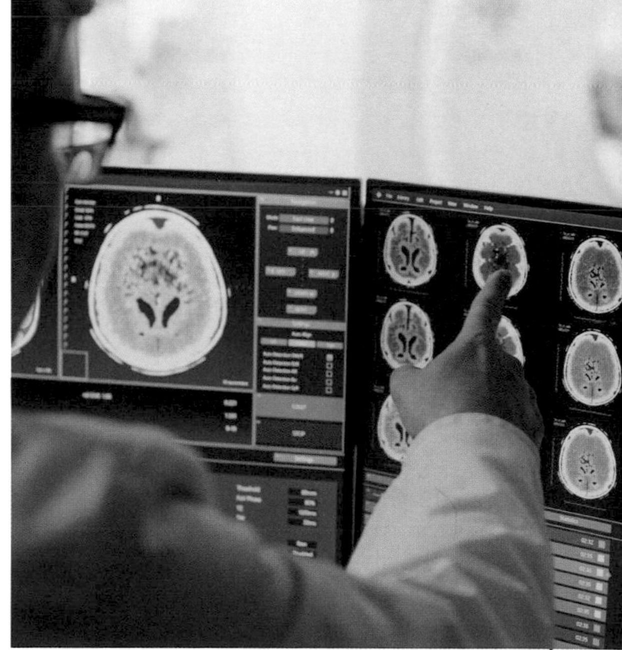

Another imaging test — this time an MRI providing a more detailed picture — showed that the stroke had damaged not only Jean's occipital lobe but also the hippocampus and thalamus. These are parts of the brain important in memory and information processing. This helped explain Jean's symptoms of dementia. Jean's doctor couldn't say for sure if she'd already had cognitive impairment that either contributed to the dementia or was worsened by her stroke.

- Test your blood pressure, cholesterol and blood sugar
- Check for thyroid problems and vitamin deficiencies
- Test your neurological health, including reflexes, muscle tone and strength, ability to walk across a room, coordination, and balance
- Order brain imaging tests to pinpoint areas of damage caused by a stroke, blood vessel disease, tumors or trauma
- Test how well you speak, write and understand language as well as work with numbers, learn and remember information, and solve problems
- Use an ultrasound to look at your carotid arteries, the arteries that run up through either side of your neck to supply blood to the brain

Although different doctors may use different criteria to diagnose symptoms of vascular cognitive impairment, doctors typically look for:

- Cognitive problems that start or get worse within three months of a stroke
- Evidence of one or more strokes or of damage to the small blood vessels in the brain (cerebral small vessel disease) on imaging tests

Telling the difference between vascular cognitive impairment and Alzheimer's disease can be challenging. For example, there may not be a clear connection to a stroke. Symptoms of vascular cognitive impairment can be similar to symptoms of Alzheimer's, and it may be nearly impossible to tell if dementia has a vascular cause. These challenges make brain imaging tests like CT or MRI key to diagnosing vascular cognitive impairment. These tests often provide evidence of stroke even in someone who doesn't show any external signs and symptoms of one.

Vascular cognitive impairment may develop as a result of dead tissue (infarcts) so small that they can't be seen even with brain imaging. Often in these cases, a person is diagnosed with Alzheimer's, and vascular cognitive impairment isn't discovered until an autopsy is done. Since it's possible to have both vascular cognitive impairment and Alzheimer's at the same time, one diagnosis doesn't necessarily rule out the other.

As with other types of dementia, vascular dementia shortens lifespan. But cognitive changes can improve, especially as new patterns of blood flow are established and undamaged cells in the brain take on new functions to compensate for brain cells that are damaged or lost. You'll learn more about helpful strategies for living with vascular dementia next.

TREATING THE DISEASE

Chronic damage to brain tissue can't be reversed, but steps can be taken to reduce the risk of additional damage. Treatment, in this case, is prevention: preventing more strokes by tackling risk factors that you can control, like lowering blood pressure and cholesterol and managing diabetes. Taking these steps can help limit the severity of vascular cognitive impairment, slow its course and prevent further decline.

Although scientists aren't sure about the exact relationship between vascular risk factors and the development of Alzheimer's disease, one appears to be related to the other. Current research suggests that the two problems add to brain damage separately, but some researchers think that vascular risk factors and disease may actually help lead to Alzheimer's disease.

WHAT DAMAGE FROM A STROKE LOOKS LIKE

Sections of dead tissue (infarcts) show up on an MRI as white, clouded areas of the brain. Where an infarct is located in the brain may correlate with a person's signs and symptoms of dementia.

The left image shows damage to the parietal lobe caused by a stroke (red arrow). The parietal lobe processes information about touch and movement. The center image reveals large areas of damage from vascular disease, causing vascular cognitive impairment. The image on the right shows the effects of cerebral small vessel disease (Binswanger's disease), a type of dementia caused by tiny, widespread areas of damage to layers of white matter deep within the brain. These changes are associated with cell damage from atherosclerosis and restricted blood flow in small blood vessels deep within the brain.

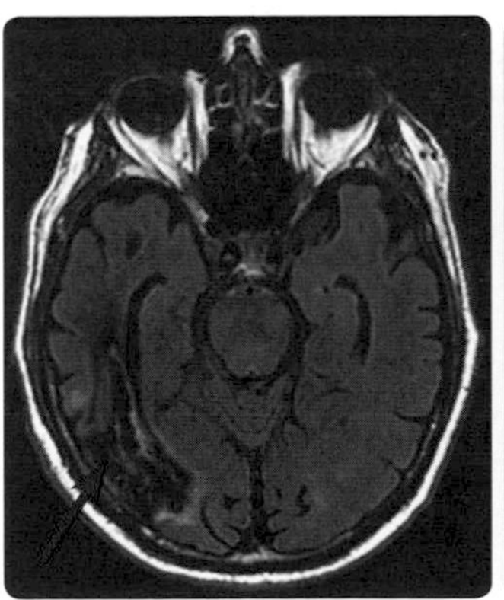

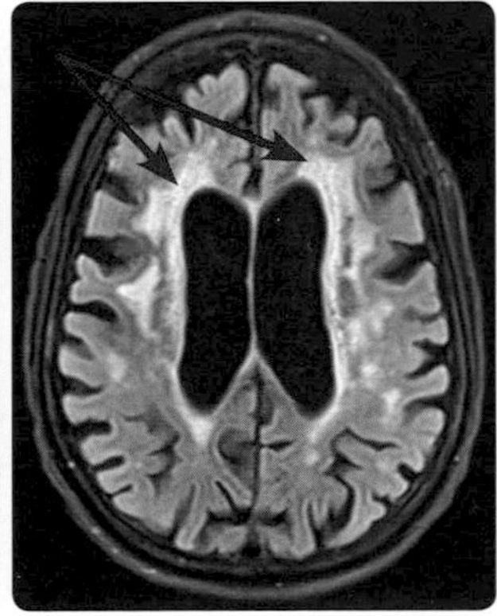

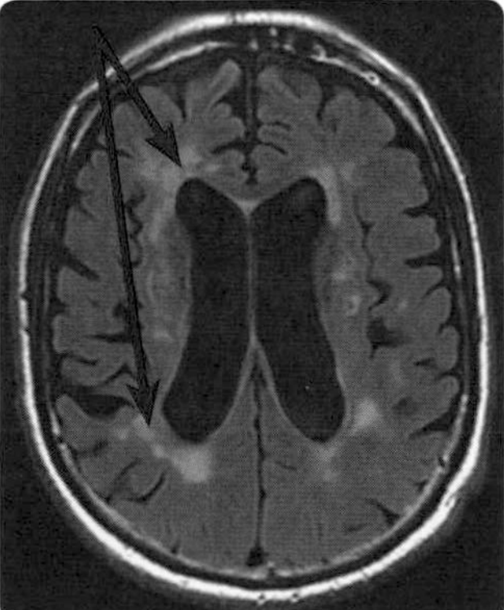

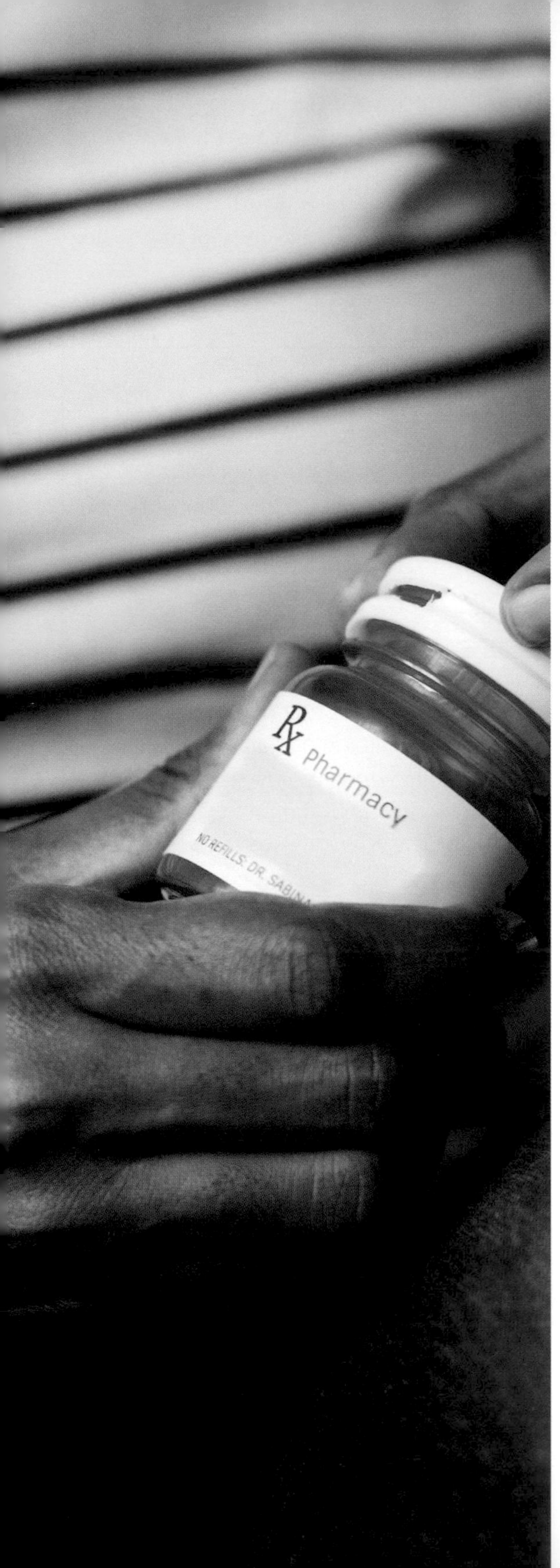

MANAGING SYMPTOMS

Medications and lifestyle interventions can help manage symptoms of vascular cognitive impairment.

Medications

No drug is approved by the FDA to treat vascular dementia specifically. However, cholinesterase inhibitors and memantine may help. You learned earlier that these drugs are used to treat Alzheimer's disease. Cholinesterase inhibitors boost levels of a brain chemical involved in memory and judgment. Memantine regulates the level of a brain chemical involved in memory and learning.

Experts recommend these drugs for people who have vascular dementia, in addition to Alzheimer's disease or dementia with Lewy bodies. But for people who have vascular dementia on its own, these drugs may still help. Some studies, for example, show that cholinesterase inhibitors may mask the symptoms of vascular cognitive impairment and improve thinking and memory. Memantine can help with apathy.

Brief outbursts of uncontrollable laughing or crying (pseudobulbar affect) sometimes seen in vascular dementia may be treated with the combination drug dextromethorphan hydrobromide and quinidine sulfate (Nuedexta). Because anxiety and depression often accompany vascular cognitive impairment, anti-anxiety drugs and antide-

"NO DRUG IS APPROVED BY THE FDA TO TREAT VASCULAR DEMENTIA."

pressants are also sometimes prescribed. Finally, aspirin therapy may be used to prevent future strokes.

Lifestyle interventions

Aside from medications, various types of therapy — physical therapy, occupational therapy and speech therapy, for example — can help people manage symptoms of vascular cognitive impairment.

Many lifestyle choices also can help. For example, managing certain risk factors can help manage symptoms and prevent further damage. Examples include getting regular physical activity, following a healthy diet, reaching and maintaining a healthy weight, engaging socially with others, and participating in brain-stimulating activities.

Experts also recommend managing blood pressure, blood sugar and cholesterol. Taking these steps can help prevent stroke and keep sections of damaged or dead tissue (infarcts) from forming in the brain.

Much can be done to not just keep vascular cognitive impairment from progressing but also prevent it from happening at all. Researchers are finding, more and more, that some of the most common components of a healthy lifestyle — reducing blood pressure, preventing or treating diabetes, lowering cholesterol, adopting a healthy diet, and getting regular physical activity — can keep vascular cognitive impairment from getting worse or starting in the first place.

In turn, adopting healthy-living approaches may also help with preventing other dementias, as you'll learn later on. Because vascular health seems to be tied to the risk of many different types of dementia, taking good care of your blood vessels may help prevent not just vascular cognitive impairment but also dementia in general.

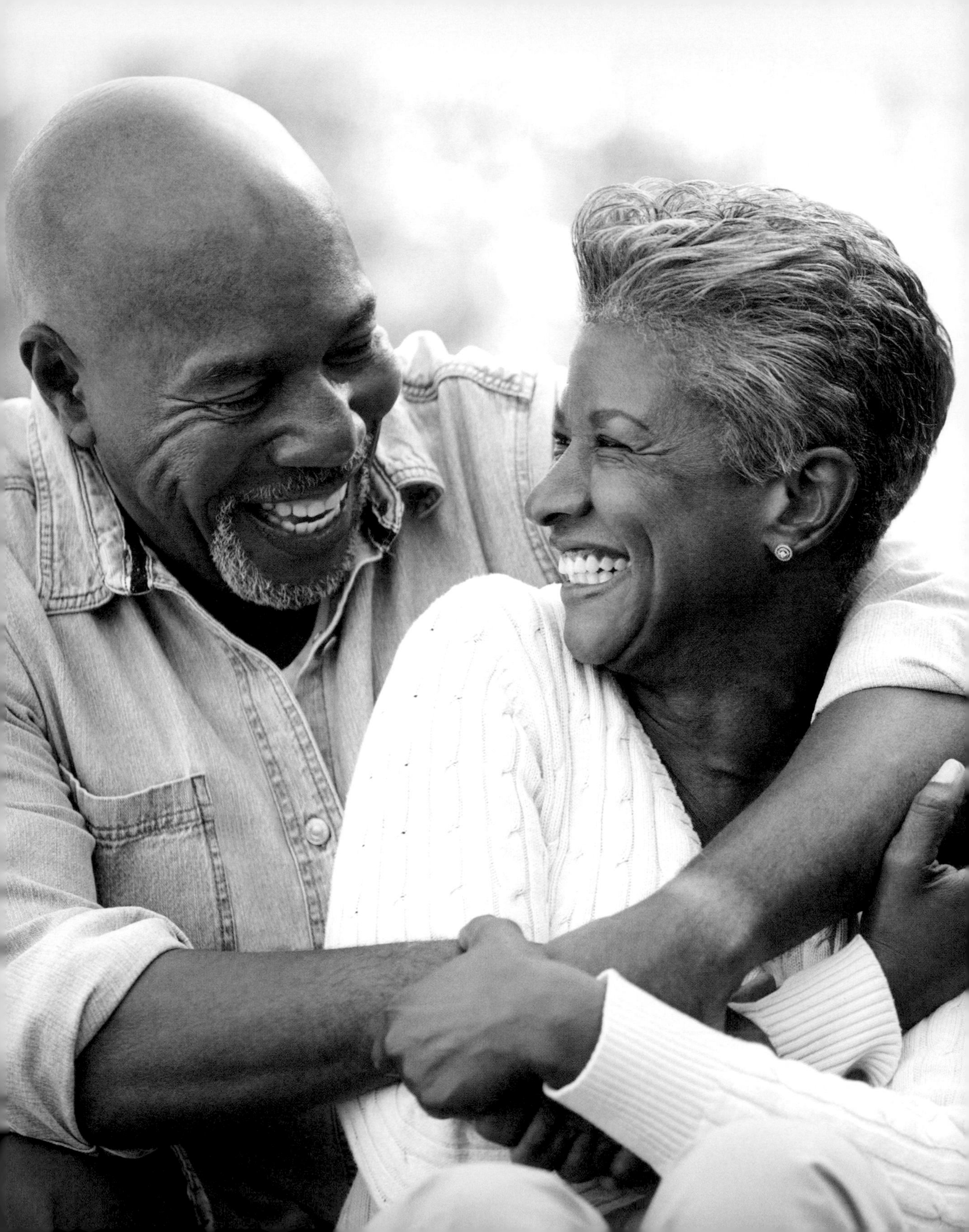

PART 4

Living a full life with dementia

MIKE'S STORY: 'GET BUSY LIVING OR GET BUSY DYING'

Editor's note: At the beginning of this book, you met Mike, who was diagnosed with dementia. Here, Mike shares how he lives a full life with dementia.

When I was given my diagnosis, my wife, Cheryl, and I were obviously shocked and confused. We sat there and listened as the doctor went over the numerous test results and then told us the diagnosis. I was given a medication to start taking and told, "I'll see you in six months." Cheryl and I walked out of his office like we were sleepwalking, not even sure what to say to each other.

The most important thing I wish I'd been told right away was that I can still have a meaningful, purposeful life.

I truly believe I'm here because of the things we've done to keep me socially engaged. It gave me back purpose and fulfillment when I thought I was useless — especially when I had to retire from work.

I no longer drive, I can no longer do some of the things I could before, and things that I used to do in minutes now can take me hours or even sometimes days. Forgetfulness and frustration abound.

But here's the thing: I don't focus on the things I can't do anymore. Rather, I focus on what I still can do.

One of my favorite movies is *The Shawshank Redemption*. There's a line in the movie that Tim Robbins' character says to Morgan Freeman's character: "Get busy living or get busy dying." I've chosen to get busy living.

“THE TERM *STIGMA* IS APPLIED WHEN LABELS, STEREOTYPES, SEPARATION, LOSS OF STATUS AND DISCRIMINATION TAKE PLACE TOGETHER.”

CHAPTER 12

Addressing the stigmas

Imagine for a moment that you're meeting someone for the first time.

Here's how she introduces herself:

"My name is Fiona. I live in the small city of Stockton, just a few miles from here. I'm 67 years old. I have Alzheimer's disease."

What do you see? Who do you see? What are you thinking?

As you look at her, do you focus on the fact that she has Alzheimer's? Do you immediately think her cognitive abilities are limited? Do you avoid starting a conversation with her because you feel uncomfortable or think she won't be able to understand you? Are you taken aback because she doesn't match your mental image of a person with dementia?

Beliefs and attitudes about dementia, as well as mental images of people with dementia, are shaped by many factors. These factors include your own experiences, as well as your understanding and knowledge of dementia. What you know about dementia has likely been influenced by friends, family, health care professionals, and the way dementia is portrayed in literature, media and film.

Because dementia is commonly associated with a range of symptoms, mostly losses, people with dementia are often stereotyped as having deficits — not only in the later stages, when some deficits are more common, but also throughout the entire course of dementia. What someone with dementia can still do is often overlooked. Not appreciating the ways that people with dementia are just like everyone else and focusing on stereotypical, negative and disturbing images of dementia contribute to stigma.

WHAT IS STIGMA?

Stigma happens when labels, stereotypes, separation, loss of status and discrimination take place together. Today, people living with dementia are speaking out about the ways in which they're experiencing these elements of stigma in their lives.

For example, a person living with dementia is often labeled as "suffering from" or "a victim of" dementia. Although people with dementia may say that they have days when they are, indeed, suffering, describing people living with dementia as "sufferers" is a generalization. In essence, it says that all people with dementia are suffering all the time — and that's a misconception.

These labels and words not only send a message to those who hear them, but also reinforce stereotypes and perceptions that influence attitudes and behavior. They devalue and disempower people living with dementia. They also divert the focus away from the person behind the disease — a person with needs, wants, desires, values, preferences, strengths and abilities, just like anyone else. And, just like anyone else, people with dementia deserve to be treated with dignity and respect at all times.

Stigmas are harmful for a number of reasons. They keep people from seeking medical treatment. They can prevent people from getting an early diagnosis — or a diagnosis at all. Stigma contributes to low self-esteem, isolation, poor mental health and a decrease in quality of life for people living with dementia and those who support them.

Often, people with dementia hide the diagnosis, which makes it harder for them to benefit from available treatments, make plans for the future, develop a support system or participate in clinical trials. Stigmas can keep people living with dementia from getting the support they need. This can lead to a transition to a care community or nursing home sooner than might have otherwise been needed.

Stigma also affects care partners, keeping them from getting the help and support that can help them most. This can contribute to increased burden, stress, depression and physical illness. Many people living with dementia and those who support them say that the stigma associated with dementia is their No. 1 concern.

Even though there's been more awareness and research on dementia-related stigma in the last two decades, more study on effective ways to reduce dementia-related stigma is still needed.

In the meantime, there are things you can do to help overcome the stigma associated with dementia. The first is to become educated and teach friends and family about the disease. Be open and direct. Be aware of the common myths that surround dementia so that you can share the truth.

5 COMMON MISCONCEPTIONS

Here are some of the most common dementia-related myths and stereotypes, followed by the truths about each one.

Myth: Memory loss means dementia

Truth: People naturally forget from time to time. But the memory issues in dementia are much more than the occasional lapse. When memory loss affects day-to-day function, it's important to visit a doctor to determine the cause. It's also important to note that for many forms of dementia, memory loss isn't the first symptom, so any unexplained changes in mood, behavior or ability should be checked out by a doctor.

Myth: Only older people get dementia

Truth: As you're learning in this book, many types of dementia can affect people at an earlier age. Alzheimer's disease, for example, can affect people in their 50s — and even in their 30s and 40s. As you learned earlier, this is known as young-onset Alzheimer's disease. Frontotemporal degeneration is another example of dementia that can affect people at an earlier age.

Myth: People with dementia become agitated, violent and aggressive

Truth: Not all people with dementia are agitated, violent or aggressive. The disease

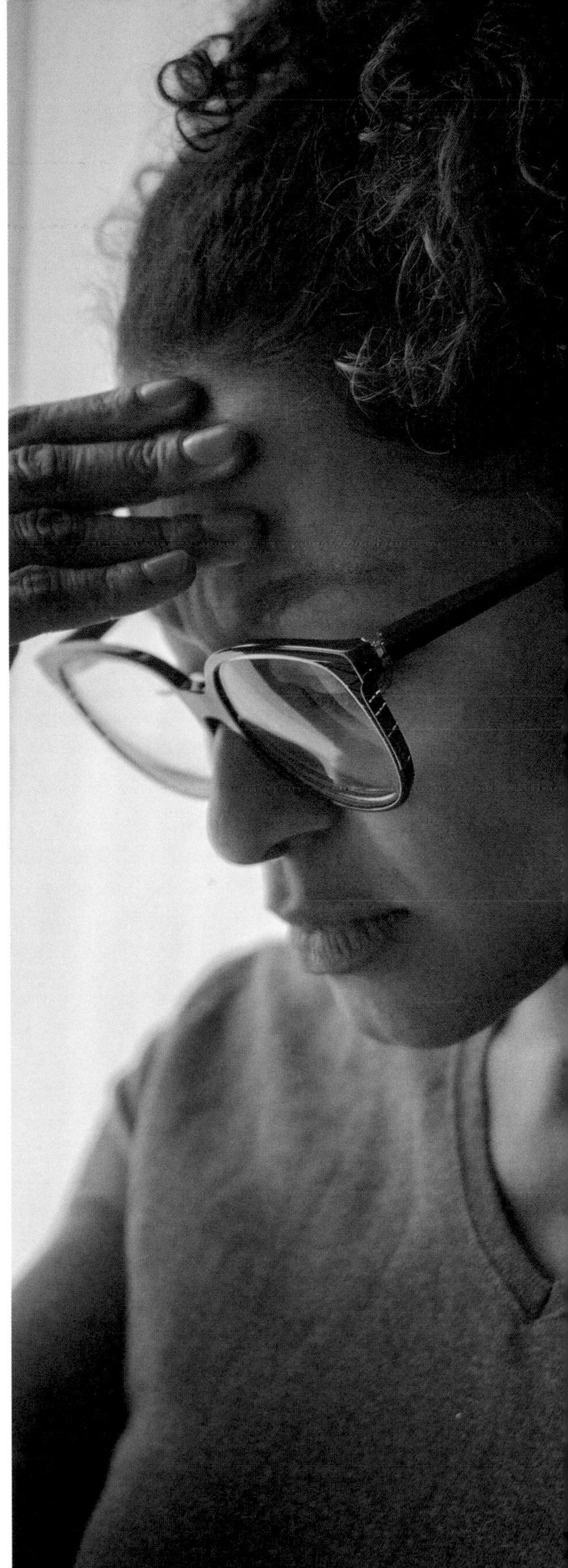

affects each person differently, and each type of dementia takes a different course for everyone living with it. Changes in the brain contribute to confusion and fear, but often, behaviors or expressions like agitation are a result of an unmet need.

By becoming knowledgeable about dementia, care partners and others can learn strategies that help eliminate or reduce distress in a person with dementia. Strategies like employing skillful communication, identifying unmet emotional needs and creating an accommodating environment are examples of ways to address dementia-related behaviors. Learn more in Chapter 17.

Myth: People with dementia can't enjoy new activities, learn new things, function or have a good quality of life

Truth: People with dementia can continue to live meaningful, active lives. People with dementia shouldn't simply stop doing what they enjoy in life. Instead, it's critical that they try to continue to enjoy their usual activities, recognizing that they may need to make some adaptations and rely on a little help from others along the way.

And don't rule out learning something new. Many people in the earlier stages of dementia — and even into the middle stages — can learn new skills, routines and habits.

Throughout all stages of disease, people living with dementia are human beings capable of giving and receiving love. They can participate in meaningful activities and can share moments of joy and laughter.

Myth: Nothing can be done for dementia

Truth: Overcoming the idea that nothing can be done for dementia is needed to help people talk about dementia rather than hide from it. The sooner there's a diagnosis, the more opportunity there is for treatments that may slow the progression.

A diagnosis also opens the door to treatments and therapies that can help with symptoms. But that's not all. People living with dementia and their families need to believe that there's still life to live after a dementia diagnosis.

Conversations with family and friends shouldn't focus only on losses and decline. They should also include discussions on what brings joy to the person with dementia. What can the person still do? How can the person contribute in meaningful ways? What things really matter to the person with dementia, and how can these things continue to be a part of day-to-day living? Some people living with dementia find it helpful to adjust routines, seek out new hobbies and interests, and simplify.

SHIFTING AWAY FROM STIGMAS

As long as myths and misconceptions continue, dementia will carry a stigma. This

GARY'S STORY: 'I'M NOT ASHAMED OF HAVING ALZHEIMER'S'

When people say "dementia" or "Alzheimer's," everybody thinks you're going to die the next day.

There is a stigma that goes along with the disease. Many people are worried about sharing the fact openly that they have this disease because of the negative stigma.

I heard someone whisper the other day, "My father has Alzheimer's." I just gave him a big hug and said, "You don't have to whisper — shout it out loud."

I'm not ashamed of having Alzheimer's. All my neighbors are aware I have a problem and there's no ridicule, no stigma, and so I wish we would get it out of our minds that we've done something; that we need to go under the table and hide.

means that people living with it and affected by it will continue to hide and withdraw in shame, fear and embarrassment.

It takes everyone — people living with dementia, their care partners and loved ones, and even those who aren't directly affected by dementia — to break down stereotypes and stigma.

The first step toward changing perceptions and breaking down stereotypes and stigma is understanding what dementia is — and isn't — and being open about the disease itself. You're already taking an important step by reading this book.

Tips for people living with dementia

If you're living with dementia or supporting someone who is, you have a powerful opportunity to help shape how people view and think about dementia. These suggestions can help deter stigma not just for you, but also for others affected by dementia.

Share your story If you're living with dementia, talk about your diagnosis as openly and honestly as you can. Talk about the type of dementia you're living with, and share your feelings and experience. There is no shame in having dementia.

Think of it this way: Most people aren't ashamed of having a broken leg or cancer. You're still you, and sharing your diagnosis and the symptoms you're experiencing will go a long way toward helping reduce stigma. It may even make you feel a little freer.

Offer information Lack of knowledge contributes to stigma. Share information you've received from your health care team or information you've found that you think is important for others to know. This can help others understand more about the type of dementia you're living with, as well as its symptoms.

Most important, let others know that receiving a diagnosis of dementia doesn't mean that you've changed and you can no longer do what you used to do. For most people, symptoms of dementia progress slowly over time.

Tips for everyone

Even if you're not directly affected by dementia right now, you can make a difference in dispelling myths about the disease. Here are several ways you can help create a supportive community for people affected by and living with dementia.

Learn the facts Share your knowledge about dementia with others, including family and friends — especially if you hear something that isn't true. Accurate information helps clear up misconceptions about the disease. Talking about dementia lessens fear and increases understanding.

Don't make assumptions There is a misconception that a person who's diagnosed with dementia automatically loses the ability to make decisions, as well as independence. This simply isn't true. Dementia is a progressive disease, and it affects each person differently. Being diagnosed with dementia doesn't mean that a person has to stop his or her daily routine or give up working right away.

Be a friend People with dementia don't want to lose their friends or stop doing the things they enjoy. Be supportive. Stay in touch and connected. Social activity helps slow the progression of the disease and lets people with dementia know you care. Do things with — rather than for — the person.

Use language thoughtfully For those living with dementia, using words or phrases that label, demean or depersonalize can have a big impact on the way they feel about themselves, impacting mood, self-esteem, feelings and actions. Just like you, people with dementia react negatively or positively to what's said to them or about them.

Language and word choice can also influence the way other people think about dementia — and can make it more likely that

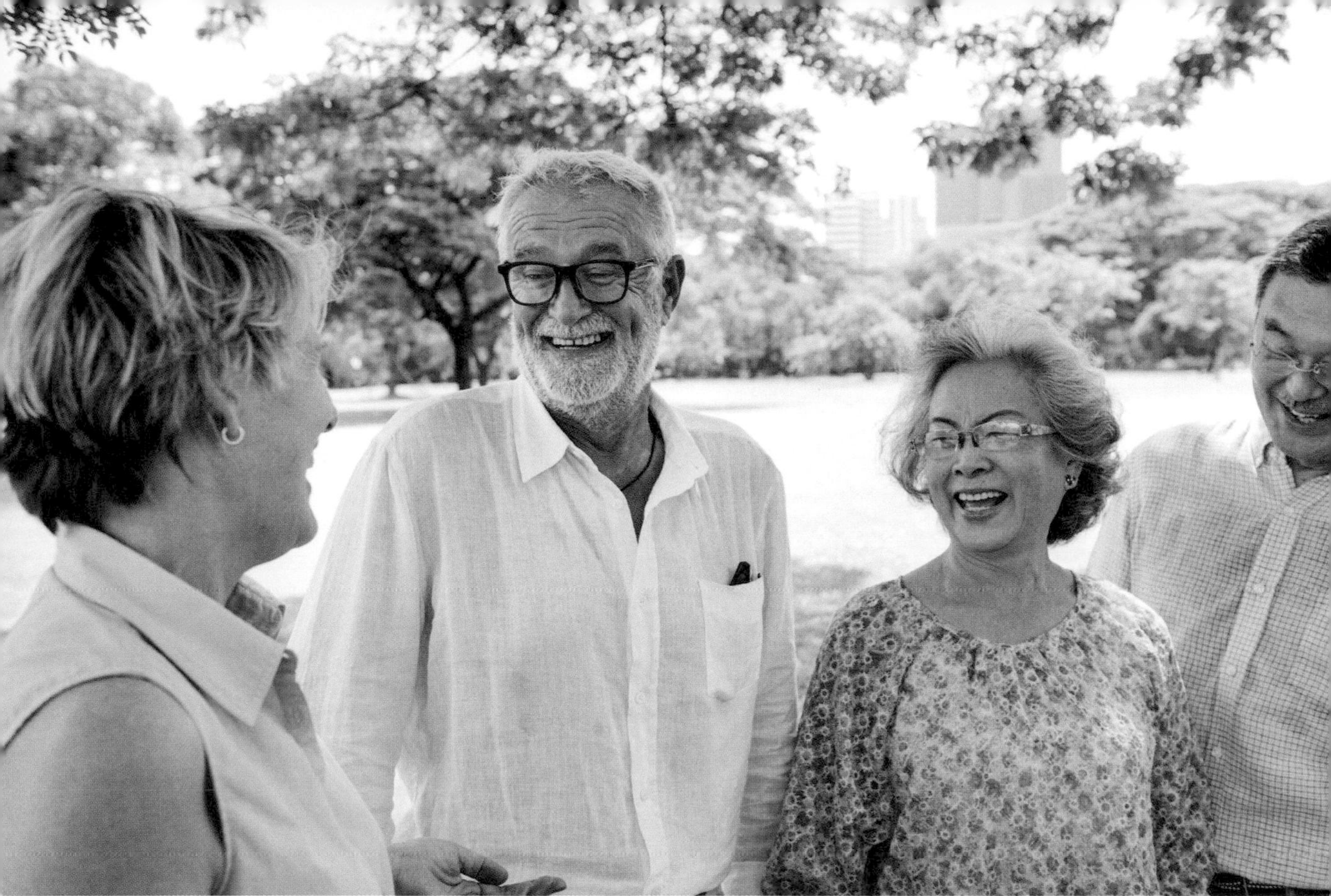

someone with dementia will experience stigma. Terms like *victim* and *sufferer* are examples of words that label people with dementia as helpless, disempowering them and inaccurately generalizing what it's like to live with dementia.

Instead, use language that doesn't highlight dementia as the defining aspect of a person's life. For example, don't describe someone with dementia as a patient. The term *patient* should only be used to refer to a person being cared for in a hospital, or in relation to seeing a doctor or another health care professional. Instead, use terms like *person living with dementia*. This puts the focus on the person instead of the condition. See the person, not the dementia.

“SEVERAL APPROACHES ARE SHOWN TO HELP PEOPLE WITH DEMENTIA BECOME MORE RESILIENT IN THE FACE OF THEIR DIAGNOSIS.”

CHAPTER 13

Adjusting to a diagnosis

Hearing the news that you or a loved one has been diagnosed with mild cognitive impairment, Alzheimer's disease dementia or a related dementia may come as a shock.

Maybe you were hoping to hear something else — perhaps that forgetfulness and confusion were due to aging or that the symptoms would disappear with a change in medication. You may be flooded with disbelief. It's hard to imagine something like this happening to you or someone close to you.

Leading up to this moment, it may have been difficult enough to acknowledge your concerns, let alone bring them to a doctor's attention. After all, the onset of dementia is often gradual, so it's easy to pass off symptoms as a typical part of getting older. Plus, the word *dementia* can stir up many commonly held beliefs, many of which aren't true. You may think, *There's nothing that can be done, My life is over, I'm going to be completely dependent on others for the rest of my life,* or have other misconceptions like those you read about earlier. These are strong emotions to work through.

This chapter offers guidance to help you adjust to and live with a dementia diagnosis, whether you're the one who's received it or you're supporting someone who's been diagnosed with dementia.

COMING TO TERMS

A dementia diagnosis is life altering. It means coming to terms with changes that, over time, cause increased challenges with memory and thinking, as well as language, physical abilities and emotions.

WHEN SOMEONE WITH DEMENTIA HAS LIMITED INSIGHT

Limited insight — when a person lacks understanding about his or her cognitive impairment — is often related to the type of dementia the person has or the area of the brain that's affected. In some types of dementia, like frontotemporal degeneration, lack of insight is common. In other types of dementia, like posterior cortical atrophy, lack of insight is rare. Loss of insight tends to be linked to shrinkage (atrophy) in the right hemisphere of the brain.

No matter what you're feeling, you're not alone. There's no right or wrong way to feel.

Some people struggle to accept the news and deny that they have dementia. It may come as a shock that symptoms aren't related to typical aging. Others have trouble understanding that they have dementia. They may lack insight about their impairment. The medical term for this is anosognosia. When someone lacks awareness of functional limitations, it can lead to risky behaviors, like driving when it's no longer safe to do so.

And finally, others say they felt prepared to hear the news, given the symptoms they'd been experiencing. For some, a diagnosis offers a sense of relief. Many people find themselves feeling several different emotions all at once.

You may worry about not being able to do the things you've always done, and about becoming dependent on others or a burden. You may be concerned about what others will think of you. How will family, friends and others who know you react when they hear the news? Will they think of you differently, treat you differently or stop coming around altogether?

You may fear that you'll no longer be seen as a person with talents, strengths and abilities, and that instead, you'll be seen only as a person with dementia. You may feel sadness and a sense of loss, uncertain about your hopes and plans for the future.

Although all of these thoughts and concerns are understandable and common reactions, you can adjust to a dementia diagnosis with both acceptance and positive action.

Several approaches are shown to help people with dementia become more resilient in the face of a diagnosis. For example, in a recent study of people diagnosed with dementia, about a third said that focusing on what they could do and on the benefits of receiving a diagnosis allowed them to maintain a positive outlook.

For many, this involves making adjustments. For example, people interviewed for the study said it helped to accept that some things may need to be done differently — but that they still could be done. When reading a book, for instance, some people found it helpful to write down character names so that they would remember them. Making lists of things to remember was also helpful.

The people interviewed for the study also said that accepting help from others was critical. Reaching out to others who will support you can help you adjust to the news of a dementia diagnosis. It can help to talk with someone you trust about what you're feeling. Reaching out to others can have practical benefits, too. For example, people in the study said that making a to-do list for the day and having someone review it was helpful.

After the initial shock and other strong feelings have worn off a little, a diagnosis is often seen as a positive event. The person who's been diagnosed with dementia and his or her family now know what they're dealing with and can start to take action and plan accordingly.

It takes time to process and accept a dementia diagnosis and everything it means. Just as there's no right or wrong way to feel

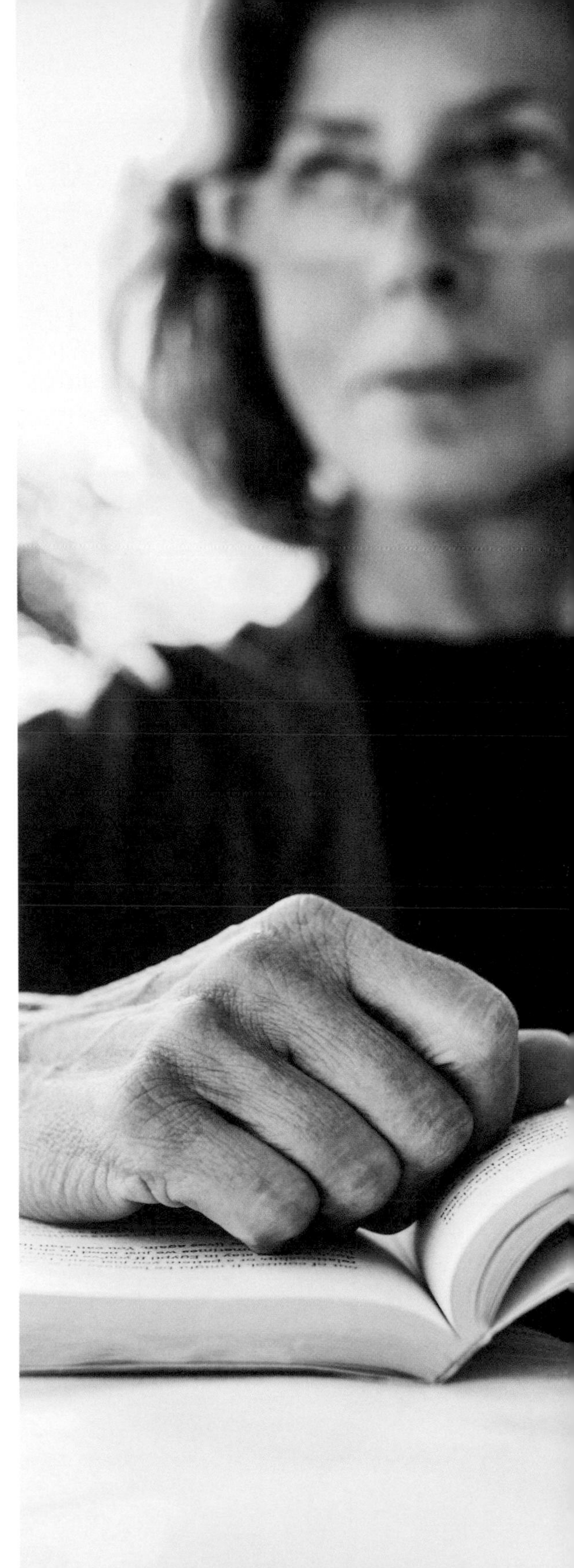

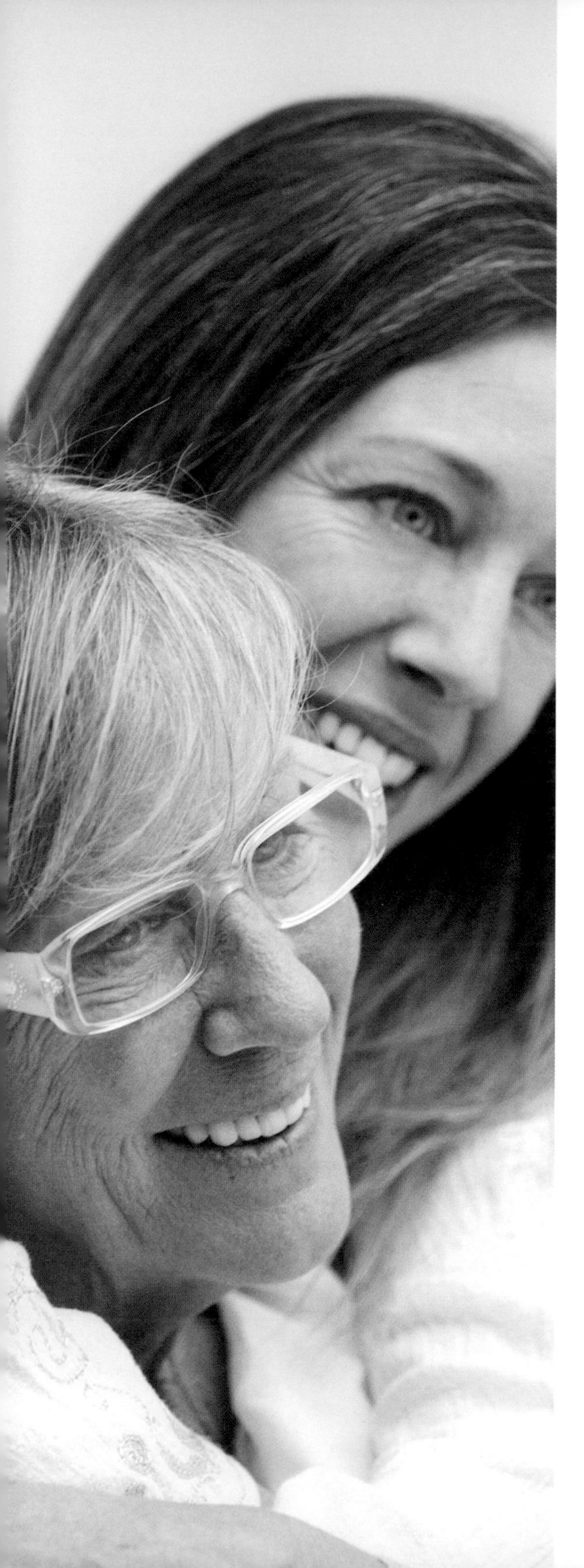

about a dementia diagnosis, every person's path toward working through and accepting it is different. Here's more on the many feelings family members may experience.

EFFECTS ON THE FAMILY

Family members often play a key role in recognizing symptoms that lead to a diagnosis. They're usually the ones who first notice the memory or other thinking changes, disorientation, changes in mood, and sometimes personality. Family members often initiate a doctor visit out of concern that something's wrong. They may also have to help provide information on the diagnosis if the loved one doesn't completely understand it or is in a state of shock or denial.

There's generally a lag between the time family members first start to notice worrisome symptoms and when an appointment with a doctor is scheduled. The delay may be due to confusion about what are typical age-related changes and what are more serious developments. Often, the delay is a part of the process — the gradual realization that symptoms aren't getting any better and may be getting worse.

Denial can be the earliest and strongest emotion that family members feel. It's a normal response to a difficult situation — as family members become aware that a loved one may have an incurable disorder, they worry about what the future holds and their ability to cope. Denial is a common response to the uncertainty that lies ahead.

Sometimes, often before a dementia diagnosis, family members experience anger. Emotions like fear and anxiety are often mixed in. They may think, *If only she would try harder, If only he would pay attention,* or *I wish he'd listened to what I said.*

Often, and over time, a diagnosis offers a sense of relief. For example, the person with the diagnosis and family members can understand why the person's memory has been so unreliable.

At the same time, a diagnosis can lead to feelings of guilt as family members realize that behaviors that perhaps made them feel angry are due to a disease and not the fault of the person.

It's important to forgive yourself when feelings of guilt arise. Getting angry or frustrated over things you didn't fully understand at the time makes sense. The good news is that with a diagnosis, you can move forward with understanding and empathy.

Even with a diagnosis, the journey from denial to acceptance isn't a straight path. The person receiving the diagnosis, family members and friends may find themselves at different places along the path at different times. You'll work through your feelings and adjust emotionally to the changes at your own pace.

If you ever feel like you're the only one in this situation, remember that you're never

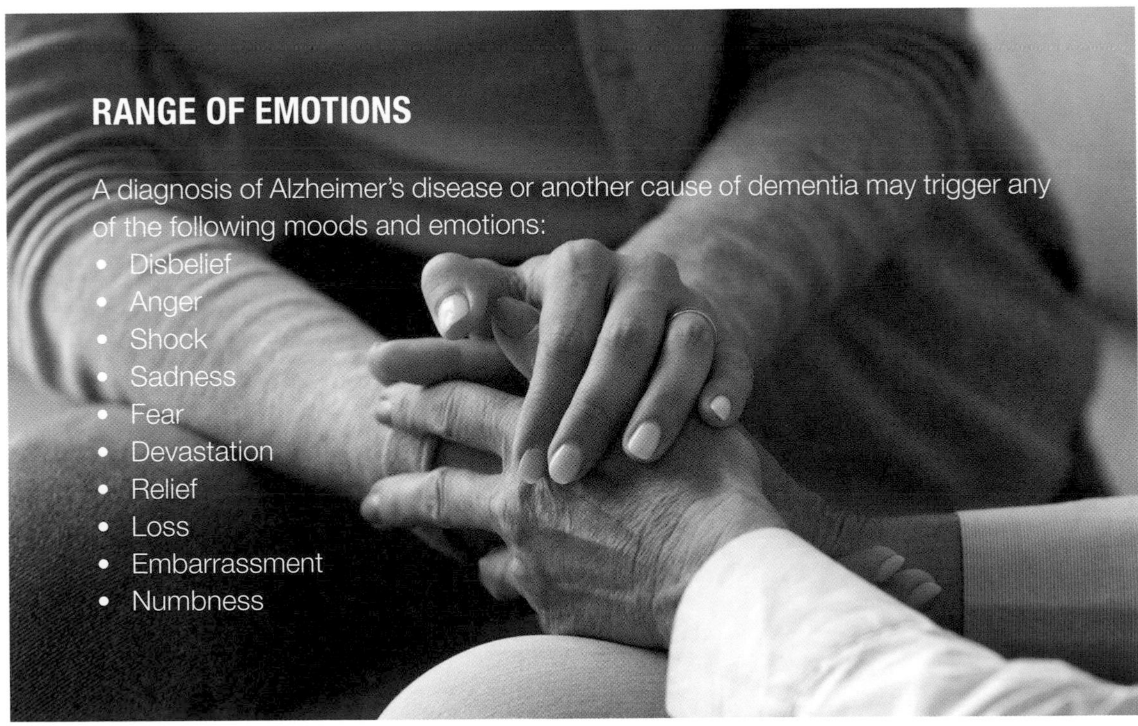

RANGE OF EMOTIONS

A diagnosis of Alzheimer's disease or another cause of dementia may trigger any of the following moods and emotions:

- Disbelief
- Anger
- Shock
- Sadness
- Fear
- Devastation
- Relief
- Loss
- Embarrassment
- Numbness

alone. Millions of people around the world are living with the impact of Alzheimer's disease and other neurodegenerative disorders. Millions more are in a caring and supportive role. The first, and sometimes most difficult step, is accepting the diagnosis and adjusting to a new normal.

NEXT STEPS

A diagnosis of dementia doesn't signal the end of living. On the contrary, a diagnosis can point you toward information, support, resources, treatments, clinical trials and services that can help. For the person living with dementia, one of the most important first steps after a diagnosis is to attend to the task of living to the best of his or her ability.

You'll learn more about this in Chapter 14; for now, here are several steps to take after a dementia diagnosis has been made.

Continue living a pre-diagnosis life as much as possible Receiving a dementia diagnosis doesn't make you any different from who you were the day before the diagnosis. One of the best things you can do after being diagnosed with dementia is to continue living your life as fully as you can. Very few people are diagnosed in the late stages of the disease, so there's a lot of living still to do. Staying engaged in life and doing things that keep you mentally and physically active is important.

Get your affairs in order Whether you have dementia or not, it's important to complete important legal documents. A living will and a durable power of attorney for health care are examples. These documents allow people to communicate their wishes about the kind of medical care and treatment they want to receive. These documents also designate someone to make medical decisions on an individual's behalf when the individual is unable to do so.

Participate in support groups People in the early stages of dementia often withdraw from friendships and social groups they once enjoyed because they're afraid that they'll make a mistake or embarrass themselves in some way.

But this doesn't mean that socializing and friendships are less important now than they were before. In fact, being with others in an easy and comfortable manner can help increase a person's ability to adapt to the life changes that are occurring. The same is true for care partners.

This is where support groups for people with dementia and their care partners can help. A common theme echoed among support group participants is that they don't feel alone when they're with others in similar situations who truly understand what they're going through.

Support groups can vary in their makeups and activities. Look for one that meets the needs your needs. For example, some groups get together in restaurants, cafés or museums — places where it's not obvious to the public who has dementia or who

"RECEIVING A DEMENTIA DIAGNOSIS DOESN'T MAKE YOU ANY DIFFERENT THAN YOU WERE THE DAY BEFORE."

doesn't. Other groups offer dementia-friendly programs such as walking groups, volunteer programs, or yoga designed for people with physical or cognitive impairments. The important thing is to find a group that allows you and your loved one to feel comfortable sharing, growing and adapting.

Consider enrolling in research programs and clinical trials The only way to develop new treatments or effective prevention efforts against dementia is through research and clinical trials with human volunteers. Participants at all stages and representing all aspects of dementia, including those who have dementia, care partners and even healthy individuals, are urgently needed. While every clinical trial has risks, and it's important to understand them, there are many benefits, as well.

By participating in a clinical trial, you can take an active role that helps future generations who might one day benefit from its results. Find links to more information about clinical trials in the Additional resources section.

Learn about treatment options After receiving a diagnosis, you may feel that since no cure exists for dementia, there's no point in taking any medicine for it. But the diseases that cause dementia are often gradual in nature, and some medications may help treat the symptoms and make present life better. In addition, services like occupational therapy, physical therapy and speech therapy can improve quality of life.

Talking about the diagnosis

If you've been diagnosed with dementia, you may wonder when and how to share the news. It can be a difficult topic to discuss with others.

A big factor is your own personality and how comfortable you feel talking about personal issues with various people. Some people are likely to share the diagnosis with only a few close relatives and friends. Others may be much more open about their experience with dementia.

Wait until you feel ready to communicate with family and friends. You don't have to tell everyone at once. Come up with a list of who you need or want to tell first and a few brief talking points. If other loved ones have

(continued on page 273)

WHEN TO STOP DRIVING

Safe driving requires attention, concentration, and the ability to follow particular steps and rules. It also requires the ability to make quick and appropriate decisions. For people with dementia, these skills will decline over time. Eventually, driving will not be an option.

People with mild dementia are at a much greater risk of unsafe driving compared with people of the same age without dementia. The American Academy of Neurology recommends that people with mild dementia strongly consider discontinuing driving. With dementia, strengths and weaknesses vary from person to person, so it's important to talk about driving safety with a doctor as soon as possible.

Signs of unsafe driving include:

- Getting lost when driving to familiar places
- Not staying in the lane
- Confusing the brake and gas pedals
- Failing to observe traffic signs
- Making slow or poor decisions
- Hitting the curb while driving
- Driving too slowly or speeding
- Becoming angry or confused while driving
- Getting into an accident or getting a ticket

People with mild dementia who are still able to drive safely may be able to drive for some time. If the person with dementia would still like to drive and his or her

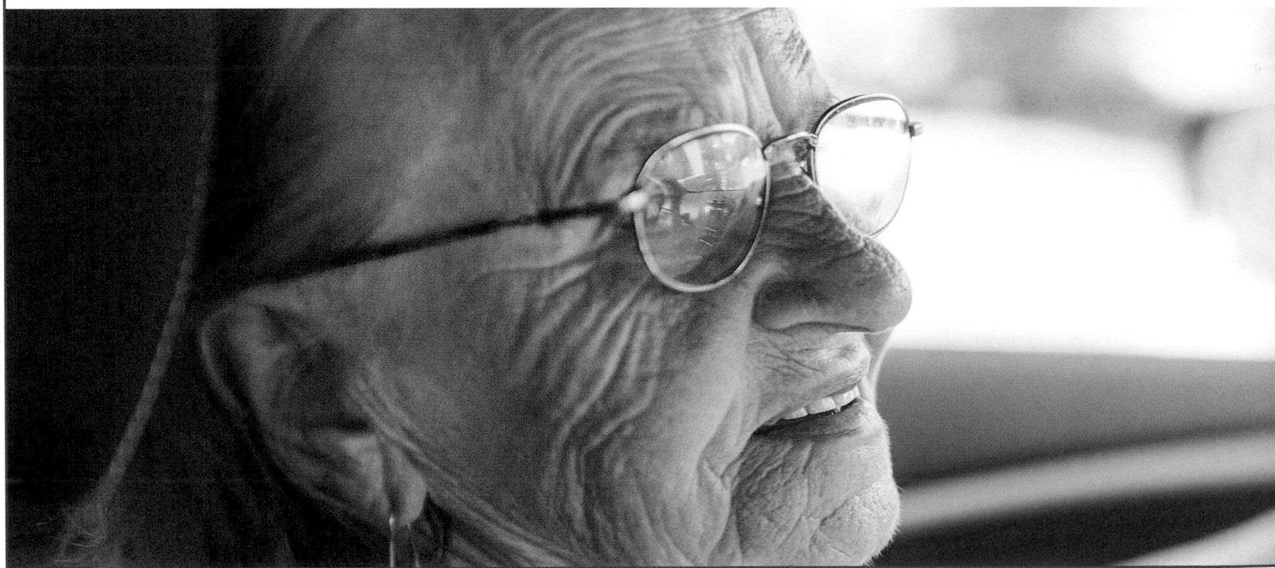

family feels it's safe to do so, a roadside driving evaluation is recommended. During this test, an occupational therapist evaluates the impact of the disease on a person's ability to drive and offers strategies for driving safely, as well as when and how to reduce or stop driving.

While giving up driving isn't a big issue for some people, for others, it's a much more difficult choice to have to make. This is especially true for people with dementia who lack insight into their limitations. In these cases, these strategies for care partners can help ease the situation, especially in cases of anger and resistance.

- Be patient but firm. With understanding and empathy, acknowledge how difficult this change likely is. At the same time, emphasize that not driving is a responsible choice to make.
- If needed, ask someone that the person with dementia respects to reinforce the reasons why not driving is the best choice to make.
- Taking away car keys and even selling the car may be needed. It's important to make sure that the person with dementia has a safe, reliable form of transportation.

If the discussion doesn't go well, keep in mind that it can be difficult for someone with dementia to understand when certain choices, like driving, are no longer safe choices to make.

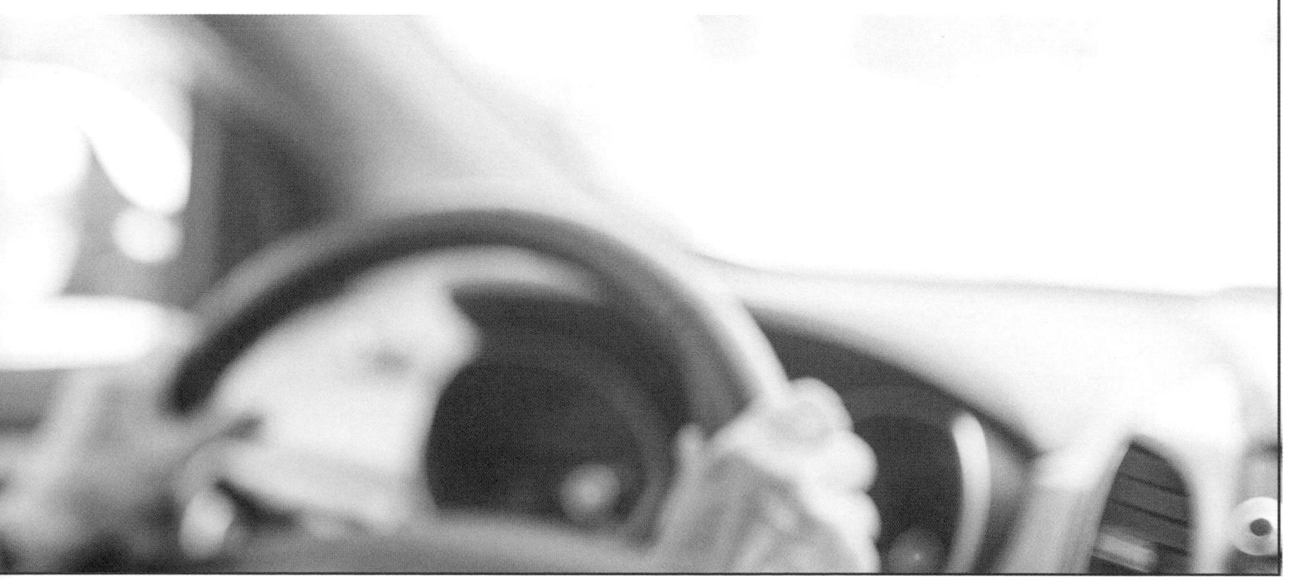

WORKPLACE TRANSITIONS

One of the messages you've read throughout this book is that life doesn't end with a dementia diagnosis. Although adjustments may be needed, many people with dementia can continue to live satisfying, active lives. This brings up a concern for many people diagnosed with dementia: Can I still work?

Whether or not to keep working — and what adjustments may be needed — are best evaluated on a case-by-case basis. Sometimes a team of experts, including a doctor who specializes in occupational medicine, can help navigate these situations. In some cases, people with dementia can continue to work in a more narrow or modified capacity.

As a first step, talk to your doctor about your symptoms and how they may affect your ability to work. This is a conversation you'll likely need to have on an ongoing basis as symptoms change over time.

Dementia is progressive, which means its symptoms gradually worsen over time. Most people living with dementia will need to transition out of the workforce if they're not already retired. Your employer may offer benefits that can help, including an employee assistance program, which may include referrals, counseling and other assistance. Short-term disability and long-term disability are other possible benefits that may help during the transition. Social Security benefits are another possible option. Learn more in the Additional resources section.

Transitioning out of the workforce can bring about feelings of uncertainty around identity and purpose. It's not uncommon for people with dementia to ask questions like, *What now? Who am I?* as they search for a new sense of identity and purpose. One way to address these questions is to explore skills you already have or take on activities that offer a fresh sense of purpose. You may look into opportunities that make use of your preserved strengths, interests and talents. If there are new activities you've always wanted to try, this may be the time to explore them. Connecting with others living with dementia may be another option.

(continued from page 269)

been through the diagnosis process with you, they can help. As you become more comfortable communicating the information, you can decide if there are others you want to tell. Or entrust a few reliable family members and friends with the job of spreading the news. What's most important is for you to feel comfortable and able to move forward with positive support.

Reactions may vary. Some are quick to provide support and offers of help. These are people who will be sensitive to your needs and want you to educate them about your condition. They're the ones who won't mind repeating themselves when you forget what they said. Or they will laugh with you when you need a dose of humor. At times, relatives and friends you least expect become the most supportive.

But some people in your life may be unable to handle the news or confront their fears of what lies ahead for you. They may steer clear of any conversation about your health or avoid seeing you. Still others may say inappropriate things. Or they ask more questions than you feel comfortable answering.

Changes in relationships are common when a serious illness is diagnosed. Learning to accept these changes and leaning on stable relationships and friendships can help lessen some of the stress you may be feeling. If you're living with dementia, one of the most important things you can do is to talk about

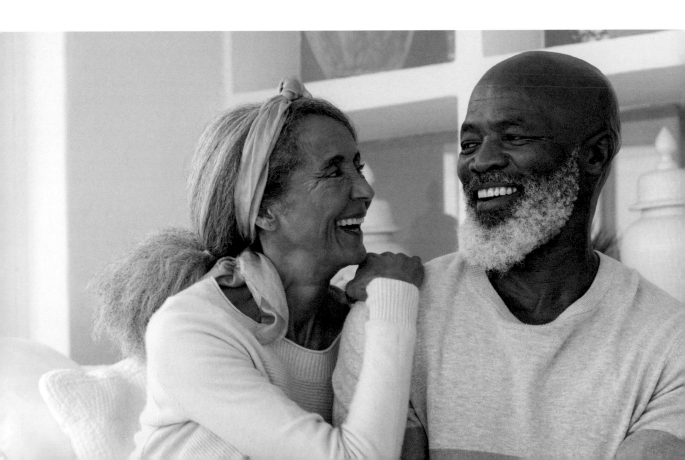

it. Let family, friends and others in your community know how they can support you. This will help put others at ease and help you stay engaged and independent.

In addition, talking about dementia increases understanding and reduces fears, which can help to address stigma.

Tips for care partners

Care partners often wonder whom to tell about the diagnosis and when to tell them. A person diagnosed with dementia may be afraid to feel "under the microscope" as people watch closely for signs of illness. You may be torn between protecting your loved one's privacy and sharing parts of the emotional roller coaster you're on.

As a first step, talk to the person diagnosed with dementia. It's important, first and foremost, to respect the privacy of someone who's been diagnosed with dementia. If the person with dementia is OK sharing the diagnosis with others, the next step is to decide how to share the news and determine who to tell.

When sharing the diagnosis with others, explain the disease and its effects. It may help to share that dementia involves a disease that causes brain cells to degenerate and die and that this causes a decline in memory and mental function. You may also explain what symptoms the person with dementia will likely have and how the disease may progress. This is where educational materials from organizations like the Alzheimer's Association can be helpful. They can help

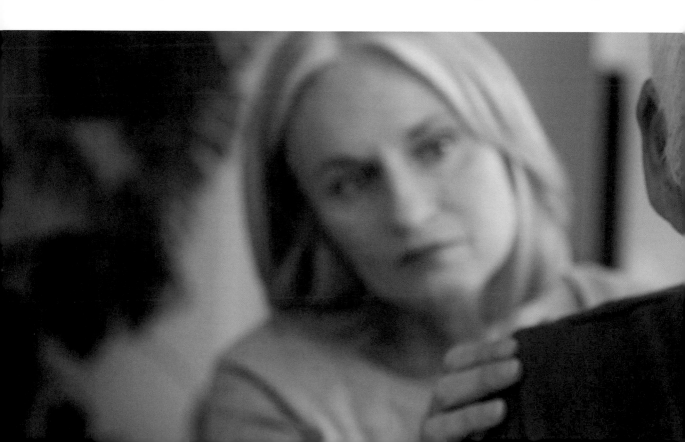

explain a disease, its effects, and its symptoms. The Additional resources section of this book offers recommendations for organizations that offer these materials.

Most importantly, emphasize that a dementia diagnosis doesn't mean someone has lost all of his or her skills, habits, passions, likes, dislikes, or the desire to be involved with life and connected with others. Let others know that the person with dementia can still do many or most things, sometimes with a little support or a few accommodations. You may also explain that social interaction is healthy for the brain and that it's important for the person living with dementia to stay engaged.

For practical needs, offer specific examples of ways people can help. The more specific you are about your needs, the better. Rather than hinting that you're uncomfortable driving across town, for example, you might say, "We're looking for help getting to doctor appointments, and here are the scheduled times." If people ask how they can help, be prepared to answer.

You may want to post updates to keep people aware of your loved one's condition. Look to your local Alzheimer's Association chapter or a related organization for ideas regarding information that may be helpful to include in updates.

Finally, as you consider the needs of the person living with dementia, remember to keep your own needs in mind, as well. Friends who can provide conversation, emotional support and assistance can be invaluable.

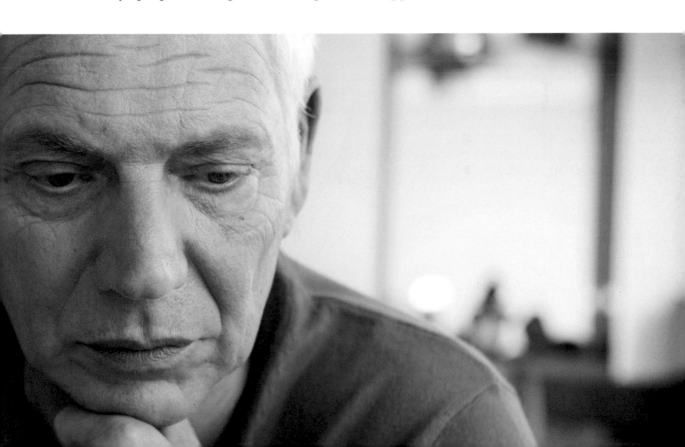

Explaining to children

Adults may choose to shield young children from the knowledge that a family member has dementia. But children generally recognize when something is wrong. Your loved one's behavior may seem confusing, especially if the children don't understand why such behavior is occurring.

Here are ways to offer simple, honest answers to several questions children commonly ask.

Question: What's wrong with Grandma?

Explain that just as children can get sick, adults sometimes get an illness that causes them to act differently and to forget things. You may add that they might look like the same people on the outside, but that their brains are changing on the inside.

Question: Doesn't Grandpa love me anymore?

Your child might feel rejected if the person with dementia no longer recognizes him or her. Remind your child that the disease makes it hard to remember things — but that the person can still feel your child's love.

Question: Is it my fault?

If the person with dementia accuses your child of a wrongdoing — like stealing a belonging — your child might get upset.

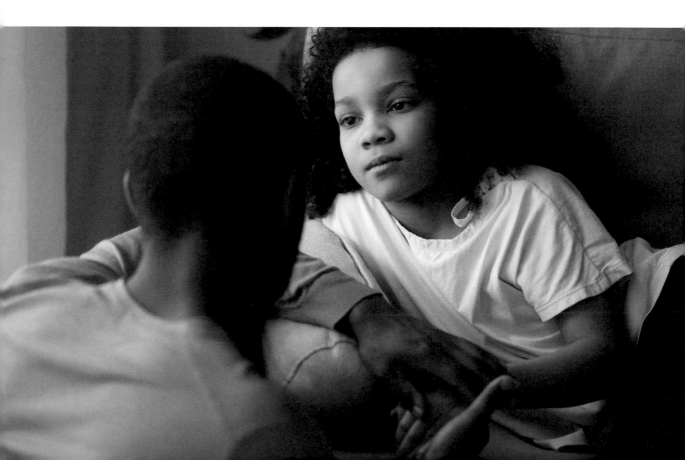

Explain that the person with dementia is confused. You might explain that it's best not to disagree with this person because it could make the person upset or frustrated.

Question: Will other family members get Alzheimer's?

Reassure your child that dementia isn't contagious. You might explain to an older child that just because a relative has dementia, it doesn't mean that every family member will get the disease.

Question: What will happen next?

If you'll be caring for the person who has dementia in your home, talk to your child about changes in your family's routine. Explain that the person will have good days and bad days.

If your child has trouble talking about the situation or withdraws from the person with dementia, open a conversation. Ask what changes your child has noticed. This might lead to a talk about your child's feelings and worries.

Tell your child it's OK to feel nervous, sad or angry. You might tell your child you feel that way sometimes too. To boost your child's understanding, seek out websites, books or videos on the disease.

A child may express emotions in indirect ways, like complaining of headaches or other physical problems. Your child might feel awkward around the person with dementia. If you're caring for the person with dementia in your home, your child may not feel comfortable inviting friends to the house or may look for ways to spend more time away from home. If you notice these behaviors, gently point out what you've seen — and offer your child comfort and support. Listen to your child's concerns.

After adjusting to a diagnosis, the next step is to find ways to optimize well-being. Well-being is critical for people living with dementia, as well as their care partners. The next few chapters offer valuable information and strategies.

"PEOPLE LIVING WITH DEMENTIA CAN STILL SENSE LOVE, EXPERIENCE JOY, AND CONNECT TO WHAT'S GOING ON MOMENT TO MOMENT."

CHAPTER 14

Road map toward well-being

"Maintaining a fulfilling lifestyle under prevailing emotional and physical circumstances, being engaged in what gives me joy as I live in the gift of the present."

This is how Sandy — a father of two, a grandfather of three, and a former dentist and Harvard assistant professor who was diagnosed with Alzheimer's at age 60 — describes what many people living with dementia want to accomplish. At the same time, Sandy's description offers a new and different way to think about well-being.

Well-being has many definitions. In a medical sense, well-being may be defined in terms of a health outcome, like successfully treating or curing a disease. In another context, well-being may refer to a number of other factors, like having enough food to eat, or having adequate housing and safety.

For people living with dementia, these descriptions may not fit their experience, and they don't they tell the whole story.

The definition of well-being differs from one person to the next. Most agree, however, that well-being includes the presence of positive emotions like joy, as well as a sense of fulfillment, as Sandy describes. In addition, well-being for a person living with dementia may need to include approaching each day with positivity.

Every person is unique. How well people live with dementia depends on who they are and the parts of the brain affected by dementia, as well as their situation, relationships and support network.

Having dementia doesn't define who someone is, nor does it predict a person's future.

However, it does mean that some things will change, and it may mean a shorter life expectancy. But people living with dementia are just like anyone else, striving to live their best life now, for as long as they can.

While dementia will affect each person in a different way, many people can and do live well. People around the world who are living with dementia are working hard to send the message that life doesn't stop with a dementia diagnosis. While dementia is a debilitating condition, life can still be lived and enjoyed.

This chapter offers insights from people living with dementia and practical advice that can help people with dementia move toward greater well-being. Because people living with dementia are unique with different needs, not everything will apply to every person. The most important message in this chapter is that a good life alongside dementia is possible.

ADDRESSING THE STIGMA

For people living with dementia, one of the biggest hurdles involves assumptions people may make about what they can or can't do. Many people with dementia say they feel that others, including family members, see them as dependent, incapable or helpless since they received their diagnosis.

"Relationships with family (and friends) may change," says Brian, who's living with young-onset Alzheimer's disease dementia. He's also a member of the Dementia Action Alliance Advisory Board.

"Family members (and friends) may not want to talk about the disease, perceive you as having little or no quality of life, or may avoid interacting with you."

In turn, negative reactions and messages from others can affect self-confidence, self-esteem and self-worth.

The first step toward living well with dementia is to ignore these misconceptions, like the ones you read about in Chapter 12.

A prevailing message from people living with dementia is that they shouldn't be defined by their condition. They don't want to be marginalized and deemed incompetent based solely on their diagnosis. Instead, they want to be seen as a whole person; a person who will need some help and support over time, but also as a person with the same needs as everyone else: to feel needed, worthy and respected as a person with strengths and potential.

Mike, whose story you read earlier, describes how he dismisses stereotypes and adopts a can-do mindset while living with dementia, this way:

"I do not focus on the things that I can't do anymore; rather, I focus on what I can still do," Mike says. "People who have been given this diagnosis can still contribute, learn, and can still live a meaningful and purposeful life. They also still have a voice even if they cannot communicate in the way they could before."

This doesn't mean that life will be as it always has been and that there won't be loss and heartache. Dale, who's living with Alzheimer's disease, explains it this way: "I am not trying to sugarcoat it. I know that the disease is terminal. I know that nobody, as of yet, has beaten Alzheimer's, but I have had to change my own mindset.

"I have had to accept my diagnosis, slow down and take an early retirement," Dale continues. "But I can also see how great life really is right now. I still am blessed with wonderful people in my life — my wife, children, grandchildren, relatives and friends. I am able to open my eyes every morning and see the wonders of the world and hear the sounds of life."

Moving toward a greater sense of well-being starts with establishing your own set of attitudes and beliefs. You may start with a list like this:

- Dementia is just one part of who I am. It does not define me.
- I can enjoy today and what I have now.
- I will maintain a "can do" mindset.
- I believe in my ability to contribute, learn and live a meaningful life.
- I will accept my disease and know that things will change, and that I will need help and support from others.
- I will treat myself with kindness and know that I am doing the best I can — and that is good enough.

With these attitudes as a foundation, the rest of this chapter offers additional information, recommendations and strategies for living well with dementia.

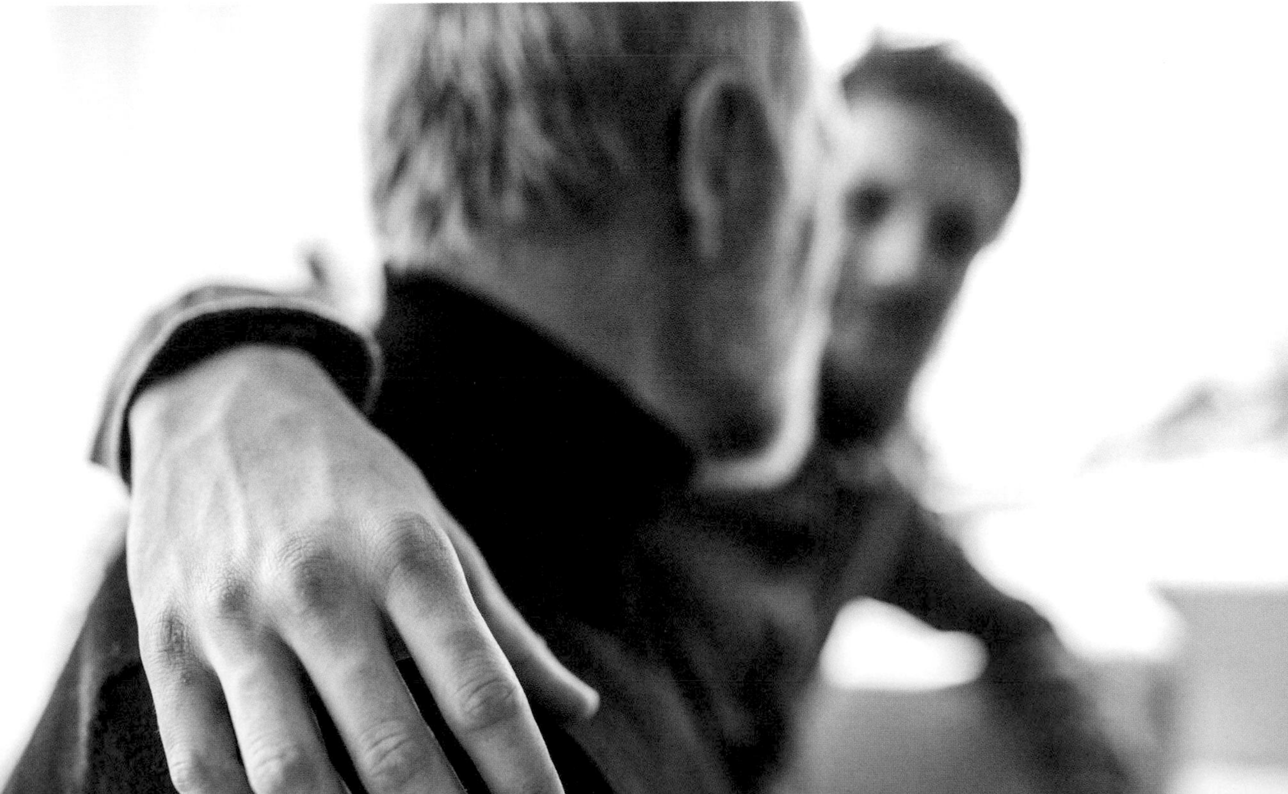

LIVING WITH DEMENTIA: GUIDANCE FOR EVERYONE

The Dementia Action Alliance offers key ways that everyone can support and promote the dignity and well-being of people living with dementia. These action items were written by people living with dementia.

- I am a person. Know me and relate to me as a person with a unique background, life history, interests and capabilities. When you call me a "patient," "victim" or "sufferer," I feel minimized.
- Understand that my autonomy, choices, dignity, reciprocal relationships, privacy and self-determination are fundamental to my well-being.
- Support my holistic emotional, social, physical and spiritual dimensions.
- Promote ways I can continue to experience personal growth and development through purpose, meaning, relationships and enjoyment in my daily life.
- Recognize that my personal goals, measures of success and interests may change over time and may not be the same as yours.
- Recognize that choice may have risks — a normal part of everyone's life.
- Partner with me, utilize my strengths and provide the right amount of support and opportunities I need to achieve my goals.
- I am trying to communicate the best I can; understand that my verbal and physical expressions are my way of communicating. I may say or do something I regret.
- Understand that my personhood may become hidden but is not lost.
- Place my needs before tasks and understand that we need to work together at my pace.
- Help me stay connected to what is important to me.

KNOW YOUR STRENGTHS

Later on, you'll read in-depth about areas of the brain that are often less affected by dementia. People with dementia can harness these areas of strength and use them to optimize their quality of life.

Having dementia doesn't automatically make people helpless and unable to do the things they used to do — or unable to learn new things. For many people with dementia, the disease progresses slowly, and they can continue to do most of the things they've always done.

As dementia progresses, gaps in memory and thinking will become more noticeable, but memory for well-established routines, habits and skills may be less affected or may not be affected until later on. For example, if you've mowed the lawn for decades or played a musical instrument since you were a teenager, it's very likely that these skills will remain for quite some time. Daily habits like brushing your teeth, walking on a treadmill or caring for a pet are other examples of things you may have done over and over. These are skills that may not be affected for quite some time.

This area of memory is known as procedural memory. As you learned earlier, it's the part of long-term memory that's responsible for knowing how to do things.

Because procedural memory is often less affected early on in dementia, this also means it's possible for people living with dementia to learn how to do new things through repetition. For example, you may be able to learn to sing a song you haven't heard before or learn your way around a new neighborhood or apartment. The key is to do the new task and repeat and practice it over a period of time. With practice, cues and reminders — like signs and notes — and help from family or friends, many people with dementia can continue to learn to do new things.

Many other strengths also may be retained for quite some time. These specific strengths are unique and based on past experiences, skills, jobs and interests.

Creativity and imagination also may be areas of strength. The ability to appreciate, produce and participate in art isn't significantly affected by dementia. That's because art involves brain functions that most dementias may not affect for quite some time, including vision, sense of touch and basic coordination. And because most art doesn't require specific memories or traditional language use, it allows people with dementia an opportunity to express feelings they may not be able to communicate verbally. This offers a wealth of opportunities.

The arts also engages intuition, curiosity and imagination, additional areas of strength for those living with dementia.

Even for people who've never been involved or interested in it before, the arts may be something enjoyable to take part in.

The following are just some of the many ways people living with dementia can participate in art:

- Listening to and enjoying music
- Singing and participating in a group sing or choir
- Enjoying movies, museums or cultural events
- Painting
- Drawing
- Sculpture
- Gardening
- Dancing
- Writing poetry
- Storytelling
- Discussing art

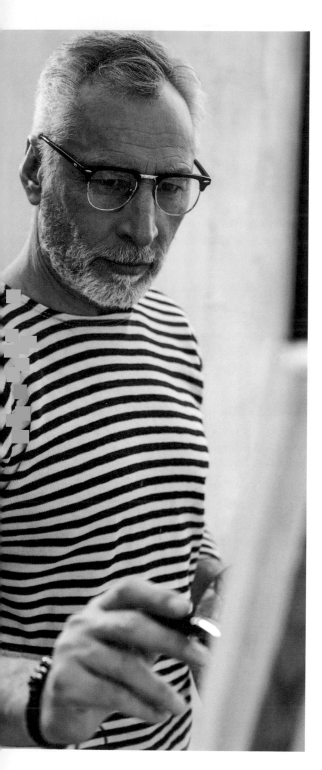

Take Mike, whose story you read earlier. Since his diagnosis, Mike has engaged in new hobbies. He's started to paint, and over time, he's developed a love of watercolor. With this new hobby, Mike now creates works of art for his grandchildren and friends. Mike's example illustrates that you can retain certain skills and learn new ones — dementia doesn't have to change that.

As dementia progresses, retained skills and areas of strength may change. Nonetheless, the person is still there. People living with dementia can still sense love, experience joy, and connect to what's going on moment to moment. Mike and others living with dementia offer an opportunity to appreciate the gift of present-moment living.

ACCOMMODATE CHANGING ABILITIES

Although having dementia doesn't automatically mean you can no longer do the things you used to do, in some cases, it may mean doing some things differently.

Here are several ways to accommodate abilities as they change over time.

Establish routine

Routine has benefits for everyone. It offers a sense of comfort, control and predictability. For someone living with dementia, all of this is extremely important. Routine can also reduce anxiety and stress, and it may help with maintaining function and promoting independence.

A daily schedule is a good place to start. It should list the activities that are consistent throughout the week, like mealtimes, medications, exercise and bedtime. Place the daily schedule where it will be easily seen. Hanging it in the kitchen and carrying it in a physical or electronic planner are two options. A care partner can help with a daily schedule, both in creating it and in offering reminders to look at it throughout the day.

Routines may also apply to the order in which tasks are completed. At night, for example, a routine may include enjoying a light snack, watching a favorite TV show, walking into the bathroom to brush your teeth, using the toilet and washing your hands. This may be followed by a prayer or meditation ritual and then going to bed.

Make changes as needed

After living with dementia for three years, Sean realized he could no longer do things in the same way he had in the past. However, he discovered that with simple changes, he could still enjoy them.

For example, Sean had always loved building things, but he could no longer make sense of a measuring tape. Instead, he uses string for measuring. Gardening is another example. Sean loves gardening, but he often forgets what he's planted or where he's planted it, so he takes photos to keep track. Sean also wears swimming goggles in the shower so that he can keep his eyes open to protect his balance.

Sean's examples illustrate how simple adaptations can make a significant difference in maintaining independence and quality of life for someone living with dementia.

Consider assistive technology

Mike uses online videos when he cooks, so he essentially has a virtual partner with him in the kitchen. The videos allow him to view each step, pause the instructions when he needs to or go back to repeat instructions. Mike is using the technology of video to help him do what he loves to do. For people living with dementia, technology can offer new ways to do things and help people do what they want to do by making the most of the skills they have. In addition, technology offers the opportunity to learn new skills.

Using technology to help people living with dementia isn't a new concept; it was first introduced about 20 years ago. Since then, many devices have been invented and revised to better meet the needs of people living with dementia.

What these devices do for people living with dementia isn't that different from how they help everyone in daily life. However, for people with dementia, these devices help make up for things that someone with dementia can no longer do, or no longer do as well, as easily or as safely.

Other assistive devices that aren't high-tech can help people with dementia, too. Sean's use of a simple piece of string for measuring is an example. Placing labels on cupboards and drawers can help people living with dementia remember where things are.

Assistive devices help people engage meaningfully in the world around them. They can boost quality of life for someone living with dementia.

Assistive devices have been created to help with a number of challenges people living with dementia face. Some devices, like calendar clocks, are low-tech; others, like automatic lighting, are high-tech.

Assistive devices can help with:

- Finding items like house keys
- Memory issues — for example, alarms and to-do lists that help people with remembering appointments and when to take medications
- Safety — door chimes, sensors and alarms; heat sensors; automatic shut-off systems for stoves; and fall monitoring systems
- Telling the month, day and time
- Self-care, including bathing and showering
- Establishing and maintaining a routine
- Finding information, including advice and support
- Preparing a meal
- Gardening
- Shopping
- Transportation and mobility

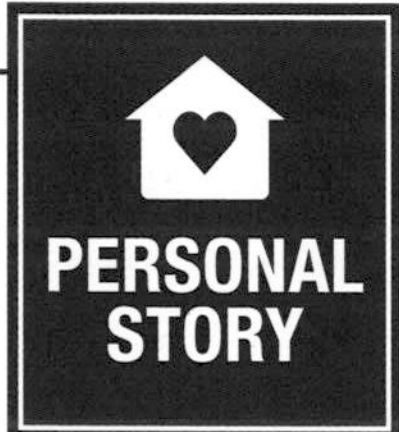

MAGGIE'S STORY

Maggie has dementia and has learned to rely on her next-door neighbor for help. Use her thoughts as encouragement to ask for help when you need it.

"My next-door neighbor is a real help," Maggie says. "She drops by every week to say hello and always has a few grocery items for me. If my husband is at work and I need help with anything, I can ask her. It's great to have someone close by to rely on."

- Communicating with others
- Making and receiving phone calls
- Answering questions — smart devices are designed for this

Set up your environment for success

A person's living environment also contributes to overall well-being. To this end, some modifications may be needed for safety and well-being.

An occupational therapist with expertise in dementia can help by offering a home assessment and recommending modifications.

Basic, but critical modifications include:

- Removing potentially dangerous items.
- Reducing clutter, which can contribute to disorientation.
- Making sure lighting is bright enough.
- Reducing excess stimulation. Too much noise from a television, for example, can lead to frustration or confusion.
- Posting visual cues like labels that identify where common objects are stored. Underwear, socks, toothbrush, coffee mugs, silverware, paper and pens are examples.
- Installing handrails along staircases and grab bars and shower seats in bathrooms to reduce the risk of falls.
- Using picture aids to serve as reminders. Instructions on to how to use the microwave or coffee maker are one example.
- Using memory aids, like message boards, that include your daily schedule and a care partner's schedule, along with contact and emergency information.

Ask for and accept help

If you need help, ask. This goes for people living with dementia and care partners. Asking for help is nothing to be ashamed of.

People with dementia can benefit from help from friends and relatives who can provide practical support and enable them to keep doing the things they've always done.

For people living with dementia, be open with others about your diagnosis — but also let people know you're still very much the same person you always have been. There's a balance to strike when it comes to help from others. If people offer to help, try to accept their offers. Doing so gives people the opportunity to show they care. At the same time, avoid letting people completely take over a task if it's not necessary. You may need to let people know it may take you a little longer to do some things.

AVOID ISOLATION

Social isolation is when a person lacks a sense of belonging, isn't engaging with others, lacks opportunities to interact with others, or doesn't have many social contacts or quality relationships.

Research highlights social isolation as a growing health epidemic, with health risks that have been compared to smoking 15 cigarettes a day. According to experts, social isolation is as harmful for health as obesity, high blood pressure and high cholesterol.

Among older adults, social isolation increases the risk of:

- Poor health practices
- Mental and emotional distress
- Neglect
- Being exploited
- Poorer health and well-being
- Depression

In people with dementia, less social contact has been linked to a more rapid decline in thinking and memory. Staying socially engaged and finding purpose are two important ways to avoid isolation. Here's more on each.

Stay socially engaged

Staying socially engaged is critically important for people with dementia. A growing body of research shows that taking part in social activities boosts self-esteem and feelings of confidence in one's own abilities. It also improves bonds with others, lessens feelings of loneliness, and can help lessen the need for medication.

Evidence also suggests that social health plays a significant role in helping people living with dementia manage their own lives. Social engagement has been shown to help people with dementia perform daily tasks, have less cognitive impairment and feel less depressed.

Earlier, Mike shared that he feels that one of the biggest reasons he's been able to live well with dementia is because he's stayed socially engaged. He believes that everyone diagnosed with dementia should leave their doctors' offices with a prescription for social engagement.

One final note on the importance of social engagement: A recent study asked more than 1,500 people with mild to moderate dementia to rate their quality of life, satisfaction with life and well-being. Researchers then compiled these ratings into what they called a living score — a reflection of their total health and quality of life. Social interaction topped the list.

Finding purpose

Connecting with others is closely tied to having a sense of purpose. Here's how one group of men living with dementia described how their needs for purpose and connection intersect:

A group of men gets together every month at the same restaurant for lunch. Each one of the men is living with dementia. When asked how they would describe their quality of life, with 1 being very poor and 10 being exceptional, not one man would give a specific number. Instead, they opted to give a range.

One said his quality of life ranges between a 3 and a 7. Another man in the group said his varies between a 2 and a 9. When asked what makes one day a 2 and another day an 8 or 9, one of the men said that a good day is

WAYS TO STAY ENGAGED

There are many ways people living with dementia can stay engaged socially. First, try to stay connected to the things you're already involved in. This may mean telling others about some of the changes they may notice and letting them know how you may need their help and support. From there, consider these ideas for staying socially engaged. The Additional resources section of this book offers more ideas, including contact information for various organizations.

- *Say yes to invitations.* Or ask friends to join you for coffee, lunch, a movie or a walk around your favorite park.
- *Make it routine.* Incorporate social connections into your routine most days of the week. Visit your children, grandchildren, friends and neighbors.
- *Volunteer.* This offers the chance to meet others who share similar interests and values. Schools, hospitals and local nonprofit organizations like your local Alzheimer's Association chapter are all options.
- *Take a class.* A local college or community education course can connect you with others who share similar hobbies or pursuits. It also gives you a chance to learn something new.
- *Join a group.* A book group or social club is a way to connect with others who share similar interests. Or you could try a support group. Support groups abound for people living with dementia, both online and in person. For example, you can search for Alzheimer's support groups in your area by visiting *www.alz.org/help-support/i-have-alz/programs-support*. Look to online resources for other specific forms of dementia that may offer similar resources. Dementia choirs offer another opportunity to connect with others.
- *Look online.* Social networking sites can help you stay connected. You may find online dementia groups that fit your needs and interests and give you an opportunity to connect with people having similar experiences to yours. Stick to reputable sites, and be cautious about in-person meetings. Find examples of online groups to try in the Additional resources section of this book.
- *Participate in your community.* Various services, social events and faith activities are all ideas. Or you may find trips sponsored by local community centers that pique your interest.

a day when he's able to contribute to someone or something in a meaningful way.

Most people with dementia say that their quality of life is less about remembering the details of an event a few days ago or remembering the name of friend. Instead, it's more about having strong supportive relationships and feeling respected, worthy and needed. This example illustrates just that.

Research on the science of well-being shows that people with a strong sense of purpose are more able to handle the ups and downs

LIVING WELL WITH DEMENTIA

Many basic, healthy habits that foster overall well-being are particularly helpful for people living with dementia. Here are several ways that people with dementia can nurture overall health.

Connect with your care team. Work with your doctor and other medical specialists involved in your care to monitor and respond to changes as they occur.

Listen to your body. Rest when you need to so that you can conserve your energy for times when you need it most.

Exercise. Regular physical activity keeps blood flowing and boosts the level of chemicals that naturally protect the brain. Learn more about the benefits of physical activity in Chapter 19.

Follow a healthy diet. Healthy-eating choices like those in the Mediterranean diet — rich in fruits, vegetables, olive oil, legumes, whole grains and fish — may help slow the progression of Alzheimer's disease and help people with Alzheimer's disease live longer. Learn more in Chapter 19.

Get regular, good-quality sleep. Getting good sleep benefits your body and your mind. Proper rest can help you respond to the challenges of living with dementia with greater perspective and understanding. Learn more about the benefits of good sleep and get tips for improving your sleep in Chapter 19.

of life. In essence, a person with a strong sense of purpose still feels good about life even in the face of difficulty. Nurturing a sense of purpose may involve activities that use skills you already have or that involve taking part in new activities.

If you need ways to reestablish purpose after a dementia diagnosis, ask yourself:

- What has brought meaning and purpose to my life in the past?
- What do I enjoy doing?
- What can I do at home or in my community that uses my strengths and taps into my interests?
- Are there new activities in my community I want to try?

Your answers to these questions are an important step toward reestablishing your purpose after a dementia diagnosis. Look to "Ways to stay engaged" on page 289 for more ideas. You may also find purpose by mentoring others, recording your life story, or writing a story, a memoir or poetry.

BE KIND TO YOURSELF

If you are living with dementia, you can — and will — experience losses, feel heartache, make mistakes and get frustrated. This is where self-compassion comes in. Being compassionate toward yourself is acknowledging that you're struggling and keeping a balanced perspective.

People with dementia can be wonderful grandparents and not remember the names of the grandchildren they adore. They can be with people they love and enjoy time together even if they can't follow the entire conversation. People with dementia can still be loving partners even if they no longer remember their spouse's birthday or can provide them the same level of support as in the past.

The key is not to blame yourself for your shortcomings and to give yourself the same kind of understanding and kindness you would a good friend. Everyone faces difficulties in life. It comes with being alive. Self-compassion is being kind to yourself when the going gets tough.

"MANY STRATEGIES CAN HELP SOMEONE WITH DEMENTIA HAVE A DIGNIFIED DEATH."

CHAPTER 15

Planning for the end of life

For many people, it's not easy to talk about death and dying. But conversations about these topics are incredibly important, not just for someone with a terminal illness, but for everyone. When someone is diagnosed with a condition that has an uncertain future, it's especially important to prepare for the end of life in ways that will honor an individual's values, preferences and wishes. It's difficult to know what someone wants at the end of life without talking about it ahead of time.

Talking about death and dying early on allows an individual the opportunity to have more control over his or her care, helps families make important decisions, and helps make the transition a little easier for everyone involved. Dementia makes these conversations even more critical — and more difficult.

In the later stages of dementia, a person's ability to think and share thoughts may be compromised. This makes it harder for someone with dementia to express his or her wishes. In turn, not knowing a person's preferences makes a difficult situation more challenging and stressful for loved ones.

For these reasons, planning for the best possible end-of-life experience, sooner rather than later, is critical. These conversations should include the person with dementia, care providers and loved ones.

Research shows that end-of-life conversations and advance care planning that's done soon after someone is diagnosed with dementia are positive and empowering, both for people living with dementia and their care partners. In this chapter, you'll learn how to have these important conversations.

STARTING THE CONVERSATION

If you're supporting someone with dementia, you may feel unsure about starting a conversation about end-of-life care. Or you may worry about how your loved one will react when you bring up the topic.

Rest assured that starting this conversation is an important way to show someone with dementia that you care. In fact, surveys show that most people *want* to talk about their end-of-life preferences and wish that loved ones would start the conversation.

Initiating this conversation shows that you share your loved one's concerns and worries and that you'll honor and respect your loved one's wishes as much as possible — especially if your loved one can no longer make decisions for himself or herself.

While surveys show that most people find it important to talk about end-of-life care and want to talk about their wishes, these conversations don't always go smoothly. Long before you start this conversation, it can help to make sure that your loved one feels comfortable talking about these important and sensitive issues with you.

For example, when a person with dementia expresses fear, sadness or loss about not being able to do certain things, this can be a natural opening to talk more about these feelings. Talking about feelings early on establishes trust and connection that can help you discuss end-of-life wishes later on. If a

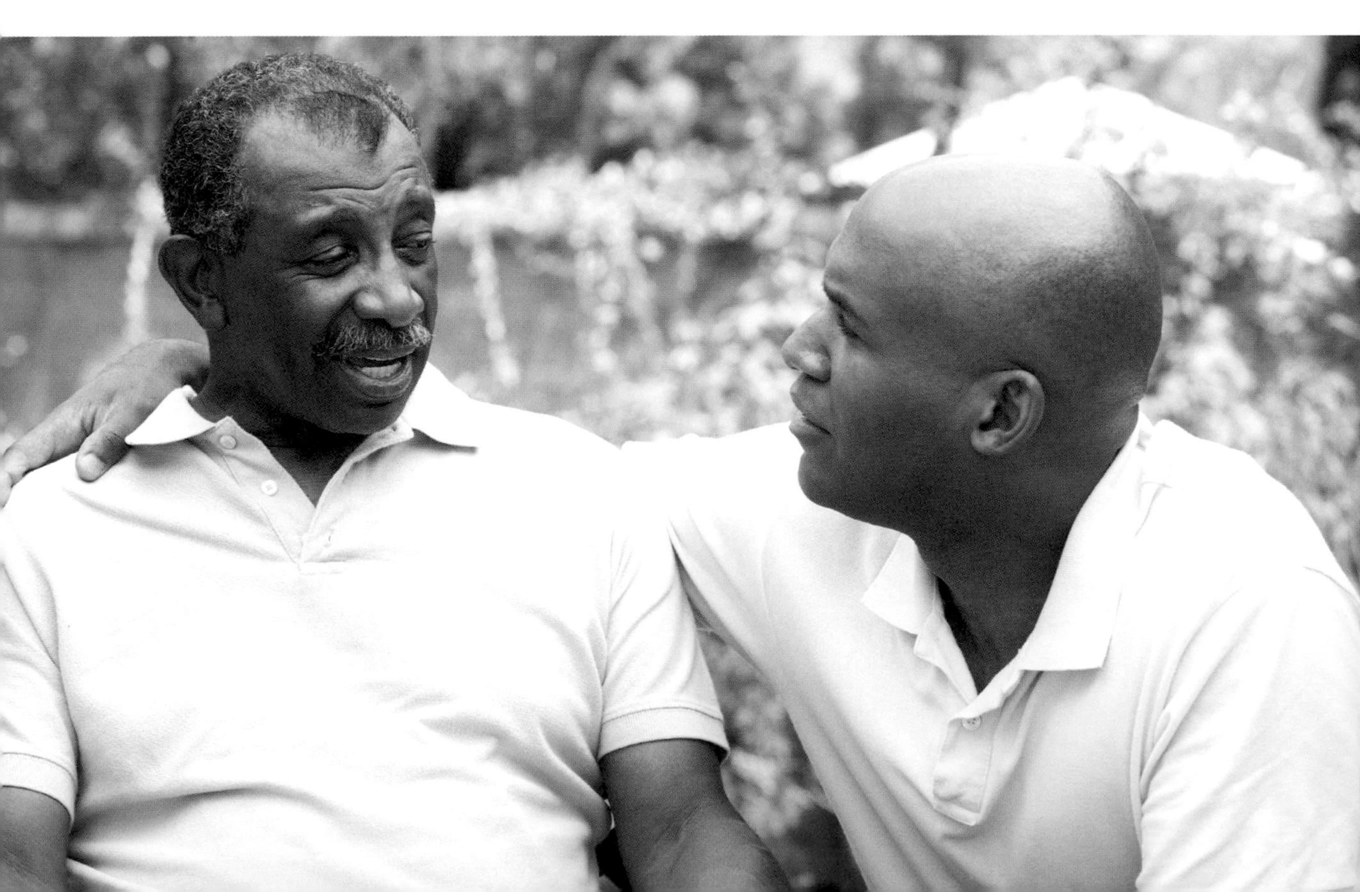

family member has recently declined in health or died, this may also open up an opportunity to reflect on that person's care or the circumstances around the death. This may help guide the conversation around what care a person may want — or may not want — near the end of life.

Even with this groundwork, it can be hard to know when and how to talk about the end of life. Adjusting your conversation style and content can help.

For example, depending on the person and the type of dementia, open-ended questions may be too vague. Instead, you may need to ask a question and then offer options or choices. You may also want to start the conversation at a time when the person with dementia is doing well with remembering things like distant memories. In this way, you could reflect on the death of a friend or a family member.

Try to understand the whole person by having conversations that explore the person's values, beliefs and preferences. Knowing a person's values can help you make decisions in the future in the event that a person's exact wishes aren't clear. It can also be helpful to have several conversations over a period of time and keep them short and simple.

Above all, make it clear that talking about the end of life is as much for you as it is for your loved one. This goes a long way in establishing a caring connection that allows you to have this important conversation.

Questions to consider

Advance care planning is a dynamic process that involves discussing and documenting an individual's wishes, values and preferences around care and treatment. These discussions are held between an individual and the individual's family members and care providers. Even people who are healthy can — and should — engage in advance care planning. It's never too soon to make an advance care plan.

Advance care planning involves:

- Sharing personal values with loved ones and care providers
- Getting information on different types of life-sustaining treatments
- Deciding what types of treatment an individual would want or not want after being diagnosed with a life-limiting illness or at the end of life
- Completing useful documents that put an individual's care preferences into writing in the event that the individual is unable to speak for himself or herself

Advance care planning also requires conversations important questions like these:

- What makes life worth living?
- Which is more important, your quality of life or how long you live?
- What does quality of life mean to you? Does it mean being able to care for yourself? Does it mean recognizing others?
- Who do you want to make decisions for you if you can't speak for yourself? Your spouse or partner, an adult child or a trusted friend are examples.

- Would you want life-sustaining measures in the last stages of dementia or as you're dying? For example, would you want CPR if your heart stopped beating?
- Where do you want to spend your last days if you're ill? At home? At a nursing home? In a hospital?
- If you knew your life was coming to an end, what would bring you comfort and make dying feel safe? Who would you want to be with you?
- What are your beliefs about the end of life? How do you want them to be respected and honored?

This may also be a good opportunity to consider funeral and burial plans. Burial versus cremation, choosing a final resting place, and details about a funeral or memorial service are all helpful topics to discuss. Choosing a brain autopsy or a brain donation may be part of this process; these decisions may affect when and how arrangements are made after death.

Putting preferences in writing

After having these conversations, it's important to document the answers to these questions. This is where advance directives can help.

Living wills and other advance directives are written, legal instructions that spell out your preferences for medical care if you're unable to make decisions for yourself. These documents help people with dementia and their care partners make decisions about end-of-life care. These documents —

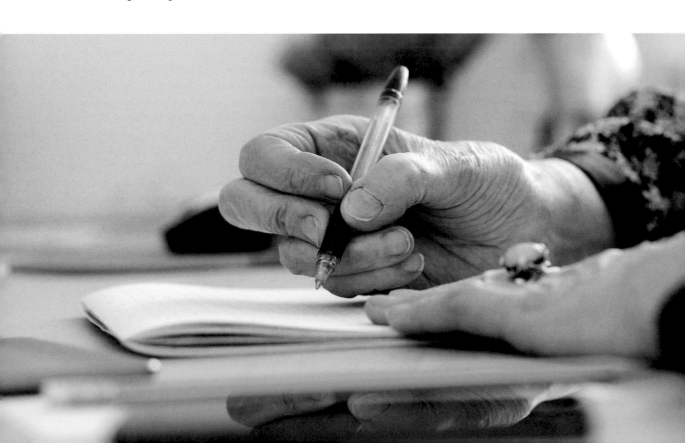

and the conversations around them — help make sure that a person's wishes are spelled out and honored.

In the U.S., each state has different forms and requirements for creating advance directives, but they must be in writing. The documents may also need to be signed by a witness or notarized. Links to state-specific forms can be found on the websites of various organizations, like the American Bar Association, AARP, and the National Hospice and Palliative Care Organization. Learn more in the Additional resources section.

Once these forms are completed, review them with family or other trusted individuals, as well as your health care team. Keep them in an accessible place and make sure your doctor and others involved in making decisions for your care have a copy. Here's more on each of these documents.

Living will This legal document spells out what medical treatments you want and don't want to be used to keep you alive. It may also include preferences for other medical decisions, like pain management and organ donation. A living will only goes into effect if you're at the end of life.

Whether you want CPR if your heart stops beating, whether you want a machine to keep you breathing, and whether you want a tube used to feed you if you can no longer eat are examples of decisions you would spell out in a living will. If you'd like your body to be donated to science for further study, you can specify it in a living will.

Power of attorney This legal document gives someone you choose the power to make decisions for you if you're unable to do so.

A living will and power of attorney are documents that ensure a person's wishes are respected. However, a power of attorney document is more flexible because the person who is named in the document can make decisions about care that a living will may not address.

The person named in the power of attorney document may be may be a spouse, another family member, a friend or a member of a faith community. It may also help to choose one or more alternates in the event that the person named in this document is unable to fulfill the role.

A person selected to fill this role should be someone trustworthy who's comfortable talking about medical care and end-of-life issues. It's important to choose an individual who can voice your preferences to your health care team and loved ones. This person shouldn't be your doctor or another member of your health care team.

PALLIATIVE CARE AND HOSPICE CARE

Palliative care and hospice care are two terms you'll likely hear in conversations around end-of-life care. It's helpful for people living with dementia and their families and care partners to understand these terms.

Palliative care

Palliative care is specialized care that focuses on providing relief from pain and other symptoms of a serious illness. An interdisciplinary health care team works together to provide medical and emotional support that allows a person with dementia to live optimally with the disease.

This type of care isn't just for people who may die soon. It can be offered to people of any age who have a serious or life-threatening illness, no matter the diagnosis or stage of disease.

Improving quality of life for people living with dementia and their families is the goal of palliative care. This form of care is offered alongside other treatments to provide an extra layer of support.

Hospice care

Hospice care is for people who are nearing the end of life. Services are provided by a team of health care professionals who maximize comfort for a person who is terminally ill. They reduce pain and address physical, psychological, social and spiritual needs. Hospice care also offers counseling, respite care and practical support to families.

The focus of hospice care is to support the highest quality of life possible for whatever time remains. Hospice care is for a terminally ill person who's expected to have six months or less to live, but it can be provided for as long as the person's doctor and hospice care team certify that the condition remains life-limiting.

Most hospice care is provided at home, with a family member typically serving as the primary caregiver. However, hospice care is also available at hospitals, nursing homes, assisted living facilities and dedicated hospice facilities.

DEMENTIA'S EFFECTS AT THE END OF LIFE

As you've learned, dementia is a syndrome that causes memory, thinking, behavior and the ability to perform everyday activities to worsen over time. Because people often live with Alzheimer's disease and related dementias for years, it can be hard to think of them as terminal conditions, but they do ultimately lead to death.

It's impossible to predict how quickly dementia will progress, and the end-of-life experience is different for every person. This can make it hard to know when someone is experiencing the symptoms of late-stage dementia. Here are several common signs and symptoms of dementia at the end of life:

- Severe memory loss, such as the inability to identify family or common objects or lost awareness of recent activity
- Inability to move around, walk or sit
- Inability to speak or make oneself understood
- Inability to perform all or most activities of daily living without help, including

bathing, grooming and going to the bathroom
- Loss of appetite, difficulty swallowing and other eating problems
- Changes in breathing, often near the end of life, including shortness of breath (dyspnea)
- Excessive sleepiness
- Seizures and frequent infections, especially pneumonia
- Restlessness

MAKING DECISIONS FOR SOMEONE WITH DEMENTIA

It can be challenging and overwhelming to have to make medical decisions for someone who can no longer make these decisions for himself or herself. In the best circumstances, you'll have written documents that spell out the person's wishes. However, even when you have written documents, decisions aren't always clear.

In these situations, it can help to put yourself in the place of the person who's dying and try to imagine what he or she would do. The other approach is to decide what's in the best interest of the person who's dying, given the circumstances and what you know about the person. In these situations, even if one family member is named as the decision-maker, it's a good idea to include the whole family and other trusted individuals in the decision-making process.

Here are some of the medical decisions you may face with advanced dementia.

Feeding tubes

Tube feeding is sometimes suggested if a person has a hard time eating or swallowing — for example, after a stroke. Tube feeding generally isn't recommended for people with dementia even though trouble swallowing may develop in late stages. Tube feeding hasn't been proved to benefit or extend life for people with dementia, and it can lead to infections and cause discomfort. Before making a decision about feeding tubes, it's best to talk with the health care team about specific plans for the use of feeding tubes.

Antibiotics

Antibiotics may be prescribed for common infections. However, they may not improve the person's condition. Again, it's best to weigh the pros and cons of using antibiotics with health care professionals, should the need arise.

Intravenous (IV) hydration

IV hydration is used to give a person liquid through a needle in a vein. Dehydration is a normal part of the dying process; it allows for a more comfortable death over a period of days. IV hydration can cause uncomfortable fluid retention and swelling and draw out the dying process for weeks, which may put a burden on the person who's dying. If IV hydration is considered, it's best if it's used for a limited time period for specific goals — and only if the family and health care team agree that it's best for the person with dementia.

Cardiopulmonary resuscitation (CPR)

CPR is emergency treatment used to restore a person's heartbeat or breathing if it stops. Many experts do not recommend CPR for people who are terminally ill, and people faced with a terminal illness who can speak for themselves often don't want CPR if their heart or breathing stops. Do not resuscitate (DNR) and do not attempt resuscitation (DNAR) orders tell the health care team not to perform CPR if the person's breathing or heartbeat stops.

Regardless of the options chosen, it's important to continue to maintain the person's dignity and privacy. Advice from a doctor, other specialists and members of a hospice team are important.

OFFERING PERSON-CENTERED CARE

For people with dementia and care partners alike, care at the end of life involves meeting a variety of physical, emotional, social, spiritual and practical needs. For people with dementia, research suggests that the most important facets of a good end-of-life experience are physical, pain-free comfort; emotional and spiritual well-being; family involvement and a peaceful environment.

Emotional support, for example, may be as simple as a gentle, reassuring touch. It also involves feeling respected, a need to be with others, a need to feel understood and reassured, and a need to feel loved. Being treated not as an object but as a person who is still aware of the world is vital.

Connection is critical. It's not only still possible for those with dementia at the end of life, but also essential. Your caring attention and presence are among the most important things you can give someone who's dying.

Continue to communicate with the person, even if you think the person doesn't understand. Communication provides stimulation and can help the person with dementia feel reassured and included. Your tone of voice, body language and facial expressions are forms of nonverbal communication that can still be understood by the person with dementia and allow you to connect even when the person's ability to understand words and language is lost.

Research shows that at the end of life, a person continues to connect to the world mostly through the senses. This makes touch, sound, sight, taste and smell all powerful ways to connect with a person at the end of life and provide comfort at the same time. Bring in a beloved item for the person to hold, play the person's favorite music, rub lotion with the person's favorite scent on the skin, brush the person's hair, or read something aloud that has meaning to the person, like certain religious passages.

Use what you know about the person, including hobbies and interests from the past. Photos, treasured objects and memorabilia can all be helpful.

Providing comfort at the end of life

Many strategies can help someone with dementia have a dignified death. For someone who's no longer eating or drinking, for example, it can help to keep a person's mouth moist with ice chips or a sponge. Applying lip balm or petroleum jelly to the lips also can help.

Other ways to provide comfort at the end of life include placing pillows behind the person's head to help with labored breathing. Incontinence pads or a catheter helps keep a person with loss of bladder control dry and clean. For cold hands and feet, turning up the heat and providing warm blankets can offer additional comfort.

While not everyone experiences pain when dying, many people do. With dementia, many people aren't prescribed enough pain relief simply because they may not be able to communicate that they're in pain. Pain medications offer another opportunity to improve the end-of-life experience for people with dementia. Experts believe that care for someone who is dying should focus on relieving pain. Pain is easier to prevent than relieve, and overwhelming pain is hard to manage. For those who can't verbally communicate, direct observation can help identify pain and pain behaviors.

A variety of signs can signal discomfort in a person with dementia at the end of life.

JIM'S LAST DAYS

Jim loved to garden and enjoyed mowing his lawn. In the days before his death, Jim had his hands in the soil in the raised flower beds he tended. The staff at his assisted living facility brought in grass cuttings so he could feel and smell the grass that brought him so much comfort. Jim died with his family surrounding him and his grandchildren playing on the floor beside him.

Signs that someone is in pain include:

- Agitation
- Increased confusion or lack of responsiveness
- Yelling or calling out
- Grimacing or teeth grinding
- Scratching or picking at skin or other body parts
- Excessive sweating
- Drooling
- Striking out or other physical gestures or distress

You may wonder if your loved one is aware of what's going on in this last stage of illness. Although the body and mind are in the process of shutting down, a person with dementia still may be aware of your presence, your care and your affection.

COPING WITH DEATH

When a person with dementia dies, it's common for a care partner to experience many emotions. Loss, depression, anxiety, guilt, frustration and hopelessness are all examples. Many of these feelings can appear even before the person with dementia dies. Emotions are often intense, even for care partners who have anticipated and prepared for the death of their loved one.

The next several chapters are dedicated to the care partner experience and offer more details on the emotions related to supporting someone with dementia. For now, here are of some of the experiences families face after the death of a loved one.

Grief

While grief happens at the end of life, it's also common throughout the dementia process. Learn more about grief in Chapter 18.

Grief can be defined as the process of adjusting to loss. While the grieving process is a gradual one, grief brings on powerfully intense feelings and emotions.

The process of allowing yourself to grieve brings about emotional healing and helps you to adjust to a new life situation. Use these recommendations to help support the grieving process:

- Don't try to rush through the grieving process. Many people say they need at least two years to begin feeling "normal" after the death of a loved one. Be gentle with yourself during this time.
- Practice good self-care. Focus on your nutrition, physical activity and sleep.
- Be open with others about what you're experiencing. Your family and friends may avoid the topic, so giving them permission to open up and talk about the loss with you may be helpful.
- Avoid making major decisions for at least a year. This is a period of time when you may still feel unsettled and in shock.
- Follow your normal routine as much as possible, but let others help you with daily tasks. People will want to help you, but they may not know how.
- Acknowledge your emotions. The idea isn't to get caught up in negative or unpleasant feelings but to see what you're

experiencing as normal. Accepting emotions helps to lessen their harsh quality and intensity.
- Reduce any guilt you may feel by trying to keep a realistic view of your past actions and present emotions. Don't focus on what you wish could have been better or what could have been done differently. Believe that you did the best you could and that what you did was enough.
- Accept fear as a normal part of the grieving process. Rather than isolate yourself, stay socially connected to help ease fear.

In the final stage of the grieving process, focusing on the past and seeking an explanation for death often dissolves. This is when you can start to focus on living life the best way possible and look for ways to grow from this experience.

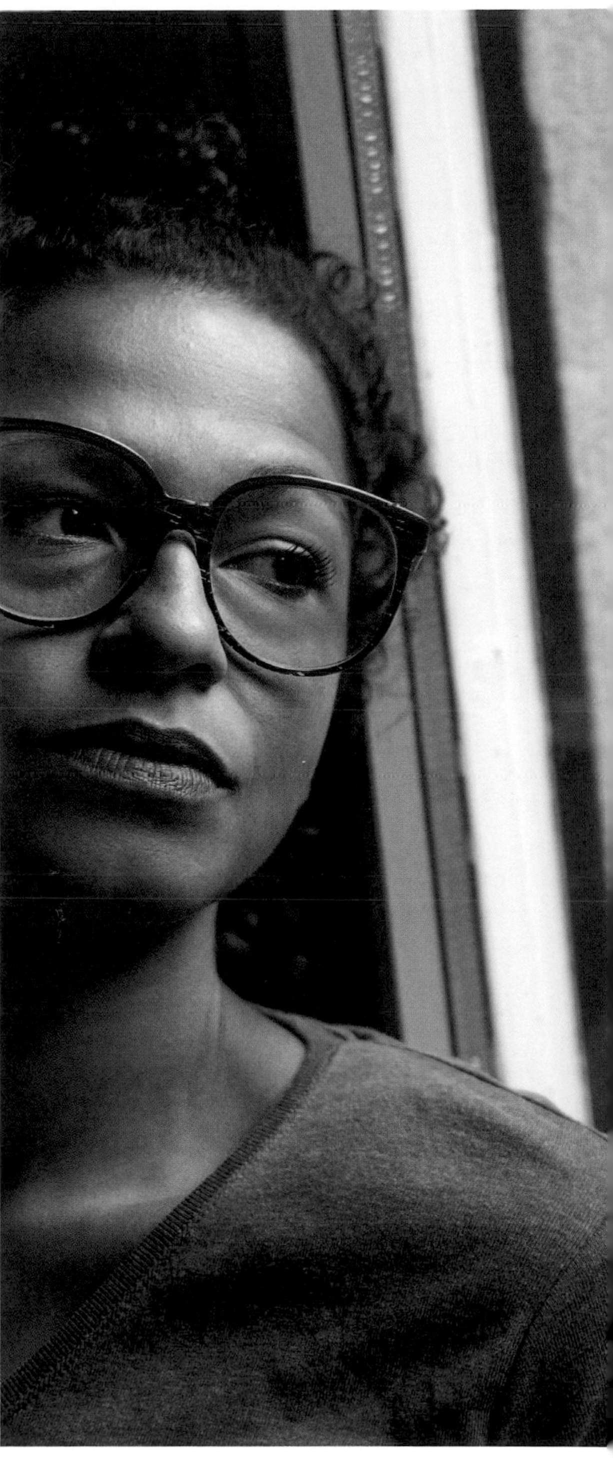

Relief

Some families and care partners experience a feeling of relief — and it's often uncomfortable. It can catch you off guard and feel overwhelming. You may feel guilty when you experience relief.

It's important to know that feeling a sense of relief is normal and natural. In fact, in one study, nearly three-quarters of family caregivers say they felt relieved when an individual with dementia died.

Feeling relief doesn't mean you didn't care about the person with dementia. Instead, relief is a natural response to knowing that the person with dementia is no longer suffering — and that you no longer have to watch someone you care about live with the losses associated with dementia.

You may also feel relief because the strain and intensity of being a care partner is lifted. The ability to return to roles you had before becoming a care partner can also bring about feelings of relief.

Feelings of relief are not only normal but also helpful. Some research shows that feelings of relief can actually help care partners grieve more effectively and adjust to life after the person with dementia has died. This is especially true for care partners who felt relatively prepared for the person's death ahead of time.

Loss of identity

For many, the caregiving role lasts several years or much longer, so when the death of their loved one occurs, life can change drastically. There can be an intense feeling of losing both the person, as well as a part of who you had become in the caregiving role. Former care partners not only grieve their loved one but also may grieve the loss of the caregiving role. Care partners may find themselves questioning their identity, asking themselves, *Who am I now? Where do I go from here? How do I fill my days and find a sense of purpose?*

In one study, care partners described the post-caregiving phase as a process of learning to live again. Accustomed to days filled with caregiving responsibilities, care partners recalled not knowing how to proceed with life as they grappled with how to use their free time. Some said they had trouble giving up their role as a care partner after years of identifying with this role.

It's important for care partners to give themselves the space, time and resources they need to adjust to yet another new normal. It's helpful to acknowledge this shift in their life and the feelings it may evoke. A care partner may find it therapeutic to write in a journal or share feelings with others in a support group.

Dementia brings life-altering changes to those who experience it, and in many ways, life will never be the same. Acknowledging these changes can offer a sense of peace and healing for care partners and families.

Although it isn't easy to move forward, people who've lost a loved one to dementia can make the choice to focus on the future and learn to live again.

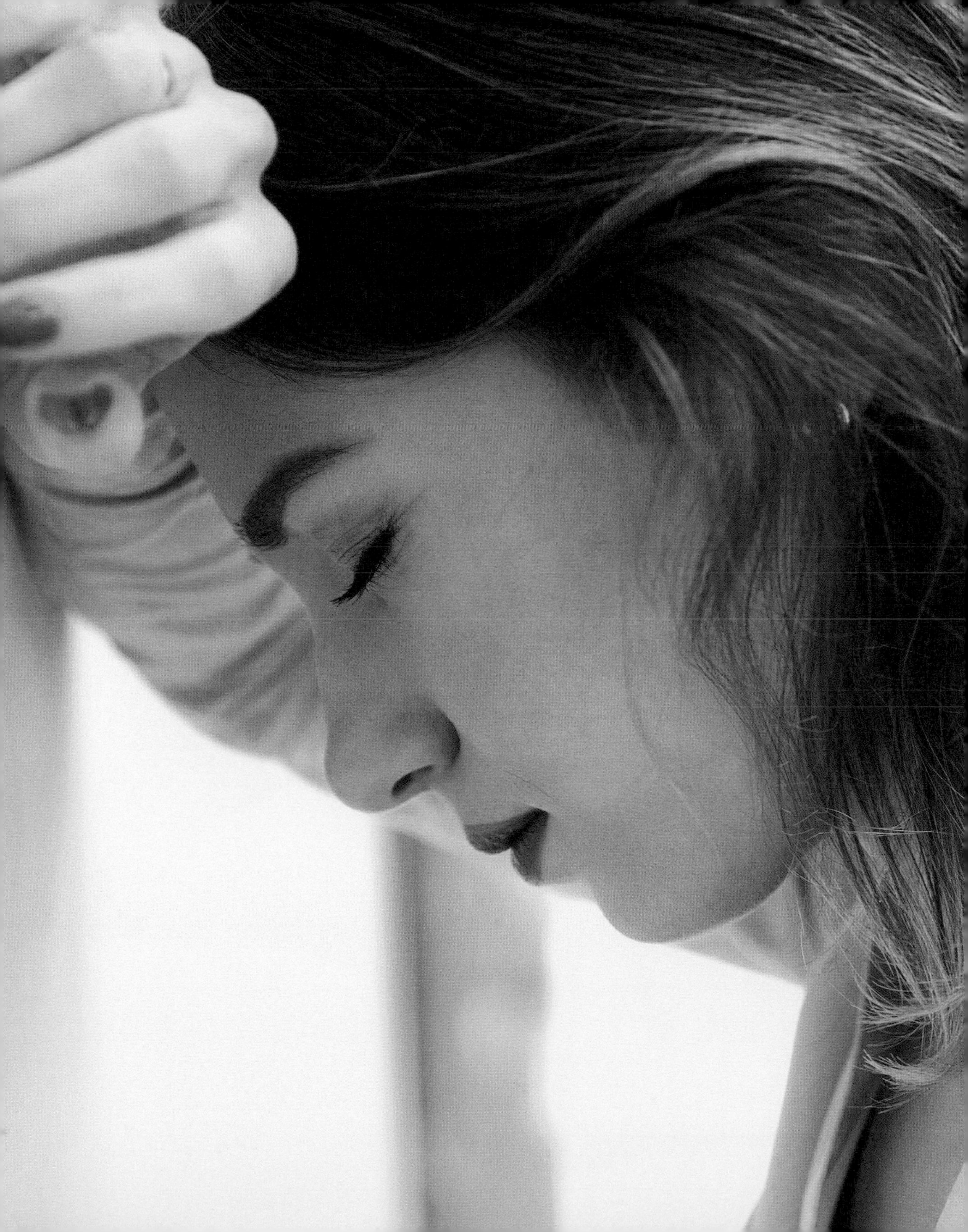

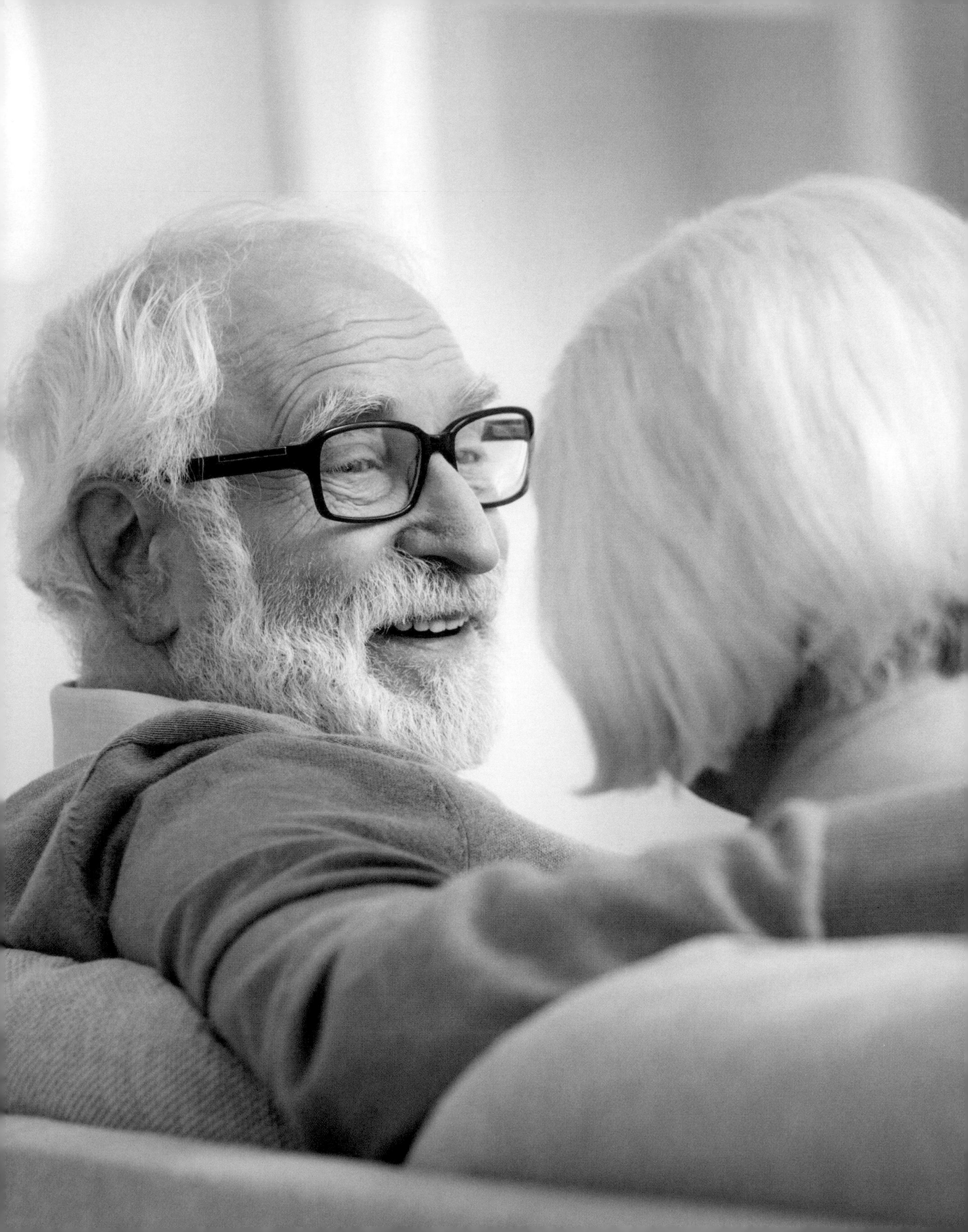

PART 5

Life as a care partner

I was 55; John was 57. The first inkling that something was wrong started with John's ability to drive. Prior to GPS navigation, he could find his way anywhere, with or without a map. He became confused when driving to familiar locations and at stop signs and traffic lights, not stopping — or stopping half a block too soon. John was also experiencing wild dreams — he would twitch, shout, toss and pound on the bed. He'd often say he was fighting off a bear.

We scheduled an appointment with John's doctor. After several days of testing, John was diagnosed with mild cognitive impairment and REM sleep disorder. Feelings of disbelief and fear overwhelmed us.

When we got home, we called our children. I was a basket case. I couldn't sleep or eat. In my head, I went directly from the mild cognitive impairment diagnosis John had received to the final stage of dementia. John and I have been happy together for years. It's not to say we've felt that way every day, but on the whole, we simply love being together. John makes me laugh. I make him laugh. Would we laugh again? I felt like I was in quicksand and couldn't find solid ground.

This short reflection from Rosalie depicts just one person's story, yet it paints a picture of the surge of emotions and uncertainty many care partners feel when a dementia diagnosis is given. What care partners may not know when dementia is diagnosed is that the road ahead can also be an opportunity for growth, with lessons in empathy, patience and acceptance.

The next few chapters address care partners directly, offering guidance and hope to lean on as care partners look after their own health and well-being.

"YOUR NEW ROLE IN YOUR LOVED ONE'S LIFE CAN GIVE YOU THE CHANCE TO CREATE A NEW — AND MAYBE EVEN BETTER — RELATIONSHIP."

CHAPTER 16

Who are caregivers?

When Nick was diagnosed with Alzheimer's disease, the doctor turned to his wife, Marie, and referred to her as his caregiver. Marie was rattled. "I'm Nick's wife," she said. "When did that change?"

When does the label *caregiver* replace *wife*? If your husband or wife is diagnosed with dementia, do you leave the doctor's office with a new label, title and role? When do spouses label themselves as caregivers?

To a large degree, people rely on labels to define themselves. Labels connect people to their identities and self-worth: wife, husband, father, daughter, artist, vegetarian.

Often, these labels don't necessarily reflect who people are as much as what they do, what their social status is, or how they function in life. In a society that puts so much emphasis on the desire to be something, each person grapples with figuring out exactly who he or she is in relation to the world. Even more important, the language or words people use to describe themselves influence their thoughts, their emotions, their expectations and their behaviors.

In Marie's case, instead of *being* a caregiver, she may choose to see herself as a wife in a caring or supportive role — a care partner or support partner. Like Marie, most people don't want caregiving to define who they are. However, identifying as a caregiver or a care partner may actually be a good thing.

By identifying yourself in this way, you start to pay attention to information, resources and services that can help you. Most importantly, you become part of a larger group of people with common issues, needs and

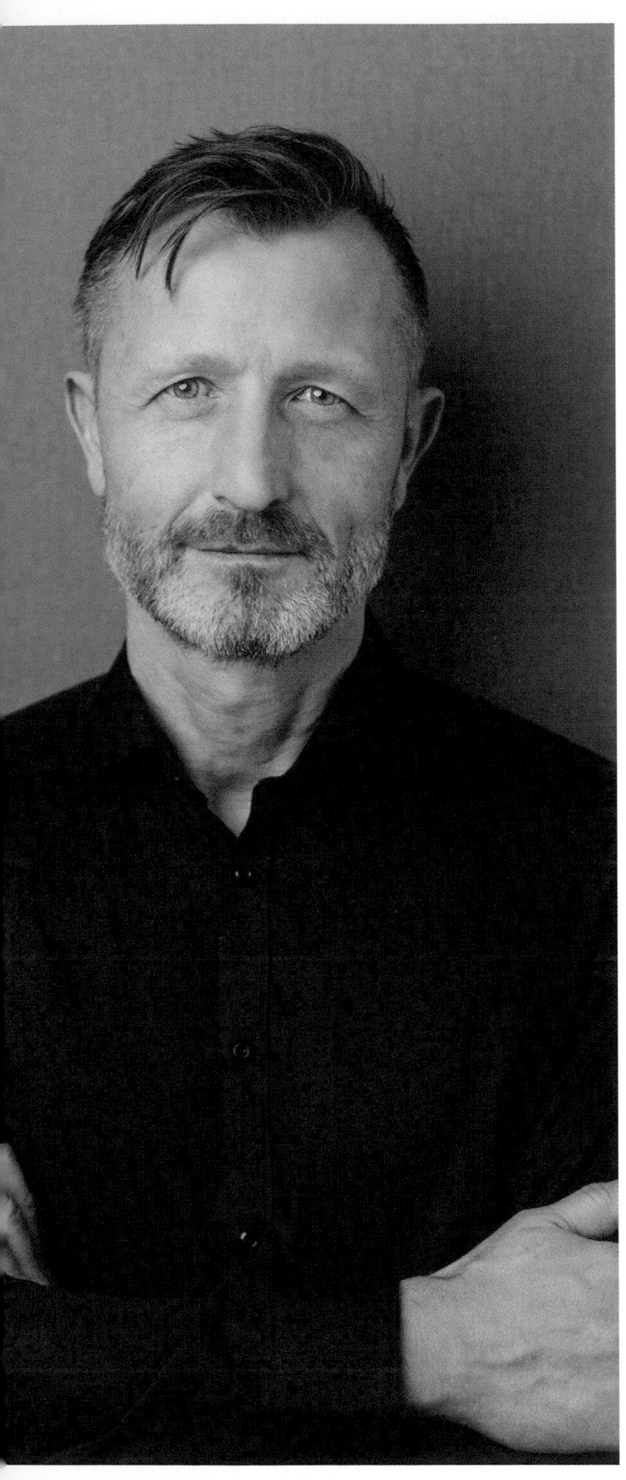

concerns. You begin to build recognition not of who you are, but of what you do. When you can name and label a role that you have, you can validate your experiences and nurture your feelings.

By calling yourself a care partner, you're saying to the world, "Here I am. Acknowledge me, hear me, support me. I matter."

CHALLENGES, POSITIVE EFFECTS

Most people who care for those living with dementia are spouses, adult children, and other relatives and friends. These people are referred to as informal or family caregivers.

Across the United States, family members, friends, and other unpaid care partners are contributing billions of hours to the care of loved ones living with Alzheimer's disease or other dementias.

Among these care partners, approximately two-thirds are women and about a third are 65 or older. Around half of all care partners are caring for a parent. About 1 in 4 belongs to the sandwich generation. People in this group are caring for both an older adult and children under 18.

Care partners provide support in a variety of ways. They may help with activities of daily living, from household chores, meal preparation and transportation to bathing, dressing and grooming. They may need to help ensure that medications are being taken correctly and other treatment regimens are being followed. They provide emotional support and may need to address changing behaviors like confusion and nighttime disturbances. Care partners may also hire and oversee paid care for their loved one in the home or in other care communities.

These supportive tasks can take a toll on a care partner, especially as the disease progresses. Compared with those who care for people living with other conditions and illnesses, dementia care partners may be more likely to experience emotional stress, anxiety and depression. This is particularly true when the person living with dementia is a spouse.

Because caring for someone with dementia can lead to chronic stress, care partners may experience a variety of health problems. Poor sleep, a weaker immune system, high blood pressure (hypertension) and heart disease are examples. Care partners may also be more at risk of developing cognitive issues, including memory decline. On the other hand, many people caring for someone with dementia say that their own health is excellent or very good.

Despite its challenges, being a care partner may have some positive effects. Playing such a vital role in a loved one's life can be deeply gratifying.

Many care partners feel a sense of accomplishment and purpose and say that they have experienced positive personal growth. In two recent surveys, most care partners said that although caring for someone with

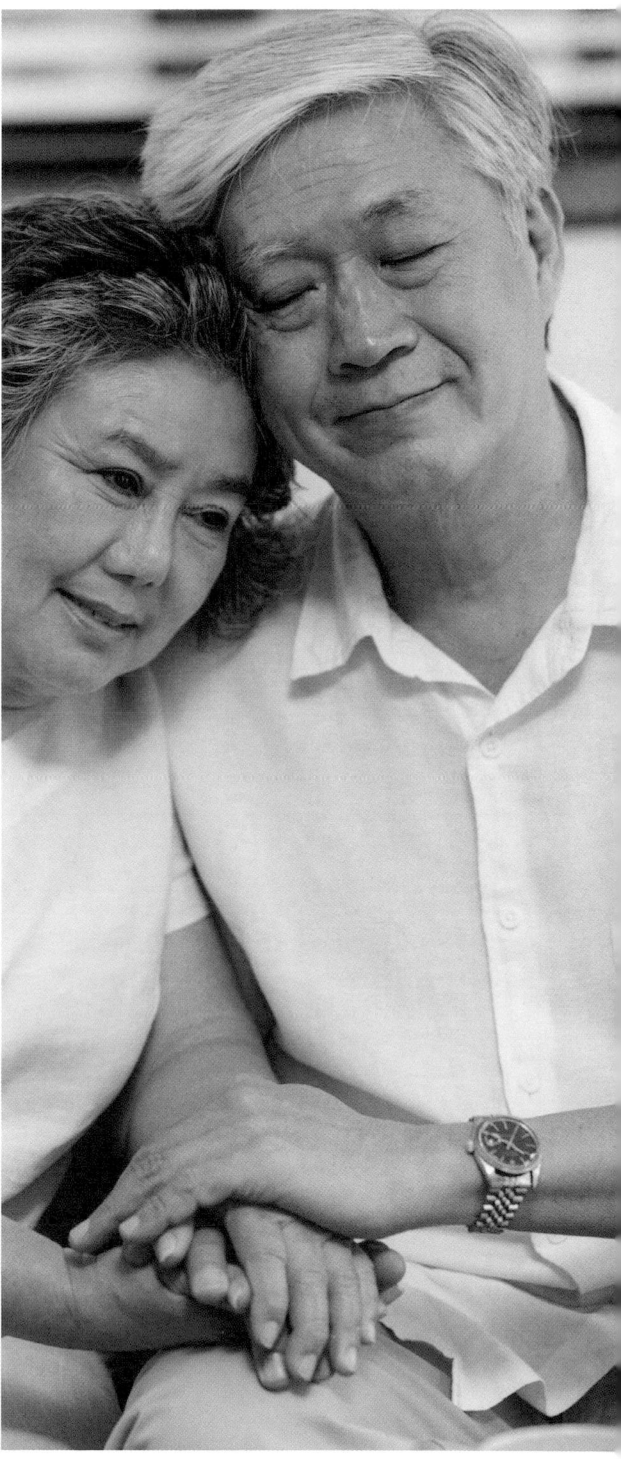

CAREGIVERS VS. CARE PARTNERS

You've likely noticed that this book often uses the terms *care partner* and *caregiver.* The term *care partner* acknowledges the reciprocal relationship that can continue to exist between a person with dementia and a spouse, partner or other relative.

Learning to approach support and caring as a partnership means seeing the person with dementia as a whole human being and not making assumptions based on a diagnosis or label. It means including the person with dementia in decision-making. It also means making adaptations so people living with dementia can continue to live life to the best of their abilities.

The term *caregiver* better describes a role in which the caring responsibility moves to a place beyond partnering and includes more "care giving." The person with dementia is just as much of an individual as before, but has become more dependent on the care of another.

LONG-DISTANCE SUPPORT

Even if you live far away, your support can be critical to a primary care partner's ability to function and cope. Stay in frequent contact with the care partner by telephone, text, email or video chat. Send cards and letters of support. Try to visit and offer some respite, if that would be helpful. Ask how, specifically, you can be helpful. The most important way to support a care partner may be by not passing judgment on his or her decisions. Listen closely and ask questions about the situation, but don't assume you know everything that's happening. Your emotional support and encouragement alone are valuable.

Alzheimer's disease or other dementias is demanding, it's also rewarding, fulfilling and meaningful. Many care partners also say that the experience has brought them closer to the person living with dementia and to other family members.

AN UNREQUESTED ROLE

When a parent or spouse develops dementia, it naturally begins to change the dynamics of your relationship.

You may feel scared, uncertain or even resentful. You may feel as if you've been plunged into a role you never asked for and don't feel prepared to take on. Your loved one with dementia is also likely dealing with this shift in roles and the impact it might have on the relationship.

Adapting to the role of care partner has many dimensions, depending on how your relationship has functioned in the past. In time, you may need to assume responsibilities your loved one has taken pride in handling. For example, you may need to start paying the bills, mowing the lawn or grocery shopping. If those tasks weren't your responsibility before, this can be a challenge.

You may also become responsible for matters that your loved one considers personal and private. Adult children, in particular, often hesitate to make decisions for parents, including moving them from a private home to an assisted-living community.

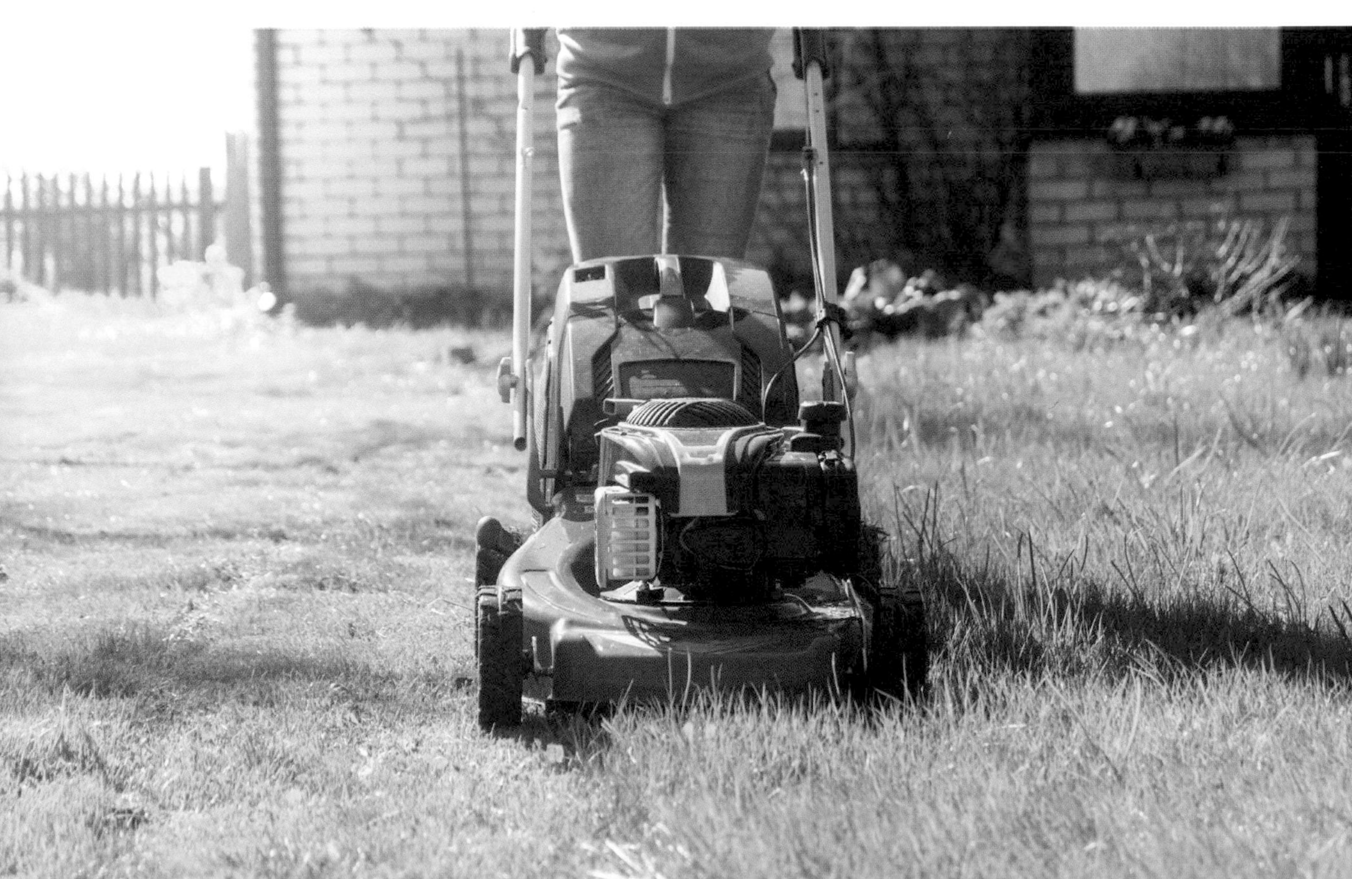

THE TERM 'LOVED ONE'

Care partners experience their roles in different ways depending on many factors involved in their relationships with someone living with dementia. Caring for a spouse you have a loving relationship with is one example of a care partner relationship. For this reason, you'll notice that people living with dementia are sometimes referred to as loved ones. In many cases, the person with dementia that you're caring for is, indeed, someone you love.

In other cases, however, the term *loved one* doesn't quite fit a care partner's unique situation. There are many other types of relationships care partners find themselves in. For example, you may be providing care and support to someone you've had an estranged or troubled relationship with.

For this reason, you'll see the terms *loved one* and *person living with dementia* used interchangeably to represent the breadth of relationships that care partners have with those living with dementia.

Taking on this new role as a care partner doesn't mean the end to a relationship, only that the relationship will change, as all relationships do over time. Adapting to these changes requires emotional adjustments. Take heart in knowing that others have walked in your shoes and experienced similar feelings. Find hope in knowing that some care partners have not only adapted to their roles as care partners but have also discovered an inner strength, patience and resiliency they didn't know they had.

What if the past relationship between a care partner and the person with dementia has been rocky? Certainly, previous differences will impact how you think about the care partner role now.

Although it's never easy, it's important to let go of the past and those feelings and thoughts that no longer serve you. They will only sap your energy and weigh you down. When you make the choice to let go of a negative past and work toward accepting the way life is today, things can improve.

Your new role in your loved one's life can give you the chance to create a new — and maybe even improved — relationship.

INTIMACY

Expressions of affection, whether sexual or nonsexual, are essential for the well-being of both you and your loved one. The need for closeness doesn't lessen with age or with cognitive decline. Yet like any relationship, the connection you share with your spouse or partner is complex and ever-changing.

You may notice that the effects of the disease or its treatment cause your loved one to experience an increase or decrease in sex drive. At the same time, you may feel a range of emotions about sexual intimacy in your relationship.

If your loved one shows less interest in sex, you might feel rejected or lonely. In contrast, you may be feeling guilt if your desire to interact sexually with your loved one wanes as the disease progresses. It's common for a caregiver to lose sexual desire for a spouse who has dementia for many reasons, including the demands of the caregiver role and the transition from intimate partner to caregiver. Caregivers should not feel guilty if their sexual desire has changed.

If you're experiencing difficult or conflicting feelings, it can help to talk about them with your spouse or partner. Build a new relationship slowly, and use your instincts to determine whether the experience is pleasurable for both of you. If you still have concerns, consider talking to a mental health provider.

Regardless of your situation, touch is a powerful tool that you can use to maintain an important sense of closeness and connection. Touch can be experienced in many ways, including holding hands and hugging.

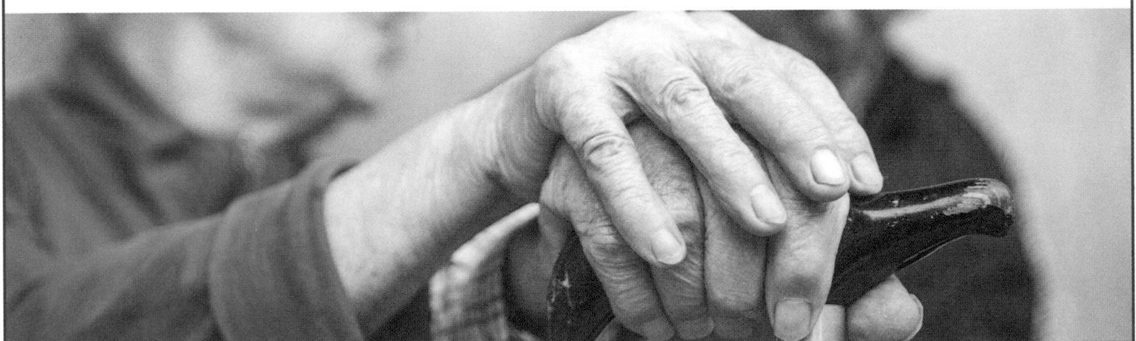

IMPACT ON FAMILY

When you become a care partner, you may find that some of the other aspects of your life are receiving much less attention. Rather than feeling guilty or trapped by these circumstances, look for ways to integrate the various aspects of your life. For example, it may be helpful to:

- Hold regular meetings to update family members about your loved one's condition and the challenges that both of you face.
- Listen closely and respond to family questions, but at the same time, make sure your voice is heard.
- Provide family members with opportunities to help if they're willing to do so. Create a list of your needs and your loved one's needs. Work with family members to delegate tasks, but only to an extent that they're comfortable with.
- Be open about the disease with young children and teenagers. They deserve explanations for the physical and behavioral changes they may be seeing.

Some families find it helpful to meet with a social worker, psychologist, nurse or other professional with specific knowledge about the disease. These specialists can assist you in planning for the future, identifying needs and making decisions.

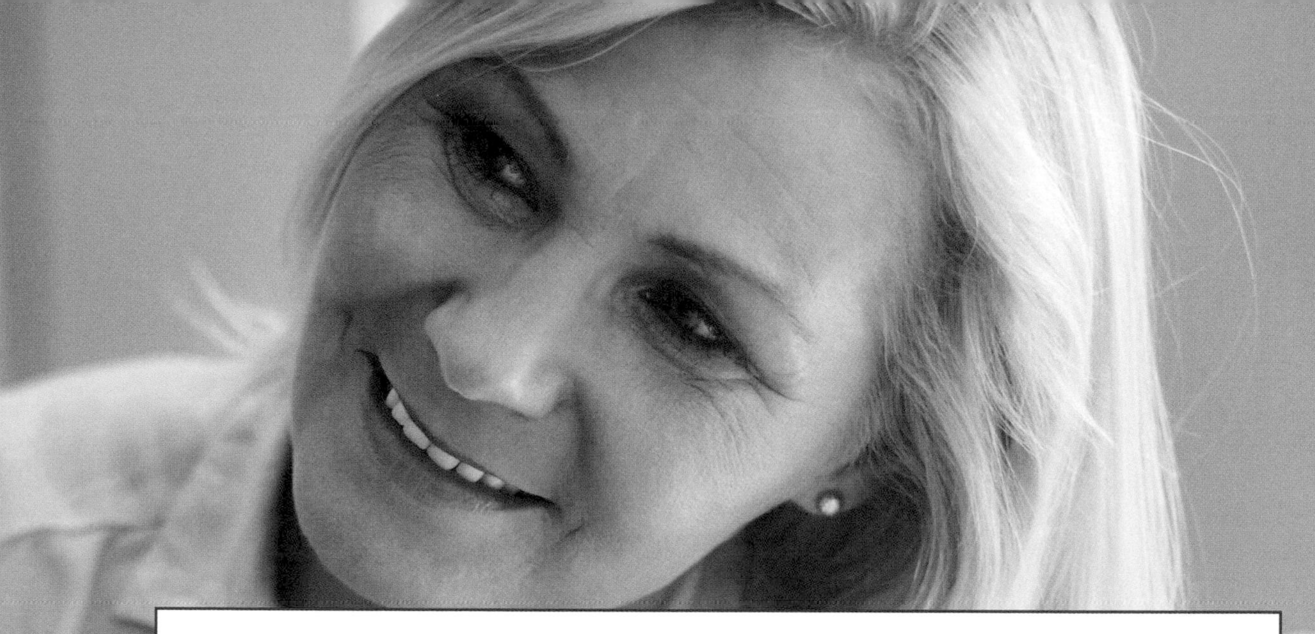

CAREGIVER'S BILL OF RIGHTS

Being a care partner comes with its share of ups and downs. It's easy to lose yourself in the needs of your loved one, pushing your own needs, feelings and desires aside. But you can't be an effective care partner if you're always putting yourself last.

Advocates for caregivers and the people they care for have developed a set of rights they believe caregivers should be entitled to. These include the right to:

- Maintain your sense of self as an individual by leading your life with dignity.
- Know that self-care is not selfishness and that it's important to nurture a life outside of your care partner role.
- Make decisions about your loved one that reflect the needs and promote the well-being of you both.
- Be recognized for the vital role you play in your family and in your loved one's life.
- Treat yourself with love and compassion so that you can reject guilt or doubt and be confident that you're caring for your loved one to the best of your abilities.

"ONE OF THE MOST IMPORTANT THINGS YOU CAN DO AS A CARE PARTNER IS TO SEEK TO UNDERSTAND YOUR LOVED ONE'S EXPERIENCE AND REALITY."

CHAPTER 17

Overcoming the challenges

I struggle to adjust and adapt to so many changes. I feel so angry. Frustrated. Everything is such an endeavor. Explaining, reexplaining and then going over it all again. I keep reminding myself to go slow, stay calm and take it easy. I am not doing so great in this role. I want to run away. I feel like I am in quicksand and can't find solid ground.

This reflection comes from Rosalie, a care partner to her husband, who has Lewy body dementia — but it could be the experience of many caregivers. The role of a care partner can be emotionally and physically exhausting. There may be many moments of frustration, anxiety and tension for everyone involved.

It's essential to keep in mind that like you, a person with dementia is a whole, multifaceted person doing his or her best in the face of challenges. There are many things you can do as a care partner to help the person you're supporting live the best life possible with dementia. This chapter offers practical advice for addressing challenging situations and overcoming obstacles.

LEARN EVERYTHING YOU CAN

Step one is to learn everything you can about dementia. The more you understand the disease, the better able you'll be to have a positive impact. Disease-related changes will seem less mysterious, and you may find it easier to adapt caregiving responsibilities so that your days feel more manageable. Knowing more about dementia can also help you feel confident about making important decisions about how to live your life and plan for the future.

This book has already given you a lot of information about different types of dementia, including signs and symptoms, changes in the brain, treatments, medications, and research. Much of what you've learned about dementia has focused on changes in the brain, deficits and the path that the disease takes — in other words, a focus on what's wrong.

While all of this information is important, it's just as critical to think beyond the disease itself and focus on the whole person, an approach defined as person-centered care.

Social psychologist Thomas Kitwood first used the term *person-centered care* in the late 1980s to define a philosophy of care that's different from standard medical and behavioral care.

Today, many experts prefer the terms *individualized care* and *personalized care*, but the idea is the same: a focus on the whole person. This means not just focusing on the disease or the diagnosis but also seeking to know and appreciate a person's past and present roles in life, preferences, beliefs, values, and needs. A person-centered approach offers a balanced perspective that can help with many of the challenges of dementia.

Relationships are especially important in person-centered care. All human beings are born to relate, connect and bond, and these needs remain for a lifetime. Having dementia doesn't change this, but dementia does make it more difficult to sustain quality relationships and meaningful engagement.

In this chapter, you'll learn how to incorporate a more person-centered approach into your life as a care partner. Doing so will open up opportunities that can improve quality of life for the person living with dementia, as well as for the care partner.

FOCUS ON WELL-BEING

Quality of life is related to a person's overall well-being. But what exactly is well-being? Well-being is a term that's used often, yet there's no agreement about what it means.

Researchers have described well-being for people with dementia in terms of comfort, inclusion, identity, occupation and attachment. More recently, Alzheimer's Disease International defined well-being as feeling content, being happy, feeling safe, experiencing pleasure and joy, and having a sense of self-worth and purpose. The opposite of well-being, in contrast, is described as suffering, pain, distress, fear, loneliness and humiliation.

To support the growing body of research on this topic, G. Allen Power, M.D., an international expert in models of care for older adults living with dementia, translates well-being into seven domains: identity, connectedness, security, autonomy, meaning, growth and joy.

No matter how you define well-being, a focus on it may contribute more to quality of life for people living with dementia than any medication available today. Despite

“DESPITE THEIR DISEASE, PEOPLE WITH DEMENTIA CAN EXPERIENCE WELL-BEING.”

their disease, people with dementia can experience well-being, and they can continue to grow and learn. Well-being is within reach when care partners, families and communities all play an active role.

The rest of this chapter offers strategies that anyone — care partners, families, friends and community members alike — can use to help improve well-being for people living with dementia:

- Offer empathy
- Recognize strengths and potential
- Understand and reduce distress
- Communicate skillfully

Offer empathy

To empathize means to imagine, as best as you can, what it's like to live someone else's life and to seek to understand another person's experience and reality.

Showing empathy can improve life for someone living with dementia, and it's good for a care partner's well-being, too. Research suggests that when people caring for someone with dementia use empathy, they're less likely to feel depressed. One of the most important things you can do as a care partner is to seek to understand your loved one's experience and reality.

Reality can be distorted for people living with dementia; trying to make them fit within your reality will cause stress for everyone involved. This doesn't mean that people living with dementia are far away or lost, but it does mean that the disease impacts the ability of a person with dementia to communicate clearly and process the world in the same way you do.

Seeing life through the eyes of the person with dementia doesn't mean you have to share the same anxiety, sadness or agitation. It also doesn't mean you have to lie or agree with the person's sense of reality (see page 334). Healthy empathy involves listening and observing with your ears, eyes and heart and means accepting that your reality of the world may be different.

Care partners can practice empathy by being authentically present. This may mean offering a touch or a look that demonstrates that you're sincerely trying to connect with the reality in which the person with dementia is living. As you'll learn in this chapter, showing empathy is also a path toward overcoming challenges.

Recognize strengths and potential

Every person living with dementia will experience dementia in a different way. Part of this experience includes retaining certain strengths and abilities. It's a myth that a diagnosis of dementia automatically means a person can't do any of the things he or she used to do, or can't learn new things.

People living with dementia have preserved abilities and areas of strength despite their disease. This is something that's not widely appreciated.

To truly help a person with dementia, it's important to focus on the person's best qualities, rather than only on what the person has lost or can no longer do. Although each type of dementia has a typical pattern of progression, people experience dementia differently. An individual's experiences, skills and interests all contribute to his or her preserved strengths. Even late in the disease, people with dementia can maintain and express a full range of emotions, including pleasure, enjoyment and affection. They often also have a sense of humor they can tap into.

Recognizing and building on strengths and abilities is an important way to nurture well-being in people living with dementia. Here are a few key areas of strength for many people living with dementia.

Strength: Procedural memory In Chapter 1, you learned the basics about memory, including how memories are formed and stored. The ability to store and recall memories is affected in many types of dementia.

Alzheimer's dementia affects the ability to form memories of new knowledge and events. For example, recalling a conversation from earlier in the day or remembering what you ate for dinner last night could be a challenge with Alzheimer's.

Asking a question that relies on this type of memory would be difficult or impossible for a person with Alzheimer's dementia. This could cause the person with dementia to feel embarrassed or frustrated.

The good news is that people with Alzheimer's dementia can make and recall new memories by using procedural memory. Procedural memory is a type of long-term memory that allows someone to perform different actions and use certain skills. It's created by repeating an activity or skill until it becomes automatic and doesn't require conscious thought. Tying your shoes, riding a bike, and brushing your teeth are examples of procedural memory.

In Alzheimer's dementia, procedural memory is more resilient than other types of memory are. Some people with dementia can maintain procedural memories for quite some time and learn new things by tapping into the way that these memories are formed.

Accountants and math teachers, for example, may retain their numbers skills longer than other people with dementia because they represent an overlearned skill — something they did daily almost without thinking. Likewise, people who played golf or bowled for decades may be able to play the game well into their disease. Overlearned skills tend to remain intact even as a person progresses into the middle and sometimes later stages of dementia. Other examples of overlearned tasks include making a bed, riding a bike, caring for an animal and folding laundry. Every individual has his or her own set of procedural skills.

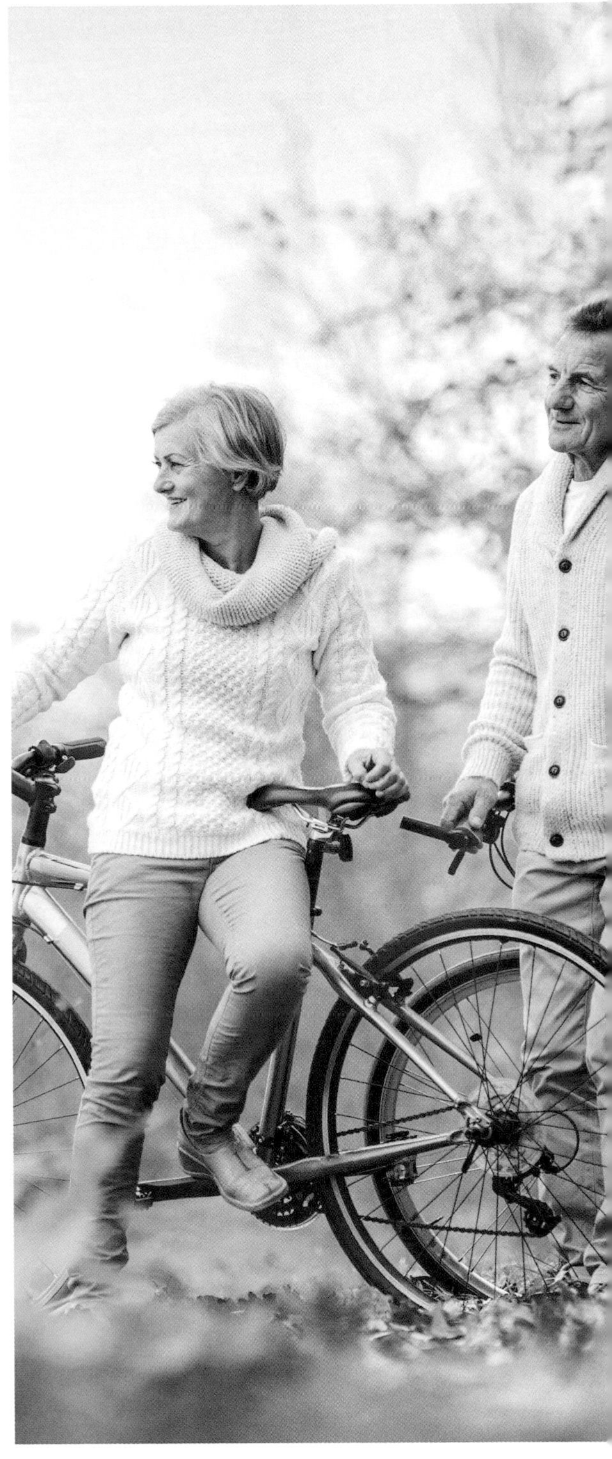

Procedural memory isn't just linked to past skills; it can also support new learning. Here's an example of how procedural memory can help someone with dementia learn something new.

Eleanor was living with Alzheimer's dementia. She and her family decided she would move from the assisted living community where she'd been for two years to a different care community a few miles away. The move went as smoothly as could be expected, and Eleanor settled into her new home. She was a bit apprehensive, but still eager to be involved in all the activities this community had to offer.

But there was a problem. Eleanor lived on the third floor, and most of the daily activities and opportunities for socializing happened on the first floor. When Eleanor left her apartment in search of something to do, she got lost. When she couldn't find her way downstairs, she became frustrated and angry. When she was offered assistance, she said she didn't need anyone's help.

HOW DOING THINGS THE SAME WAY CAN HELP

Typically, you learn by a process of trial and error. However, this process doesn't work as well in people with dementia because dementia affects a person's ability to remember making an error in the first place. This is where a technique called errorless learning can help.

Errorless learning is the opposite of learning through trial and error. It allows people with dementia to learn in a way that taps into the part of the memory that's unaffected — procedural memory. By using errorless learning, a person with dementia learns by doing things the same way, in the same environment, with the same cues. This makes mistakes less frequent and may eliminate them entirely. This approach allows people with dementia to learn by doing things rather than by thinking about how they're doing them.

After a couple of days, staff members came up with a plan. They applied large, adhesive footprint decals on the floor leading from Eleanor's apartment door to the elevator. Inside the elevator, they placed a sign next the first floor button that read, "Activity room, press here." At the elevator opening on the first floor, more footprint decals were placed, leading to the activity room. Eleanor was able to successfully follow the footprints to and from her apartment every day, sometimes several times a day.

The fact that Eleanor could find her way by using these simple visual cues may not come as a surprise, but what happened next might. After about six weeks, the staff removed the footprint decals and waited to see what would happen. At her usual time, without any sign of frustration, Eleanor arrived in the activity room like she had every day for the past six weeks.

Eleanor was able to find her way, without the assistance of the footprint decals, by using procedural memory. Repeatedly and successfully going back and forth between her apartment and the activity room for six weeks helped Eleanor learn this route, which essentially imprinted a new memory in her brain.

Eleanor's story highlights the overall benefits of repetition and establishing a daily

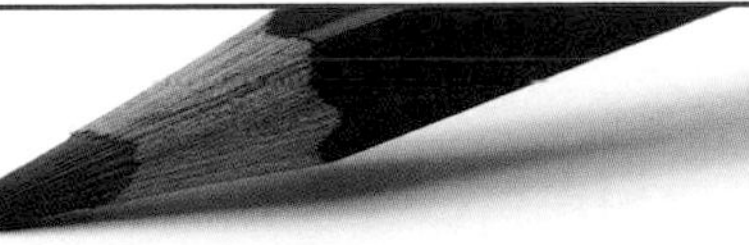

KEY TAKEAWAYS: PROCEDURAL MEMORY

- Procedural memory is a different kind of memory that doesn't rely on recalling knowledge or events.
- Procedural memory, also known as learned habits, can remain intact until later in the disease.
- New learning occurs by doing things repeatedly and consistently over time.
- Establishing a daily routine can help support new learning.

routine. These habits support new learning and can help someone with dementia remain more independent and feel less frustrated and anxious.

Strength: Emotional memory Everyone feels emotions, even without recalling what sparked them. The ability to experience and maintain emotions, as well as to accurately perceive others' emotions, remains intact for many people with dementia throughout the stages of their disease. This is particularly true for people living with Alzheimer's dementia.

In a study from the University of Iowa, researchers asked individuals living with Alzheimer's dementia to watch film clips that were intended to make them feel either sad or happy. The researchers collected emotion ratings at three different points, and after each point, they gave a memory test. Participants had trouble recalling details about the film clips; some couldn't remember a single detail about the film. However, feelings of happiness and sadness evoked by the film weren't forgotten.

This study is consistent with other research suggesting that people living with significant memory issues can still be emotionally affected by an event even if they can't recall the event itself. These emotions can last long after memories have faded.

This offers an important lesson for care partners, friends and community members alike. People living with dementia may not remember your name, recognize your face or recall how they know you, but that doesn't change how much your visits and interactions matter.

With the right communication, you can create a meaningful visit that leaves a positive, lasting emotional impact. (Learn more about communication skills starting on page 332.)

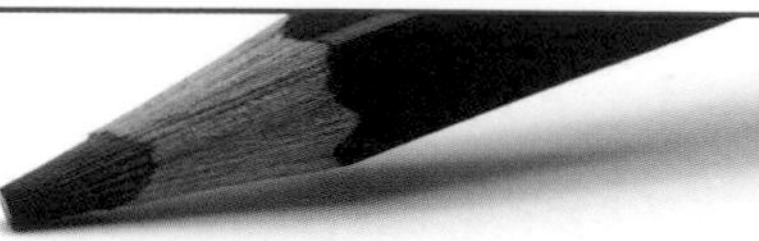

KEY TAKEAWAYS: EMOTIONAL MEMORY

- The emotion caused by an event may be remembered even if the event is forgotten. This relates both to positive emotions and negative emotions.
- Everyone plays an important role in creating the emotional imprint left on someone with dementia.

That being said, emotional memory also includes bad memories. If you say or do something that causes emotional distress for a person with dementia, those emotions can persist long after the situation that triggered the distress is forgotten. This may explain why certain people or places cause a negative reaction in someone with dementia. The person may be responding to something that happened days, weeks or even months ago.

If you think it won't be worthwhile to visit a person with dementia simply because the person won't remember it, think again. People with dementia live in the moment and will enjoy the time you spend together. Your visit can generate positive feelings that may linger well past your time together.

Strength: Art and creativity "The arts are a way of being in relationship that can ensure that we are more than our diagnosis." This quote comes from Anne Basting, Ph.D., a scholar, author and artist whose work focuses on how the arts can transform the lives of those living with dementia. Her words describe the impact that the arts can make on people with dementia.

More and more evidence points to the benefits the arts have for those living with dementia. Whether it's visual art, music, dance, storytelling, poetry, or anything else that evokes creativity and imagination, the arts can reduce stress and improve quality of life for those living with dementia and their care partners.

There are many reasons for this. For one, intuition, creativity and imagination are areas of strength for people with dementia. The ability to appreciate, produce and participate in art isn't affected by their disease. And because most art doesn't require specific memories or traditional language use, it allows people with dementia to express feelings they may not be able to communicate verbally.

Research shows that in people living with dementia, art therapy can engage attention, bring a sense of pleasure, improve symptoms like agitation, aggression, depression and apathy, and improve self-esteem and social behavior. Creativity can even emerge in people with dementia. In fact, depending on how and where dementia affects the brain, artistic ability may even be enhanced in people with a certain type of frontotemporal dementia as the disease progresses.

Music is another example of how the arts can benefit people living with dementia. Despite profound memory loss, individuals with dementia often show a remarkable memory for music. That's because the areas of the brain that process and remember music are typically less damaged by dementia than other regions are. Music also tends to arouse emotions and influence mood. For many, music retains this power throughout the disease.

Research suggests that listening to or singing songs can offer benefits for people with dementia. Music can relieve stress, reduce anxiety and depression, and lessen agitation. Certain types of music can be calming, while other types can help boost mood.

Worldwide, organizations like the Giving Voice Initiative use music to bring people living with Alzheimer's and their care partners together to sing in choruses that foster joy, well-being, purpose and community understanding. You'll find groups and organizations dedicated to the arts listed in the Additional resources section of this book.

Understand and reduce distress

Human beings all need to feel respected, worthy and connected. Although these

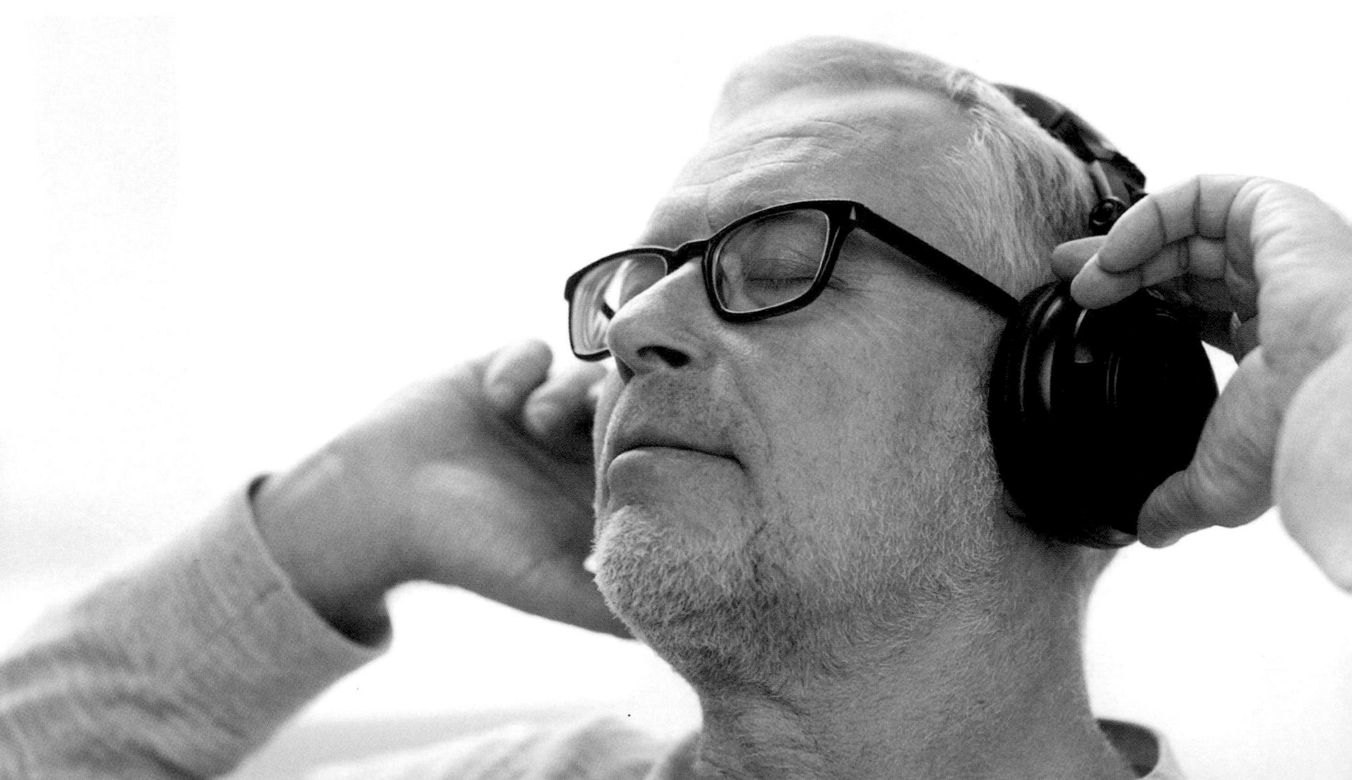

emotional needs are universal, people with dementia struggle to have these needs met.

Imagine what it would feel like to wake up one day and discover that you could no longer take part in the things that give your life meaning and purpose. Or think about how you'd feel if people suddenly started telling you what you could and couldn't do. How would you feel if you could no longer make basic choices for yourself, like choosing when to have your morning cup of coffee or with whom you share a meal?

These are examples of the reality that many people with dementia face — a reality that understandably leads to feelings of apathy, anger and frustration.

Many dementia advocates are working to improve social and emotional health for people living with dementia. You can help in your own way, too. Use the checklist on the next page to gauge how well you're helping fulfill the emotional needs of someone living with dementia. The next time you notice anger, agitation, apathy, frustration or any type of distress, this list may provide clues as to the cause.

Decoding distress Many people find changes in behavior to be the most challenging aspect of dementia. Depression, apathy, anxiety, agitation, aggression, sleep disturbances, and poorly controlled emotions or actions (disinhibition) are all examples. Anywhere from a third to nearly all people with dementia will experience some or most of these symptoms.

What causes these behaviors — and how to address them — isn't always clear. But part of the answer lies in understanding the changes in the brain. Certain brain circuits have been linked to a tendency toward certain symptoms, like apathy, delusions and agitation. Not everyone with dementia will develop these symptoms; more study is needed.

Over time, dementia changes how well people can communicate their needs and provide for themselves. Behaviors become a way to communicate. Anger or agitation, for example, are expressions of distress and can be a way for people living with dementia to say they're in pain or feeling misunderstood, confused, disrespected or bored.

For understanding the exact cause of distress in someone with dementia, empathy becomes essential. As you learned earlier, empathy is the ability to imagine, as best you can, what it's like to live with dementia. Earlier, you gave thought to what it would feel like to no longer make basic choices for yourself, like choosing when to have your morning cup of coffee or with whom you share a meal. Here are several other scenarios to help you step into the shoes of someone living with dementia.

Imagine the following:

- Having someone you don't know show up and tell you that he or she will be giving you a bath.
- Feeling bored and no longer able to do the things that give you a sense of worth or purpose.

EMOTIONAL WELL-BEING CHECKLIST

Like all people, people living with dementia have the need to:

- *Feel respected.* Treat someone with dementia as an adult at all times, under all circumstances. This includes your actions, as well as your verbal and nonverbal communication.
- *Feel needed and have purpose.* Find ways to help people with dementia feel valued and productive by helping them to engage in things that have meaning to them. Ask for their help, advice and opinions daily.
- *Feel connected and have a sense of belonging.* Recognize the importance of having strong, supportive relationships. Play a role in helping the person living with dementia maintain friendships or find new opportunities for support and belonging.
- *Feel good about themselves.* Offer honest appreciation and praise every day for traits and accomplishments large or small.
- *Have choice and control.* Involve the person with dementia in decisions every day. Think about doing things *with* rather than always doing *for* the person with dementia. Ask the person with dementia for permission.

- Someone with a grimacing face talking at you in a patronizing tone, in a language you can't understand.
- Being uncomfortable or in pain, or needing to find the bathroom, and being unable to find the words to ask for help.
- Feeling tired and wanting to find your way home so you can rest. Instead, you're stuck in a confusing, cluttered space with chatter, sounds and dozens of people you don't recognize.
- Being treated as if you can't do something that, with a little more time and patience, you could probably do just fine.

How would you feel in any of these scenarios? Would you feel agitated, angry, anxious, scared, hopeless or sad? If you said yes, know that someone with dementia feels this way, too.

Decoding distress means operating from the belief that most behavior is reasonable based on the circumstances. There's meaning behind it, and it's often triggered by something or someone. Start by asking yourself, *I wonder what could be causing this distress?* Instead of assuming that a behavior is an expected symptom of dementia, think

KEY TAKEAWAYS: ART AND CREATIVITY

- The arts can offer a path toward well-being and a higher quality of life for people living with dementia.
- The arts engage areas of strength for people with dementia that can remain accessible despite memory loss.
- The arts can reduce agitation, aggression, depression and apathy, enhance self-esteem and social behavior, and bring about a sense of pleasure.
- Arts and creativity offer the same benefits for care partners.

of the behavior as an attempt to express distress or communicate an unmet need. You may feel like a detective looking for clues, but with a little effort, you can often uncover the cause. Once you can identify the likely cause, solutions become possible.

Distress is often explained by physical issues, challenges caused by the environment, unmet emotional needs and communication problems. Here's more on each of these causes of distress and ways to spot them.

Physical needs A common physical problem is pain. This may be caused by a urinary tract infection, constipation, an aching joint or a broken bone. Other physical issues may include:

- Needing to go to the bathroom
- Not seeing or hearing well
- Feeling tired
- Hunger
- An uncomfortable position
- Constipation
- Itching
- Stomach problems
- Dental problems
- Feeling too hot or too cold

People may be able to say when they're in pain in the early stages of dementia. Later on, people with dementia still communicate pain, but through behaviors or expressions rather than with words.

Nonverbal signs of pain may include:

- Grimacing
- Gestures
- Moaning
- Restlessness
- Crying
- Expressions of distress, like agitation or aggression

The environment People living with dementia face a number of challenges that influence how well they see, feel and respond to the world around them. A person's surroundings can increase agitation and other reactions. On the flip side, the environment can promote comfort, independence and overall well-being.

Environmental factors that can cause distress include:

- Feeling too hot or too cold.
- Lack of structure or routine.
- Too much noise or overstimulation. For example, being exposed to a lot of stimulation for too long can cause stress for someone with dementia. It can cause an overload on the senses — in particular, vision and hearing.
- Too much clutter.
- Too much quiet.
- New or confusing surroundings.
- Poor lighting.

Decoding distress means looking around and putting yourself in the place of the person with dementia to see if the surroundings could be a cause.

Emotional needs Earlier, you read about several emotional needs, including the need to feel respected, worthy and connected. Everyone has these needs, but people with dementia struggle more than people without dementia to have these needs met.

Expressions like agitation or apathy may stem from emotional needs that aren't being met. A person with dementia may be feeling bored, unworthy, or disconnected from the people and things that provide purpose. When these needs aren't met, overall well-being and quality of life decrease.

In Chapter 14, you learned ways that people with dementia can engage in things that are important to them so that they continue to feel valued and productive. Communication also plays a role in fulfilling emotional needs. You'll learn about communication strategies for care partners next.

Communication Changes in the brain caused by dementia make communication more difficult over time. However, communication is still possible — and can be improved — when care partners and others tap into a person's retained abilities.

Communication can be difficult for care partners because it requires letting go of some of the ways they've communicated in the past. You may notice that the old ways of communicating don't work like they used to. Early on, you may notice your loved one having trouble finding the right word and leaving thoughts hanging in mid-sentence. These are generally minor frustrations that can be overcome, and you and your loved one can continue to communicate fairly well.

But in more moderate stages of dementia, it can be increasingly difficult to understand what someone with dementia is saying. Words, sentences and thoughts become jumbled. You may find it challenging to communicate to your loved one in ways that he or she understands. This situation may frustrate your loved one, leading to embarrassment, anger or agitation. As the disease advances into the late stages, verbal communication may be replaced by nonverbal communication, including behaviors, sounds, facial expressions and gestures.

Communicate skillfully

The good news is that you can develop new and effective ways to communicate with your loved one. Along the way, you may even learn some things about yourself and strengthen qualities like patience and acceptance. Effective communication is essential to everyone's well-being.

The basics Here are basic strategies for good communication.

- Talk to a person with dementia as an adult, in an adult tone of voice and with words that are respectful.
- Face the person before you communicate. Look directly at the person and make eye contact.
- Speak at a normal volume or a little louder if listening conditions are difficult.
- Slow the pace of your conversation. It takes more time for people with dementia to process information.
- Use words that are familiar and easy to picture in your mind (concrete) rather than abstract words. Be clear and concise; keep your message short.
- Pause after a statement or question. Allow plenty of time for a response.
- Avoid leading questions that include the answer with it. "You're comfortable, aren't you?" is an example. This kind of question can be demeaning, and in some cases, the person will agree with anything you say.
- Use nonverbal cues, like smiling or giving a reassuring touch.
- Give instructions one step at a time. After one step is completed, give instructions for the next step.
- Don't interrupt. People with dementia may need extra time to express what they want to say. If the person is struggling to express a thought, gently offer a word or phrase.
- Take note of facial expressions and hand gestures. They may offer clues to forgotten words.
- Use gestures and show the object you're talking about if your words don't seem to be understood.
- Avoid criticizing, confronting or arguing. People with dementia experience the world in a different way, so it's unlikely that they'll see things the way you do all the time.
- Do not speak in the presence of a person with dementia as if he or she is not there.

Aside from basic communication strategies, here are ways to communicate with someone living with dementia that tap into abilities that aren't affected by the disease.

Nonverbal communication How you present yourself is critical. Are you nervous or frowning? Are you speaking clearly and simply? Is your facial expression or body language sending a negative message? The words you use are only part of the message you communicate.

Body language, facial expressions, posture, gestures and tone of voice also are factors that affect how your message is received.

People living with dementia understand nonverbal communication very well. Body language is an especially powerful way to send a message to someone with dementia.

Offer choice and sense of control A sense of control is important for everyone. Yet people with dementia often feel as if they're being told what to do or that they're not capable of making their own decisions. This is another area where effective communication can make a difference.

Consider the following examples:

A. It's time for you to take your medication.
B. Would you like me to get you a glass of water so you can take your medications?

A. I need you to stay here while I get the car.
B. Would you like to stand here or sit in that chair while I get the car?

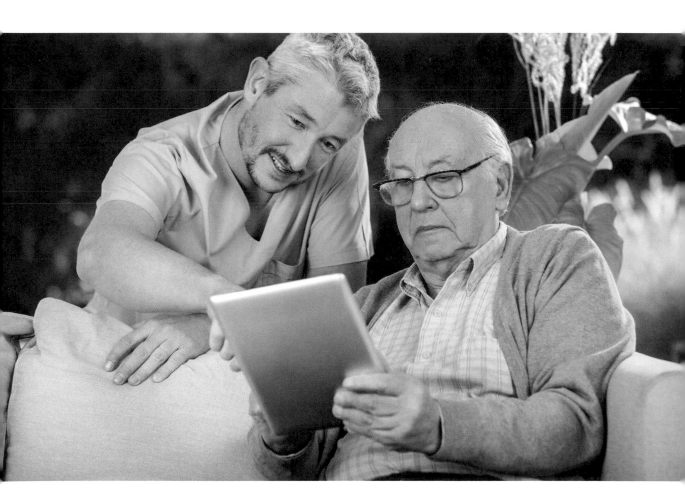

TO LIE OR NOT TO LIE

When someone with dementia believes something that's inaccurate or false, it can be hard to know what to do or say.

For example, let's say your mother has dementia and repeatedly asks where her husband is. The truth is that he died a year ago. Do you repeatedly tell her the truth, knowing that her reaction is going to be shock, grief and fear every time? Each time, it will be as if she's learning this news for the first time. Which is worse: telling a lie, or offering the painful truth?

This is where an approach commonly called therapeutic fibbing may come into play. While this can be an effective strategy, it's also controversial. It means going along with or not correcting a misconception. The idea is to decrease worry, sadness, agitation or anxiety in someone with dementia.

For the situation described here, therapeutic fibbing may involve a response like, "When the weather is nice like today, your husband sometimes stays out in the fields after dark." This statement isn't necessarily an overt lie, and it's something the woman with dementia can relate to; in her reality, this makes sense.

Most experts agree that the truth should always be the intent. Avoiding an unpleasant reaction shouldn't be the only reason to lie. Likewise, a lie shouldn't be told simply because it's more convenient. But for people who can't make sense of the truth — and in situations in which the truth will cause harm or distress — a therapeutic lie may be the better option.

A. Let's go the bathroom, Dad.
B. Dad, may I help you get to the bathroom?

A. No, that's not how you do it.
B. Here's another way.

Each of the A statements competes with a person's need for choice and control. When they're heard over and over again, these statements can cause someone with dementia to lose self-confidence and feel angry, agitated and even hopeless.

The B statements, on the other hand, offer choice, consider a person's preferences and preserve a person's need to feel respected.

Ask the right questions As memory loss becomes more noticeable, avoid asking questions that depend on memory or that have only one right answer. Never ask, "Do you remember … ?" Instead, ask questions that tap into your loved one's strengths.

Asking questions about a person's ideas, thoughts, feelings and preferences allows you to take full advantage of the areas of the brain that are less affected. It's important to keep in mind that not everyone will need the same adaptations in communication.

Here are several examples of questions you might ask. Based on what you've just read, which questions do you think are most helpful to ask someone with dementia?

A. Do you remember what I told you to do this afternoon?
B. You agreed to rake the leaves this afternoon. Can I grab a rake for you?

A. This is a big menu. What do you want?
B. Both the fish special and the meatloaf look good tonight. What do you think?

A. How many grandchildren do you have?
B. How do you feel about having 14 grandchildren?

In these examples, the A statements rely on memory or require abstract thinking. The B statements, on the other hand, eliminate the need for remembering. They also offer clarity, give limited choices and ask about preferences.

Focus on feelings Sometimes, even the best attempts to understand what someone with dementia is saying will fail. If you can't understand what your loved one is trying to communicate, you may not know how to help. In these cases, empathy and reassurance go a long way.

If someone with dementia shows signs of distress and you don't know why or what to do, keep the nonverbal skills you've read about in mind. Stay fully present in a way that shows you care. If it seems OK, touch the person's hand, arm or shoulder. Make sure your body language and facial expressions communicate concern and caring, and that you're affirming the person's reality. Communicate with words that affirm the feelings you're noticing. For example, you might say, "I'm sorry you're feeling sad (angry, frustrated)," and then offer a reassuring message, like, "I'm here for you," or "I care about you."

These strategies validate a person's emotions and support well-being. Although you may be tempted to skip this step and move toward redirecting or distracting the person, you likely won't achieve the outcome you're hoping for. In most cases, it's only after you validate the person's feelings and reality that your redirection can succeed. Having feelings acknowledged, whether they're good or bad, is a universal need. Sometimes it's all that's needed.

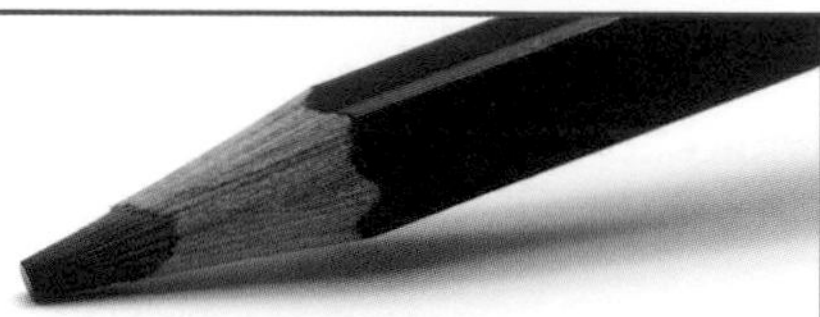

KEY TAKEAWAYS: DECODING DISTRESS AND COMMUNICATING WELL

- Trying to see things as someone with dementia does (empathy) is essential to understanding what's causing distress.
- All actions and behaviors are meaningful and reflect a desire to communicate something, including an unmet emotional need.
- How you communicate can either take away a person's sense of self-worth or preserve it.
- People living with dementia can respond to questions that tap into ideas, thoughts, feelings, preferences, curiosity and imagination.
- Providing daily opportunities to make choices and offer opinions boosts self-esteem, self-worth, sense of purpose and overall well-being in someone with dementia.
- How you communicate affects your well-being, as well as the well-being of the person with dementia.

BE COMPASSIONATE TO YOURSELF

I recognize that caregiving is now the major chapter in my life. My future holds other chapters. But for now I'm being remade and reformed by my role of caregiving into a gentler, more compassionate, more patient, kinder person.

This reflection comes from Rosalie, whom you heard from at the start of this chapter. When she wrote this, she had been on her caregiving journey for a number of years.

As you've read many times throughout this book, each care partner will have his or her own experience; no two are alike. In addition, no care partner should feel the need to become some kind of superhero. For some, like Rosalie, the experience can be transformative, and for others, not so much.

In this chapter, you've gained information, approaches and strategies for caregiving. Take what makes sense and fits your unique situation.

If you find that there's no solution for the challenges you're facing, turn to self-compassion. Sometimes this is all you can give yourself. You'll learn more about self-compassion and other self-care strategies for care partners in the next chapter.

ASKING 'BEAUTIFUL' QUESTIONS

Asking questions that depend on memory can cause feelings of shame and embarrassment for someone with dementia. That's where taking a different approach to the questions you ask — one that taps into the freedom of imagination — can be valuable.

- What is the greatest gift you could receive?
- What is the most beautiful sound in your home?
- How would you welcome a new friend to your home?
- How does painting make you feel?
- What do you wish for?
- What are you thankful for?

These are all examples of "beautiful questions," a creative way of using arts and imagination to ask questions that engage people with dementia. This concept comes from Anne Basting, Ph.D., founder and president of the nonprofit TimeSlips *(www.timeslips.org).* The TimeSlips website offers hundreds of prompts to inspire creative engagement.

Say you're visiting with someone with dementia and looking out the window, and you spot a bird outside in a tree. Your conversation may go something like this:

You: What do you see?
Response: A bird.

You: Do you want to give it a name?
Response: Robin.

You: What sounds do you imagine it makes?

Asking open-ended questions like these allows you to shift away from depending on memory and instead harness the power and freedom of imagination. This approach is designed to allow for greater engagement and to connect people with their loved ones who are living with dementia.

“WHEN YOU’RE FEELING LOW OR YOU’RE IN THE MIDST OF A PAINFUL SITUATION, TALK TO YOURSELF IN THE WAY YOU WOULD TALK TO A GOOD FRIEND.”

CHAPTER 18

Road map toward well-being

Becoming a dementia care partner is an unrequested role, and each care partner experiences this role in a different way. Many factors impact the caregiving experience, including your relationship with the person you're caring for, other roles and responsibilities in your life, and your personal coping strategies and social support.

For some, the role of caregiving can feel like a heavy, ever-increasing load. For others, caregiving is deeply fulfilling, rewarding and meaningful. Most agree that being a care partner to someone with dementia is one of the hardest "jobs" they've ever had.

According to a recent report, nearly half of all family caregivers say they feel somewhat stressed, and more than a third say they're highly stressed. Care partners juggle many responsibilities. They often feel that their loved ones are depending on them to help with daily living as well as for emotional support, comfort and a sense of security.

As a care partner, you're managing these daily demands while also living with the knowledge that your loved one has a disease that will worsen over time. You may have difficulty accepting this and adapting to changes that are beyond your control. Each change along the way may feel like a new loss to be mourned.

In the face of these challenges, it's natural to feel a range of powerful and conflicting emotions. You may feel sad, angry, guilty, overwhelmed, exhausted or lonely. All of these feelings and experiences are normal.

You will encounter frustrations and losses. You will make mistakes. Many things won't go the way you'd hoped. But the more you open your heart to this reality instead of fighting against it, the more likely you are to find inner strength and peace.

This chapter offers suggestions for addressing the ups and downs of being a care partner. You'll also learn ways to develop the inner strength you need for the days ahead. The most important thing to remember is that you're not alone. You're part of a large family of dementia care partners — each one unique, but all sharing in the struggle.

MOVING TOWARD ACCEPTANCE

Maybe a loved one was recently diagnosed with dementia and you're struggling to adjust to this life-changing news. Or maybe you thought you'd reached a kind of acceptance, only to feel the rug pulled out from

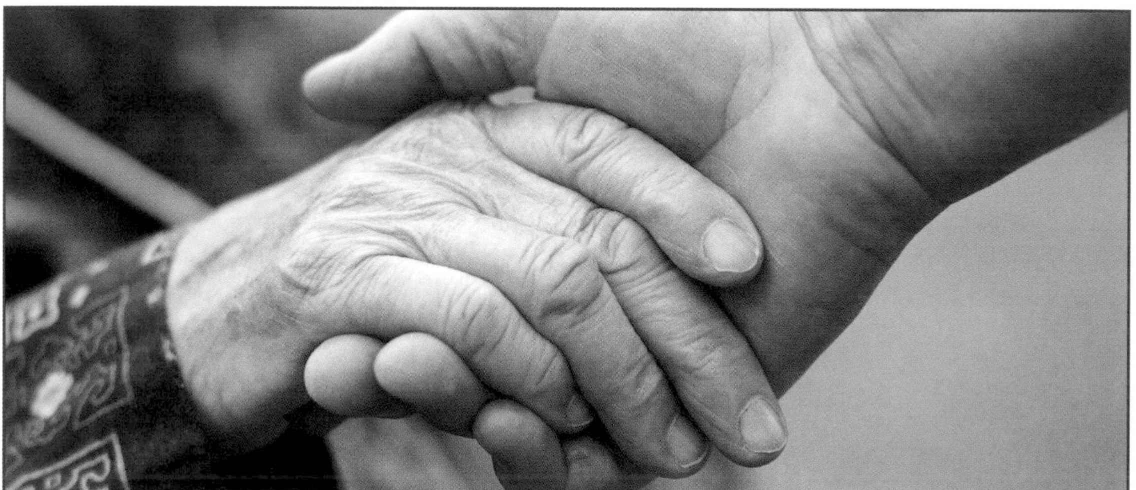

A POSITIVE SIDE TO CAREGIVING?

Although caregivers can have both positive and negative experiences in their roles of providing care and support, well-being is often measured in terms of how much stress, burden, depression or anxiety someone feels. However, this may be shifting. A recent article in *The Gerontologist* shows growing evidence that if caregivers can identify positive aspects of providing care, doing so may be beneficial to their well-being.

under you when your loved one loses a skill or shows a noticeable decline in memory. Rather than face the uncertainty that comes with a diagnosis or an unwanted change, you may unintentionally be in denial.

On some level, you may be holding out hope that your loved one will stay the same or even get better. You may look for signs that your loved one isn't truly ill, tell yourself that the changes you see are part of normal aging or convince yourself that a good day is a sign that your loved one is improving. You may reject the fact that the disease will significantly affect your relationship. These are all examples of denial. Anything that makes you feel afraid or vulnerable or threatens your sense of control can cause feelings of denial.

Occasional periods of denial are normal and entirely understandable. In some cases, initial, short-term denial can even be a good thing. It can give you time to adjust to a painful or stressful issue. But a persistent state of denial can be unhealthy. Research shows that when care partners avoid painful emotions and engage in denial and wishful thinking, they experience more stress. Those who accept their situation and allow for the emotions that come with it, in contrast, tend to experience better mental health.

Denying the reality of your situation can keep you from using the tools, skills and support you need. Accepting your situation offers opportunities that can help you and the person living with dementia. This is what makes acceptance so powerful.

Acceptance is a choice to be with your situation just as it is. Developing an attitude of acceptance doesn't mean you're supporting the unfairness of the situation. It simply means that you accept what you can't change. When you're willing to accept things as they are, you're demonstrating humility, courage and compassion — qualities that give you strength.

Acceptance also means giving your full attention to what's happening now. As one care partner said, "I had to stop dwelling on the way my dad used to be and be fully present for who he is today." This is an example of acceptance.

Acceptance is about reality, but it's also a turning point toward change and transformation. Acceptance can lead you down a path toward greater well-being. Following are four ways you can harness the power of acceptance.

Realize that you can't control everything

To find some relief from caregiving stress, try to recognize the difference between what's within your power to change and what isn't. Trying to change something you can't control leads to negative feelings like anger and resentment.

No matter what you do, you can't change your loved one's disease. While you know this on some level, the way you think, feel and respond may be a way of rejecting this

"BE WILLING TO SEE ANY ACCOMPLISHMENT AS A SUCCESS."

basic truth. This is where having realistic expectations can help, like being honest about what you can and can't control.

For example, you can't control how your loved one's disease will progress or whether or not extended family members or friends agree with your decisions. However, you can control your efforts to seek support, the caregiving skills you build and how you choose to respond to a challenging situation.

Over time, many care partners learn to let go of what they can't control, including not being able to "save" someone living with dementia or make the person better. Letting go of the expectation to "fix" someone with dementia can lift a burden from your shoulders. When you don't feel the pressure to fix the things that are out of your control, you may discover that you can engage with your loved one — and yourself — with greater empathy and compassion.

Be a good-enough care partner

As dementia progresses, you'll need to offer more help to your loved one. You'll likely take on responsibilities for things you may not have done before, like certain household tasks, yardwork or bill paying. You may also become the primary source of emotional support for the person living with dementia. He or she will likely be taking cues from you on how to react or what to do next in certain situations.

This is a lot of pressure, especially when you also have your own life to manage.

While you may want to believe that you can do it all — and do it all perfectly — this simply isn't possible. You may also think you need to sacrifice your own needs and be as available as possible for your loved one at all times. This isn't healthy for you or for your loved one. These high expectations lead to exhaustion and feelings of guilt.

Instead, choose to be a good-enough care partner rather than striving to be great or perfect. Set realistic limits for yourself. Be willing to see any achievement as a success. Instead of dwelling on the "shoulds," tell yourself, *I can only do my best, and my best is good enough.*

Forgive yourself

Guilt is often the result of refusing to accept that some things are out of your control. It's helpful to release yourself from that burden by forgiving yourself.

If you were irritated with or critical of someone living with dementia before you knew the diagnosis, forgive yourself. If you made a promise early on to keep someone with dementia living at home but that's no longer the best choice, it's OK. You didn't know then what you know now.

Whether it's making a difficult decision or making a mistake, remember that you're human and you're doing the best you can. No family or care partner can plan for every situation or anticipate every challenge.

There are no perfect families and there are no perfect solutions. This is where self-compassion comes in. Instead of judging and criticizing yourself, be easy on yourself and forgive, even when you're faced with what feels like a personal failing.

Feel what you feel

Your emotions — grief, sadness, anger or all of the above — are a normal part of being a care partner and a human being. All of your emotions provide insight and can help you through tough times.

It's normal to resent being a caregiver but love the person you're caring for. Rather than label your feelings as "bad" and push them away, remind yourself that these feelings are natural and even healthy.

This expression of openness toward whatever you're feeling at that moment is actually helpful. Research suggests that being aware and accepting of thoughts and emotions gives them less power and can lessen the stress you feel.

When you're open to noticing negative emotions, without judging them or judging yourself for having them, you're also creating space for positive emotions, like joy or relief, to enter in.

In this way, you're more likely to find greater pleasure in the quiet, unrushed moments, like when you're sitting on the porch with your loved one or sipping a cup of tea at the end of a long day. Feeling joy in life doesn't mean you're not taking your responsibilities seriously. It means you're taking care of yourself.

GUILT AND GRIEF

Two common emotions dementia care partners feel are guilt and grief.

Guilt is a normal emotion woven throughout the care partner experience. While guilt can be useful when it pushes you to make amends for something you've done wrong or for harm you've caused others, it's often an undeserved emotion for care partners.

Grief is a deep and sometimes complex emotion people feel when they experience a loss. It's both a universal and a personal experience. For dementia care partners, grief can be an ever-present part of the journey. Here's more on guilt and grief, including ways to cope with both emotions.

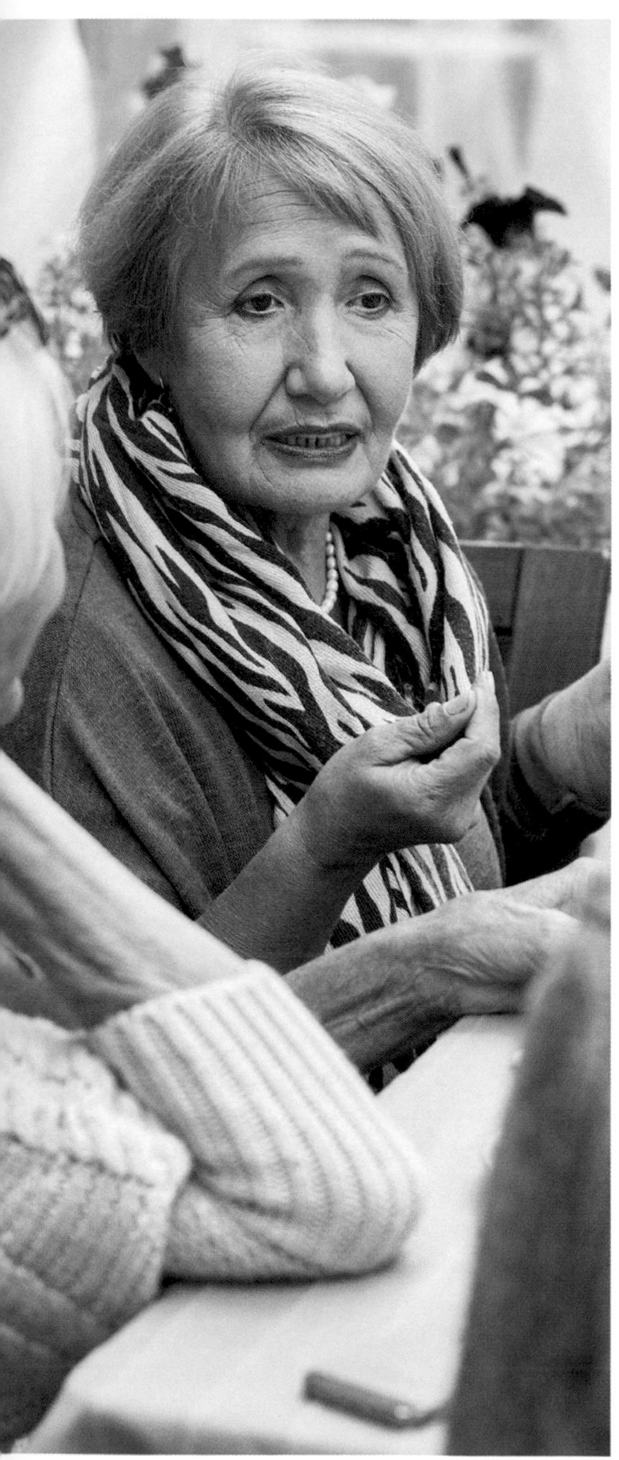

Coping with guilt

As a care partner, you may struggle with guilt for a range of imagined failings:

- Feeling anger or frustration toward the person living with dementia
- Feeling trapped in the care partner role, or wishing the person with dementia wasn't a part of your life
- Feeling that you fall short in comparison with other care partners
- Needing a break from your role as a care partner
- Moving your loved one out of the home and into a care community, like a nursing home
- Needing help from others and not being able to do everything yourself
- Feeling that you've failed to meet every one of your loved one's needs perfectly
- Feeling guilty for experiencing happiness and enjoyment in life

If, like many other care partners, you're struggling with guilt for these or other reasons, try taking steps toward adopting a more balanced and realistic perspective. Here are several suggestions that can help.

Notice it Acknowledging that you're feeling guilt is an important first step. If you try to ignore feelings of guilt, you may experience even more negative thoughts and stress. It may sound counterproductive and even unpleasant, but in order to move on from guilt, you first have to acknowledge it.

Once you've done that, you can address guilt in a more rational way.

Start by asking yourself, *Am I feeling guilty for things that are outside of my control?* From there, you have several options:

- Forgive yourself and let it go. It will pass if you let it.
- Forgive yourself and make a decision about how you will act in a similar situation next time.
- Forgive yourself and take some action that could benefit yourself or others.

Talk to others Don't keep your guilt bottled up. Talk to someone who will really listen and understand what you're going through, like a trusted friend or another care partner. Sharing your feelings with others will help to normalize the feelings and give you a more balanced perspective.

Remember that guilt is common Many other care partners have likely experienced every reason you can think of to feel guilt. It's natural to experience moments of anger or frustration, to yearn for time away, and to need the help and support of others.

Experiencing grief

Some people start to grieve soon after a loved one receives a diagnosis. Others may begin to grieve as the disease progresses or after a loved one has died. You may grieve for the person who is changing, and for the changes that being a care partner has brought to your life.

Attending to your grief as a care partner is essential. Grief can weigh you down and show up as anger or depression. Being with your grief can bring a renewed sense of peace and ease to your life. It's a necessary part of the full human experience.

Types of grief Although the process of grieving differs from person to person, it can be comforting to know that certain experiences are common among care partners. If you've experienced any one of these types of grief, you're far from alone.

Disenfranchised grief Early on, you may struggle with two conflicting realities: On the one hand, your loved one is alive and well and may seem unchanged to family members and friends. On the other hand, you've started to notice small but increasingly frequent changes in your loved one that signal bigger and more painful changes to come.

Without the full understanding and support of those around you, it may seem as if what you're experiencing doesn't matter and that you don't have the right to grieve. This type is sometimes called disenfranchised grief.

Ambiguous loss This type of grief happens when you feel a sense of loss or mourning for someone who's still there physically but mentally and emotionally no longer present in the way you need or want him or her to be. A spouse, parent or friend may be right there in front of you, for example, yet you mourn not being able to exchange advice, share emotional support, cook meals together or talk about the news of the day in the ways that you used to.

"ADJUSTING TO THE CHANGES AND LOSSES IS A PROCESS."

Ambiguous loss can vary based on the type of dementia.

In Alzheimer's disease, for example, care partners may experience losses related to changes in thinking and memory, like the ability to have meaningful conversations. Behavioral variant frontotemporal degeneration causes someone to lose the ability to have appropriate emotions and empathy for others. This is very painful for care partners and families. And Lewy body dementia can cause fluctuations in thinking that can make it seem as if someone's moving back and forth from one stage of dementia to another, but in reality, these fluctuations happen at every stage of the disease. This can cause a similar back and forth of emotions for care partners and families.

Anticipatory grief As you learn about dementia and plan for the future, you may become consumed by thoughts of future changes and challenges and start to grieve losses that haven't happened yet. For example, you may mourn a time when your loved one no longer recognizes you or needs to move out of the home and into a care community. This kind of grief is known as anticipatory grief.

Being with grief Adjusting to the changes and losses is a process. Like the practice of acceptance, addressing grief happens in several ways.

Here are three important steps to take in addressing grief.

Acknowledge your pain Rather than shove grief aside, allow yourself to acknowledge and feel your grief and the other emotions that can come with it. You may be surprised when strong feelings like anger, guilt, frustration and resentment arise. Try to be with these feelings with openness and kindness.

Share your grief Know that people may not understand your grief. Most people think grief happens when someone dies. Talk to someone you trust about your feelings. This can be a good friend, another care partner, an understanding professional or a supportive member of your family. For some care partners, support groups can be helpful. Look for a group where you feel safe sharing your experience and your emotions.

Be prepared for multiple moments of grief Because dementia worsens over time, you may experience many moments of loss over time. What triggers your grief may seem small, like the first time you attend a caregiver support group. Or it may feel overwhelmingly big, like the day your loved one enters memory care.

WHAT YOU FOCUS ON MATTERS

As you've learned, it's important and healthy to notice guilt and grief and other feelings that are distressing or negative.

However, it's *not* healthy to focus on these feelings for so long that they crowd out positive experiences and feelings. For the right balance, it's best to give painful or difficult emotions the attention they need when they come up, but then actively work to embrace positive experiences and emotions.

Embracing the good may be easier said than done. It's actually much easier for the brain to pay attention to bad things and overlook good things. This is a result of how human beings have evolved. For early humans, paying attention to dangerous and negative threats was a matter of life and death. Those more attuned to danger and bad things around them were more likely to survive.

Today, this focus on the bad is known as negativity bias. Research shows that the brain is more active when it's responding to something negative. As a result, the brain tends to be influenced more powerfully by bad news and negative experiences, as opposed to good news and positive experiences. Often, positive experience pass you by without your even noticing them.

Here's an example of negativity bias: Imagine that you're spending an afternoon with your daughter. You laugh, share stories and enjoy great conversation. You feel truly connected and joyful for this rare time together. As you're about to part ways, your daughter says that she doesn't think you should be taking her dad (your husband) to the adult day program he usually attends. "His dementia isn't that bad," your daughter says. "He doesn't belong there."

You're instantly annoyed. As you drive home, you think about her opinion over and over. By the time you're home, you're angry, exhausted and drained. You feel as if your daughter doesn't appreciate the respite you receive — and need — by taking your husband to the adult day program. You go to bed feeling that the day was ruined.

What happened to all those good feelings from the day? Your positive experiences were drowned out by the negative ones — this is how negativity bias works. In short, the bad emotions are stronger than the good ones. As a result, you think about the bad experiences for longer periods of time, and they weigh more heavily on you.

Fortunately, you can overcome your negativity bias and focus more on positive emotions by taking these steps.

Address negative self-talk

Self-talk is the way you talk to yourself in your head. These automatic thoughts can be positive or negative, but more often than not, they're negative. For care partners, negative self-talk may include thoughts of self-doubt and criticism, regret, worry, and guilt. Forms of negative self-talk include:

Filtering This is when you magnify the negative aspects of a situation and filter out all of the positive ones. In the example you just read, you had a great afternoon with your daughter, filled with connection and joy. However, your visit ended with a short conversation in which you had a disagreement. The rest of the day and evening, you focused only on your disagreement and forgot about the wonderful time you spent with your daughter.

Personalizing This is when something bad happens and you automatically blame yourself. For example, your coffee group canceled its gathering for tomorrow, and you think it's because no one wanted to be around you and hear about your struggles.

Catastrophizing Automatically believing the worst is going to happen is known as catastrophizing. Maybe you're having a bad morning and tell yourself that as long as you're a caregiver, your life is going to be one miserable day after the next. This is an example of catastrophizing.

Polarizing Polarizing happens when you see things only as either good or bad, with no middle ground between the two. Maybe you feel like you have to be perfect or you'll be a total failure. For example, if you can't convince your spouse to shower, you tell yourself you're the worst caregiver ever.

Using 'should' statements A "should" statement is when you think you should think, feel or behave in a certain way. Maybe you think you *should* be able care for your loved one by yourself, or that you *should* keep your promise to not move your loved one to a care community.

It's important to notice when you're engaged in negative self-talk so you can learn to change the pattern. From there, try to explore what's causing the negative feelings. Is your anger stemming from a sense of feeling overwhelmed, scared or lonely? Is it coming from the impossible expectations you've set for yourself or that others have placed on you? Questions like these can help you pause and see your situation in a more balanced way.

The next time a negative conversation starts playing out in your head, try asking yourself the following questions:

- Would I talk this way to my good friend?
- What am I really (angry, frustrated, concerned) about?
- Is what I'm angry or worried about just my thought at this moment? Remember, thoughts are real but they are not necessarily true.
- Do I really need to be concerned or worried about this?
- What will happen if I ignore this?
- Why am I doing this? Is this someone else's expectation?
- Can I settle for a good-enough-for-now solution?

Savor the positive

Because the brain naturally gravitates toward the negative, it's important to give extra time and attention to good things when they happen. While negative experiences can be quickly transferred and stored in the brain, positive and pleasant experiences take more of an effort to get the same effect. When something good happens, take a moment to really focus on it, be with it and savor it. Replay the moment several times and focus on the positive feelings the memory evokes.

What you focus on determines the parts of your brain that eventually strengthen over time. In other words, if you pay more attention to positive or pleasant experiences, no matter how big or small, your brain can become more wired for resilience, optimism, gratitude and positive emotion.

You may find this approach helpful as you look for moments of connection with the person living with dementia, appreciating whatever strengths and abilities he or she possesses. Pay attention to any aspect of life that you're grateful for, even if it's simply the ability to enjoy the morning sunrise and sip a cup of your favorite tea.

PRACTICING MINDFULNESS

You already know about the physical, emotional and psychological stress caused by caring for a loved one with dementia. The side effects of caregiving can put your body, mind and overall health at risk. This is where mindfulness can help; it can address the negative impact of stress and help you be kinder to yourself and others.

Mindfulness is a type of meditation in which you focus on being intensely aware of what you're sensing and feeling in the moment, without interpretation or judgment. Practicing mindfulness can help you reduce stress, make better decisions and be truly present with the person living with dementia. It can also enhance your capacity to experience the joys of everyday life.

A growing body of research shows that mindfulness is helpful for dementia care partners. One study found that people who care for family members with Alzheimer's disease and other dementias were less stressed and their mood was more stable when they practiced a type of meditation called mindfulness-based stress reduction (MBSR). Another study suggested that MBSR is more helpful than caregiver education in terms of improving mental health, reducing stress and relieving depression. A more recent review found that MBSR may help with anxiety and depression in people caring for family members with dementia.

Experts believe that mindfulness works, in part, by helping people accept their experiences, including painful emotions, rather than avoid them.

Mindfulness also offers unique benefits for care partners, according to Marguerite Manteau-Rao, a licensed clinical social worker. Manteau-Rao developed the Mindfulness-Based Dementia Care approach to training dementia caregivers at the Osher Center for Integrative Medicine at the University of California, San Francisco.

ADOPTING A GRATITUDE PRACTICE

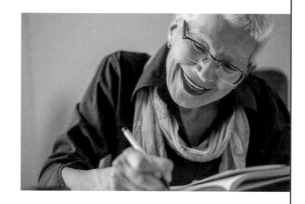

Gratitude plays an important role in well-being. For dementia care partners in particular, research shows that adopting a gratitude practice can improve coping skills and relieve feeling of distress.

Here are three ways to start a gratitude practice, from *The Mayo Clinic Handbook for Happiness:*

Keep a gratitude journal. Write in it every day. What you write can be as simple as a kind gesture from a stranger at the grocery store. Any positive thoughts or actions count, no matter how small.

Use gratitude cues. Place photos of things or people that make you happy where you'll see them often. Or post positive notes or inspirational quotes on your refrigerator door or by your computer to reinforce feelings of gratitude.

Make a gratitude jar. Keep an empty jar, with scratch paper and a pen next to it, in an accessible place at home. Write on a piece of paper one thing that you're grateful for every day and drop it in the jar. Encourage family members to do this, too. At some point during the day, take a few notes out of the jar and read them.

In her book, *Caring for a Loved One With Dementia,* Manteau-Rao says that mindfulness:

- Helps care partners spend less time in a stressful state of mind, which is usually associated with thinking too much about the past or worrying about a future event or situation.
- Trains care partners to take the time to pause in the heat of a difficult situation.
- Helps care partners to be more aware of the person with dementia, helping them to notice nonverbal signals.
- Helps care partners shift from a rushed, task-driven mode to a state of simply be-

‘ANY MEDITATION IS GOOD MEDITATION’

If meditation is new to you, it may be best to start by simply setting aside time each day to quiet your mind and focus on just one thing, according to Brent A. Bauer, M.D., founder of Mayo Clinic’s Integrative Medicine and Health program.

When he talks with patients, Dr. Bauer emphasizes that it’s OK to try different meditation practices until they find the ones that work for them.

“Sometimes patients tell me they’re worried that if they try to sit still and meditate, they’ll fail. For these individuals, meditation was one more thing they felt bad about not doing. For some people, it’s really a struggle to keep very quiet, and they get frustrated and think they’re not doing it right. I encourage these individuals to try different practices until they find one that works for them,” says Dr. Bauer. “Whatever you can do to try to quiet your mind and let the thoughts flow by, that’s what works for you. Any meditation is good meditation.”

ing. This can help the person with dementia feel recognized and respond more positively.

- Promotes a calm, centered presence.
- Increases sensory awareness. This helps care partners anticipate environmental stressors and make appropriate changes that help the person with dementia.
- Teaches ways to connect with and signal to the person with dementia that you’re attuned to his or her present state even if the person is no longer able to speak in ways that you can understand.

Use the practices on pages 353 and 354 to get acquainted with mindfulness.

SHOWING COMPASSION – TO YOURSELF

Self-compassion is closely linked to mindfulness. During the practice of mindfulness, you build a sense of self-awareness around your thoughts, feelings, sensations and surroundings.

Self-compassion is an attitude you can add to your mindfulness experience. It involves being kind to yourself, especially when you’re caught up in harsh self-judgment or you feel as if you’ve failed. Self-compassion helps you remember that all humans are imperfect, and that’s OK.

In *The Mindful Self-Compassion Workbook*, psychologists Kristen Neff, Ph.D., and Christopher Germer, Ph.D., describe self-compassion as:

Treating yourself with kindness When you're feeling low or you're in the midst of a painful situation, talk to yourself the way you would talk to a good friend. For example, you may tell yourself, *This is really stressful, and I'm so sorry. You're doing your best right now. It will be OK.* Give yourself the kind of support you need to hear most in that moment.

Accepting that humans are flawed Rather than beat yourself up for what you see as imperfections, remind yourself that all humans are imperfect. Everyone experiences failure and a sense of not being good enough at times. Acknowledge your failures and imperfections with nonjudgmental compassion. Remind yourself, *I'm flawed, and that's what makes me like everyone else.*

Being mindful of negative thoughts and feelings You've already learned that paying attention to your thoughts can help you respond more effectively to difficult emotions and situations. This kind of mindfulness is also a key element of self-compassion. Instead of resisting or pushing away negative thoughts, feelings and sensations, let them be and acknowledge them as something that's momentary and passing.

Self-compassion is essential to health and well-being. The first step toward believing that you can be a compassionate care partner is to be compassionate and caring toward yourself.

OPTIONS FOR SUPPORT

Practicing acceptance means that there will be times when you'll need assistance beyond what you alone will be able to provide your loved one. But asking for help may not come easily. You may worry that your loved one won't feel comfortable with other people. Or maybe you think no one else can provide care as well as you can.

The truth is, receiving help can make being a care partner less burdensome, both physically and emotionally. The right assistance can offer resources and skills that you may not have and give you a chance to recharge your batteries. This boost can help you be a more effective, patient and compassionate care partner.

Sources of support fall under two broad categories: informal and formal. Here's how they differ, as well as examples of these two valuable sources of support.

Informal support

Informal support includes family, friends, neighbors and faith communities. These groups often consist of people who knew your loved one before onset of the disease.

You may count on them, for example, to make visits or take the person you're caring

MINDFULNESS BREATHING PRACTICE

Focusing your attention on your breath is a common mindfulness practice. Since your breath is always in the present, this practice becomes a way to stay, as well as return, to the present moment.

1. Find a comfortable position, seated on a chair or on the floor on a cushion. Your eyes may be open or closed; you may find it easier to maintain your focus if your eyes are closed.
2. Take three full breaths in and out. Then return to your natural breathing.
3. Tune in to your natural breath. Feel the natural flow of your breath — in and then out. You don't need to change anything about how you breathe. Notice where you feel your breath in your body; it may be in your belly, or you may notice it in your chest, throat or nostrils. Become aware and curious about the breath, noticing its pattern, sounds and any other sensations.
4. When you find that your mind has wandered and you're no longer paying attention to your breath, this is a time to stop yourself and gently guide your focus back to your breath.
5. Practice this exercise for five to 15 minutes. Follow your breath, notice when the mind wanders and then return back to the breath, over and over. The intention is not to stop the mind from wandering but to notice when your mind wanders.

for to an activity. Their visits may be as valuable for you as they are for the person living with dementia because they keep you both socially connected.

Although these informal sources of support are well meaning, some care partners say that over time, they can drift away, leaving the care partner without the support they need. To maintain your connection with the people in your informal support network, be as specific as you can.

Through a phone call, letter, email or personal visit, talk to them about the diagnosis as well as the symptoms and changes you're seeing in the person living with dementia. Also let them know the ways in which the person is still very much the same and the things he or she continues to enjoy. Describe

THE STOP PRACTICE

In addition to formally scheduling a time and a place to practice mindfulness, you can practice mindfulness during everyday activities, like when you're stopped at a red light in your car, washing your hands or sitting down to eat a meal. One way to do this is with a practice developed by Jon Kabat-Zinn, Ph.D., called STOP.

This practice helps you to take a step back from the stressors of the day and the worries that may be circulating in your mind. It brings you back into the present so you can regain perspective and better regulate your response to pressure.

First, identify various activities you do regularly throughout the day. Any of the activities listed above are good examples. Use these activities as cues to pause. This practice can help you reduce your stress and invite more calm into your day. Over time, STOP may become a habit and a consistent part of your mindfulness practice.

Here's how it works:

S Stop. Whatever you're doing, just pause momentarily.
T Take a few breaths.
O Observe your thoughts. Where has your mind gone? You may notice that you are engaging in a lot of negative self-talk. What do you feel? Research shows that just naming your emotions can turn the volume down and have a calming effect. What is happening around you? Observe your surroundings.
P Proceed and resume your activities, or use what you've learned during this practice to change course.

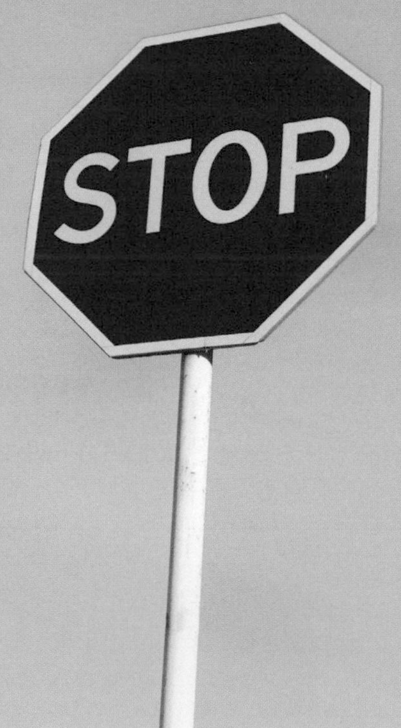

THE SELF-COMPASSION BREAK

Like STOP, a practice called the self-compassion break from Kristen Neff, Ph.D., can help you be kinder to yourself. You can use it anytime, but it can be especially helpful when you're facing difficult or painful situations.

Here's how it works:

1. Acknowledge what you're feeling, and tell yourself, *This is a moment of suffering.* Instead of the word *suffering*, you may use the word *painful* or any other word that feels right to you to describe what you're feeling.
2. Tell yourself, *I am not alone. We all struggle and feel pain and suffering.*
3. Put your hands over your heart. Feel the warmth of your hands and the gentle touch of your hands on your chest. If there's another soothing touch that feels right for you, use that instead.
4. Say one of the following to yourself:
   - May I be kind to myself.
   - May I give myself the compassion that I need.
   - May I learn to accept myself as I am.
   - May I forgive myself.
   - May I be patient.
   - May I feel ease.

your current needs for assistance and offer specific suggestions for the kinds of activities that may be helpful during visits.

Prepare a list of things that routinely need doing and let the people in your informal support network choose tasks that are right for them. Or you may take a different approach, listing the routine tasks you do in a typical day and assigning these tasks to certain individuals based on their qualities and the resources that they can provide. Family and friends often find it rewarding to help — it's a way to show they care.

Formal support

Formal support includes any nonprofit or for-profit agency that provides assistance to individuals in caregiving settings. Home health agencies, community programs like

USING YOUR INFORMAL SUPPORT SYSTEM

When someone says, "Let me know if you need something," consider this list as a starting point:

- Provide transportation to doctor appointments
- Call or visit once a week
- Help organize and process medical bills
- Provide a meal
- Take care of shopping or other errands
- Do housecleaning, laundry or yardwork
- Ask occasionally about how I'm doing
- Be a listener

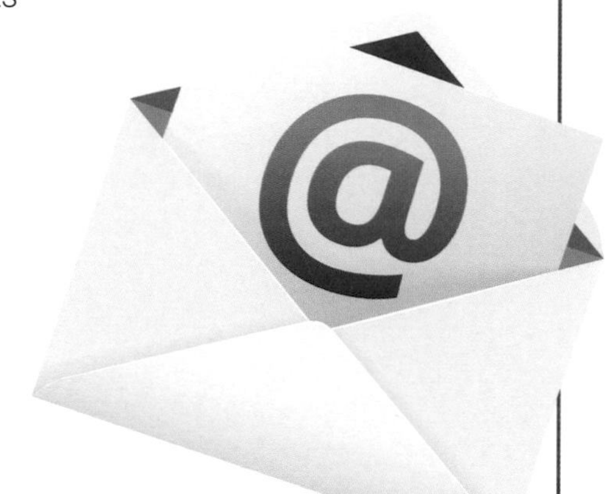

classes, day programs and elder care centers are all examples. Formal support also includes support groups.

A support group typically consists of other care partners in situations like yours. Support groups regularly meet to share experiences and emotions. Meetings are usually led by a professional or a trained volunteer.

Attending a support group can offer an opportunity for you to hear from others who have dealt with issues like the ones you've experienced. There may also be times when you aren't looking for new ideas or advice — you just want to be among people who understand what you're going through and can relate. Support groups come in many varieties:

Disease-specific groups These can be groups for care partners of people with dementia, but they can be more specific, like a group for Lewy body dementia or frontotemporal degeneration care partners.

Relationship-specific groups These groups might bring together people in specific caregiving situations or relationships. Examples include people caring a spouse or partner, adult children caring for a parent, or men who are caregivers.

Peer-led support groups These groups are led by current or former care partners who share the same experience of caregiving.

Groups led by a trained facilitator The facilitator may be a social worker, wellness coach,

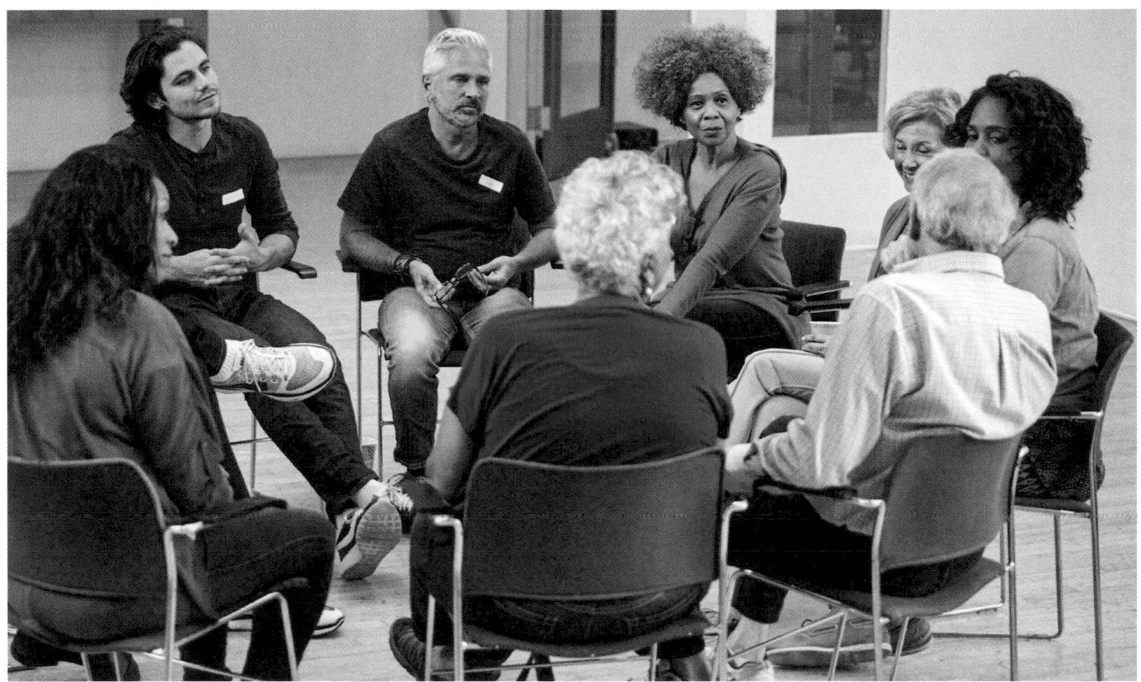

clergy person, elder care provider or another professional.

Online and telephone caregiver groups These groups offer support to people who can't travel to a face-to-face meeting, or who need to talk to someone during off hours. You may find a variety of chatrooms, blogs and support groups on the internet.

Use your own good judgment about the internet or get recommendations from a trusted medical professional.

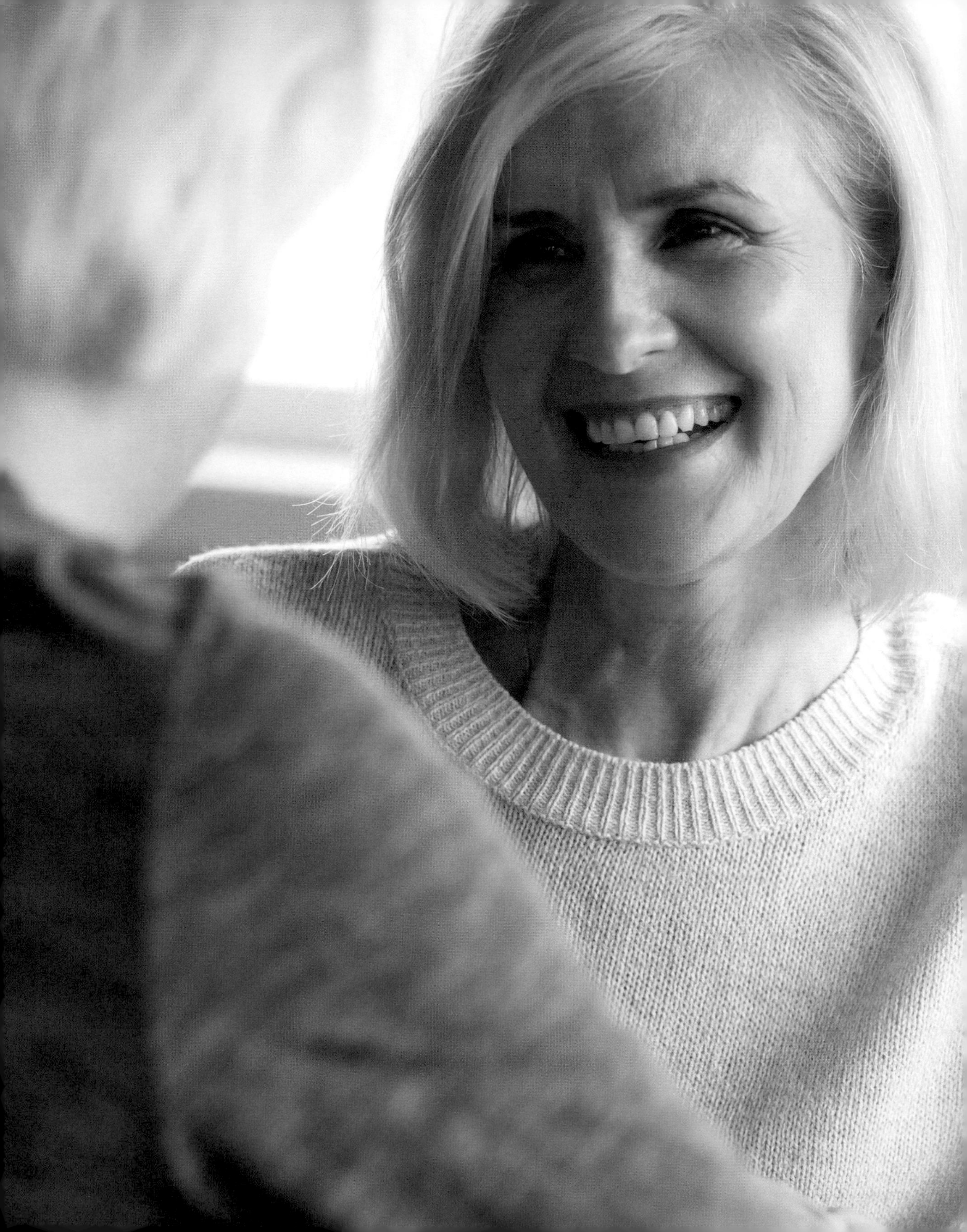

PART 6

Brain health for everyone

Brain health is a lifelong process. Throughout your life, your brain has the capacity to adapt and grow in many ways, and you can strengthen it at any age.

You can strengthen your brain much in the same way you use exercises to strengthen the muscles in your arms and legs, for example. Learning new skills, taking a class and expanding your vocabulary are all examples of ways you can improve your brain health and keep the nerve cells in your brain firing long into your life.

The choices you make every day also help keep your brain working at its best, no matter how old you are. Aside from exercises that target your thinking skills, many habits that are good for overall health support good brain health, too. Think healthy eating, regular exercise, getting enough sleep and connecting with others.

In the next two chapters, you'll learn what research shows about steps you can take to optimize brain health — and possibly prevent dementia.

"ALTHOUGH DAMAGE TO THE BRAIN CAN'T BE REVERSED, TAKING CARE OF YOUR BRAIN AND THE BLOOD VESSELS THAT NOURISH IT CAN HELP."

CHAPTER 19

Healthy aging

Early on in this book, you learned about many common changes that take place with aging, including those that involve your brain. For example, as you get older, it may get harder to multitask or it may take longer to provide an answer to a question. Most people notice at least some subtle changes in how well they think and remember as they age.

Although normal age-related changes in the brain don't mean that dementia is in your future, taking steps now to protect your brain can help it stay healthy as you age.

KEYS TO GOOD BRAIN HEALTH

Researchers have found that about a third of the time, dementia is caused by risk factors that you can control. This means in theory if you can control these risk factors you may be able to reduce your risk of developing cognitive issues.

While there's no one way to reduce the risk of dementia or slow down cognitive decline, research suggests that a combination of lifestyle habits and treatment can help. Researchers think that taking certain steps may delay or prevent many cases of dementia. Overall, these measures provide a road map for better brain aging.

Studies show that keeping your brain healthy is a lifelong process; this is a fact that's often overlooked. Take childhood education, for example. This early learning likely lays the foundation for cognitive reserve — in other words, how well you can withstand harmful changes to the brain (learn more on the next page).

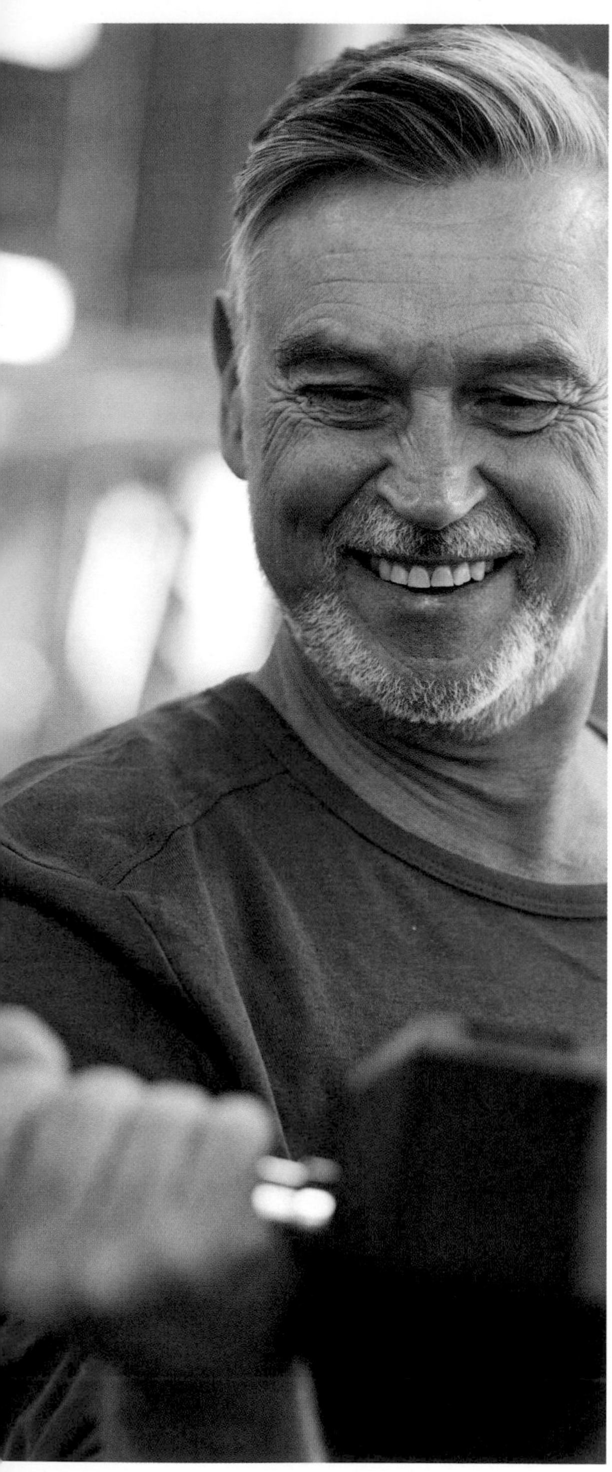

Cognitive reserve is often measured by years of formal education. By continuing your education throughout your life, you may increase your cognitive reserve and the brain protection it offers.

Likewise, addressing general health issues like diabetes, high blood pressure, physical inactivity and smoking has been shown to be helpful for brain health. While addressing these issues is important at any age, it's especially important in midlife. Taking care of your health can help protect your blood vessels, which can help prevent cognitive decline later in life. Promoting good blood flow is good for your heart and your brain.

Here are more details about what researchers have found most helpful in promoting brain health across the life span.

Cognitive reserve

If you were told that you had physical changes in your brain, like shrinkage in key areas involved in memory, and that these changes are often seen in someone with dementia, you might think the worst. But not everyone who has brain changes associated with dementia shows signs of the disease. Why is this?

Two people can have similar amounts of the hallmark plaques and tangles of Alzheimer's disease. Yet, one may have debilitating symptoms while the other has no issues with memory at all. Experts think that the difference between these two people comes

A WORD ON 'BRAIN TRAINING'

What about formal activities that stimulate the mind? There's been some buzz around brain (cognitive) training as a means of helping improve certain brain functions like memory, language and brain-processing speed. This type of structured program uses repetitive memory and reasoning exercises. They may be computer-assisted or done in person, one-on-one or in small groups.

According to researchers, there's not much proof that these activities help. Brain-training products that are widely advertised as a way to give the brain a boost may offer short-term benefits in the specific areas that are addressed. Reasoning, decision-making and language are examples. But at this point, no evidence shows that they're helpful beyond the short-term, or that they can help keep dementia from developing.

Experts say you'll get the most benefit from doing activities that stimulate your brain throughout your life. Getting a good education, working in a mentally stimulating job, and taking up mentally engaging pastimes or social activities are all good options.

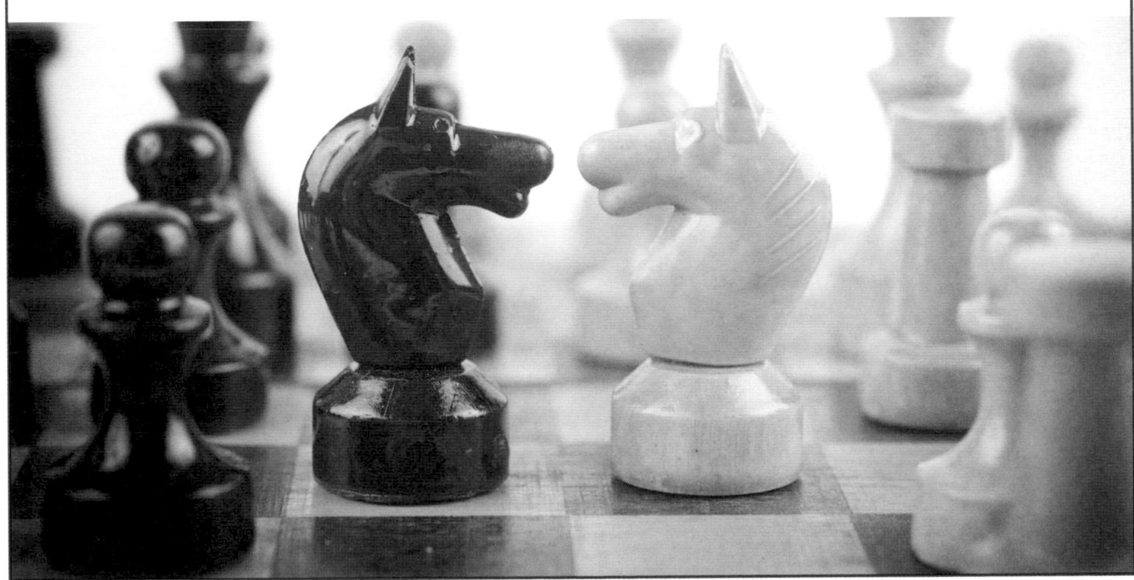

down to cognitive reserve. Simply put, cognitive reserve is how well your brain is able to cope with — or adjust to — physical changes in the brain like those brought on by dementia.

A person's cognitive reserve capacity can be developed throughout life; this may help offset some of the changes in the brain that lead to dementia. Experts think that certain activities help develop more cognitive reserve. This may make up for the loss of diseased parts of the brain. Activities that are at least moderately challenging to the brain seem to help most in building this reserve.

Whether you're born with a good cognitive reserve or not, you can build it through education and activities like learning a new skill, reading, learning music and even practicing mindfulness. It seems that people who spend more time engaged in learning throughout their lives develop more robust networks of neurons in their brains and bolster the connections between them. A strong network of neurons is better able to handle cell damage that can happen in the disorders that cause dementia.

Physical activity

Although researchers don't know yet how well physical activity can improve memory or slow cognitive decline, they do know that it's helpful.

In one study, researchers divided participants into two groups. They had one group get aerobic exercise. They had the other group do stretching and balance exercises. After one year, researchers noticed that the people who got aerobic exercise had a larger hippocampus — the part of the brain that makes new memories.

In another study, researchers found that people with a gene that causes Alzheimer's disease who exercised for 150 minutes or more each week delayed the disease by several years. People in the study who had an Alzheimer's gene but exercised for less than 150 minutes a week developed Alzheimer's disease more quickly. While it's unclear if exercise can reduce the risk of Alzheimer's disease, this research suggests that it may.

What is it about physical activity that makes it so important? Experts think exercise keeps blood flowing, which helps the brain. It also boosts the level of chemicals that naturally protect the brain. And physical activity helps make up for the connections between nerve cells in your brain that are lost as you age.

Mental function is less likely to decline in people who are physically active on a regular basis. This makes physically active people less likely to develop dementia. Physical activity helps improve other risk factors for dementia, too, like high blood pressure, diabetes and high cholesterol. It may also give the immune system a boost and combat inflammation.

Exercise alone doesn't seem to improve how well healthy older adults think, however, and it's likely most helpful when it's part of a larger wellness plan. It's also important to note that not all studies have made the connection between exercise and a reduced risk of dementia. However, the benefits of physical activity are many and go far beyond brain health.

For good overall health, the U.S. Department of Health and Human Services recommends that adults work toward getting at least 150 minutes of moderate aerobic activity, 75 minutes of vigorous aerobic activity, or a combination of the two every week. Strength training is also important; the latest guidelines recommend doing activities that strengthen all of the body's major muscle groups at least twice a week.

If you're looking for added benefits, aim for at least 300 minutes of moderate aerobic activity, 150 minutes of vigorous aerobic activity, or a combination of the two each week.

Walk with a friend, try a group exercise class or sign up through a community center to learn a new dance — all of these count toward meeting your physical activity goal. And remember, every little bit of activity is better than nothing at all.

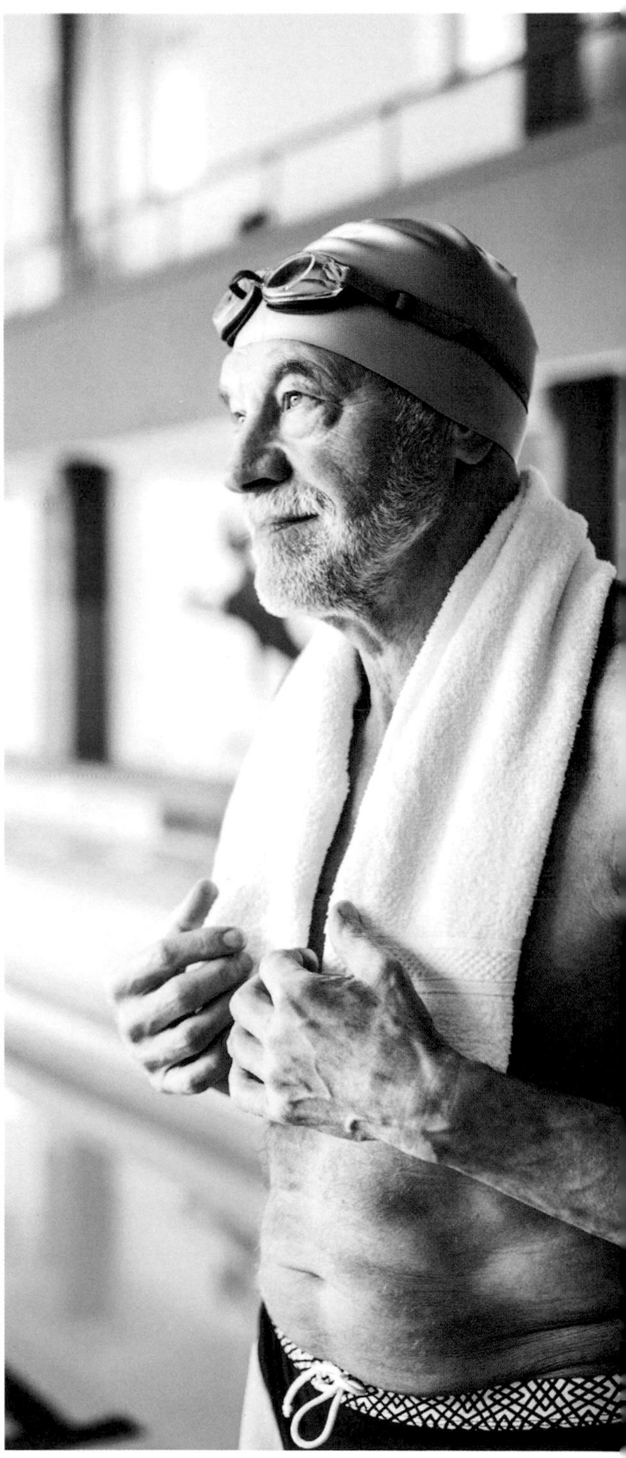

Managing high blood pressure

High blood pressure in middle age is linked to a higher risk of dementia later in life. Managing high blood pressure helps keep blood vessels healthy. This is important for preventing vascular dementia, in particular.

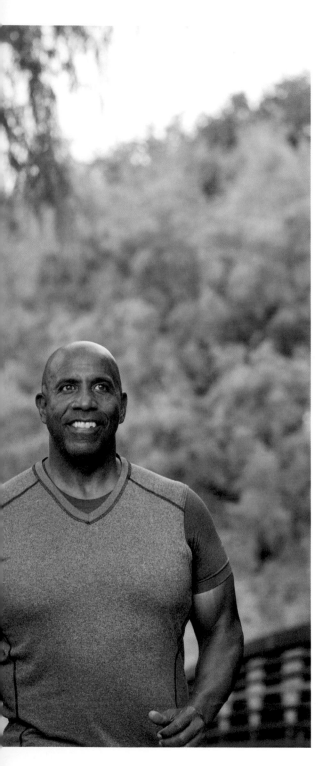

Vascular dementia happens when the arteries that keep blood flowing to the brain become narrow or get blocked. It can also be caused by a stroke that interrupts blood flow to the brain. In either case, high blood pressure may be to blame.

High blood pressure weakens the arteries that keep blood flowing through your body. It can cause a stroke, but it can also cause so-called silent strokes that you may not notice.

Over time, strokes can cause scarring in the blood vessels. This scarring leads to problems with blood flow in the brain, which can cause problems in how different parts of the brain work. It can also cause parts of the brain to stop working completely. In fact, researchers have found that people over age 65 who have high blood pressure have more scarring in their brains than do those who don't have high blood pressure.

This is why the health of your blood vessels is so important to brain health. If blood vessels weaken, they can't get nutrients and oxygen to the nerve cells in the brain that need them to function. Managing high blood pressure can help keep this cascade of effects from taking place.

Although current standard guidelines recommend aiming for a blood pressure of less than 130/90 millimeters of mercury (mm Hg), you learned earlier that reaching an even lower target can help prevent dementia. In fact, researchers have found that lowering systolic blood pressure — the top

"HIGH BLOOD PRESSURE WEAKENS THE ARTERIES THAT KEEP BLOOD FLOWING THROUGH YOUR BODY."

number in your blood pressure reading — to 120 mm Hg can reduce the risk of cognitive impairment.

To lower blood pressure, lifestyle measures like a healthy diet and regular physical activity are good places to start. In some cases, medication may be needed. Several studies have shown a reduced risk of cognitive decline in people who treat high blood pressure with medications.

WHAT ABOUT SOCIAL ISOLATION?

Social isolation has been tied to poorer health for decades. Different from loneliness, social isolation means having little or no contact with others or not having many social contacts, like a spouse, family, friends and co-workers.

Social isolation increases the risk of having poorer thinking skills and memory. It also makes Alzheimer's disease more likely. This may be in part because it can lead to brain inactivity and result in faster mental decline. In addition, it may increase the odds of developing conditions linked to Alzheimer's, like high blood pressure, heart disease and depression.

Social isolation has also been tied to unhealthy behaviors, like smoking and not getting enough exercise — behaviors that can put you at a higher risk of cognitive impairment. And like other risk factors for Alzheimer's disease, social isolation may also be a symptom of the disease.

Staying socially connected helps the brain in many ways. It boosts the cognitive reserve that helps buoy the brain against age-related changes. In addition, people who have larger social networks and spend more time engaged with the people in them perform better in terms of their thinking skills. They also show less decline in thinking skills as they age.

In fact, people who have many social contacts and engage with them regularly may be half as likely to have memory problems.

Research also shows that engaging with others has a positive effect on chemicals that protect the brain from dementia, especially dementia caused by Alzheimer's disease.

How many people you have in your social network, how diverse your connections are, and how often you're in touch with the people in your social circle all play a role in how well your brain functions. That makes staying connected with others, especially later in life, an important way to keep the brain healthy and help prevent changes in the brain that can lead to dementia.

Social interaction is an area where anyone can make a change at any time, and it will likely have positive cognitive benefits. Interacting with others — family, friends, neighbors, co-workers, community members — can lift your mood, improve your outlook and engage your brain. All of these positively affect your cognitive abilities. Social engagement is seen as such a strong predictor of well-being that some experts think it should be included as part of a dementia-prevention plan.

DOES SLEEP MAKE A DIFFERENCE?

It's not news that getting enough good-quality sleep is important for overall health and well-being. But in terms of dementia risk, good sleep seems to be especially critical.

Research is starting to suggest that not getting enough good sleep over a number of years may increase the risk of dementia. In one analysis, researchers found that people whose sleep is interrupted over many years are more at risk of developing dementia. Researchers have also found that those who didn't get enough sleep may be twice as likely to develop Alzheimer's disease.

What makes sleep so important?

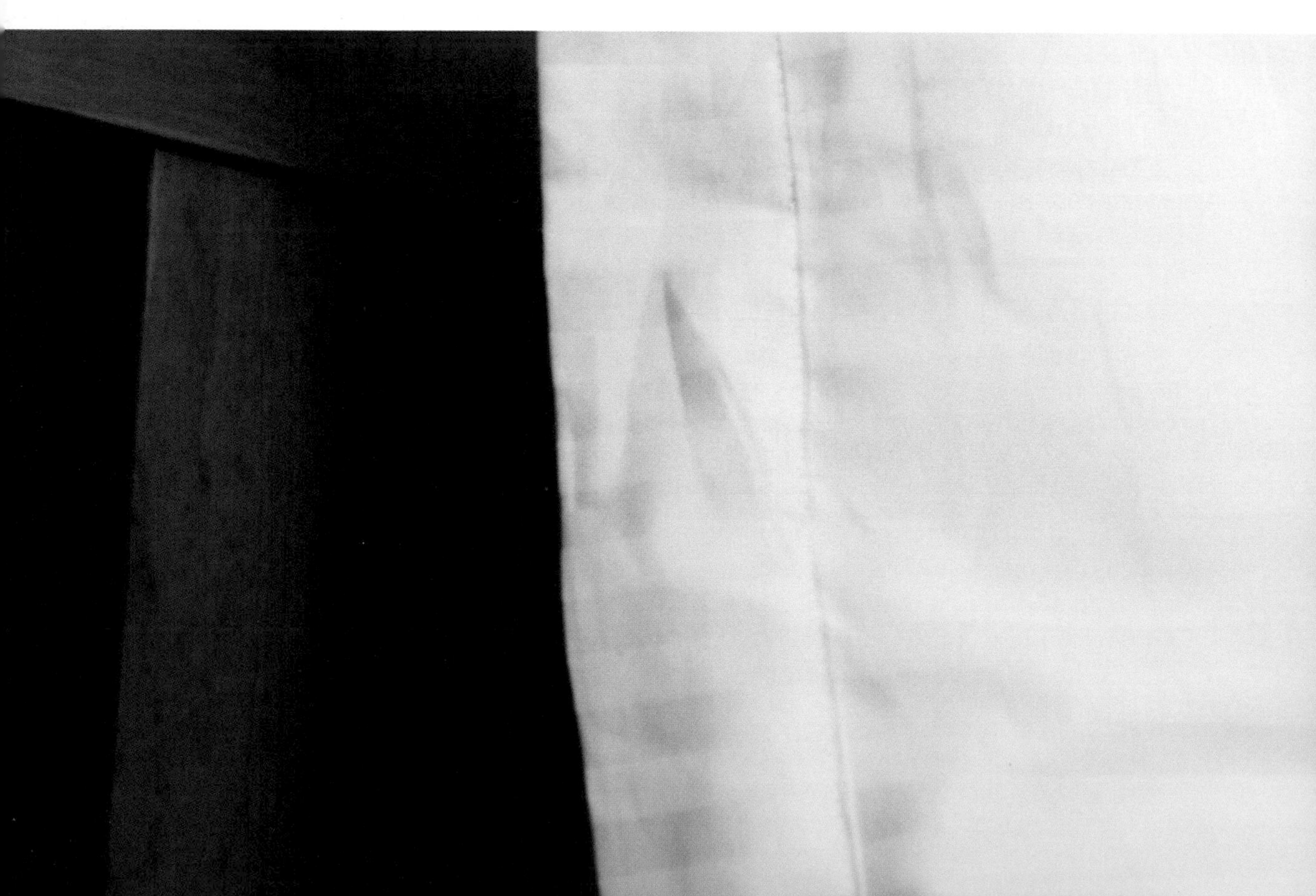

Earlier, you learned that clumps of the protein beta-amyloid harden into plaques. These plaques cause nerve cells in the brain to die. This is the process that's thought to lead to Alzheimer's disease, a common cause of dementia. Beta-amyloid and other toxins are cleared from the brain during sleep. Without good sleep, especially over a long period of time, this process may not work as well.

A lack of good sleep can increase the risk of dementia in other ways, too; namely, by increasing the risk of conditions like high blood pressure and diabetes. These conditions can make dementia more likely. Sleep apnea provides another possible link. Sleep apnea is a disorder that causes breathing to repeatedly stop and start during sleep. Snoring and feeling tired even after a full night's sleep are two common signs of sleep apnea. Sleep apnea causes oxygen levels in the body to drop, which means the brain doesn't get enough oxygen. As a result, the hippocampus — where memories are made — shrinks.

For all of these reasons, addressing sleep issues and improving sleep quality may help with cognition. Researchers are still determining if improving sleep can reduce the risk of developing Alzheimer's disease, but given all of its potential benefits, regular, good-quality sleep is a good step to take. The following are several simple steps to ensure good-quality sleep.

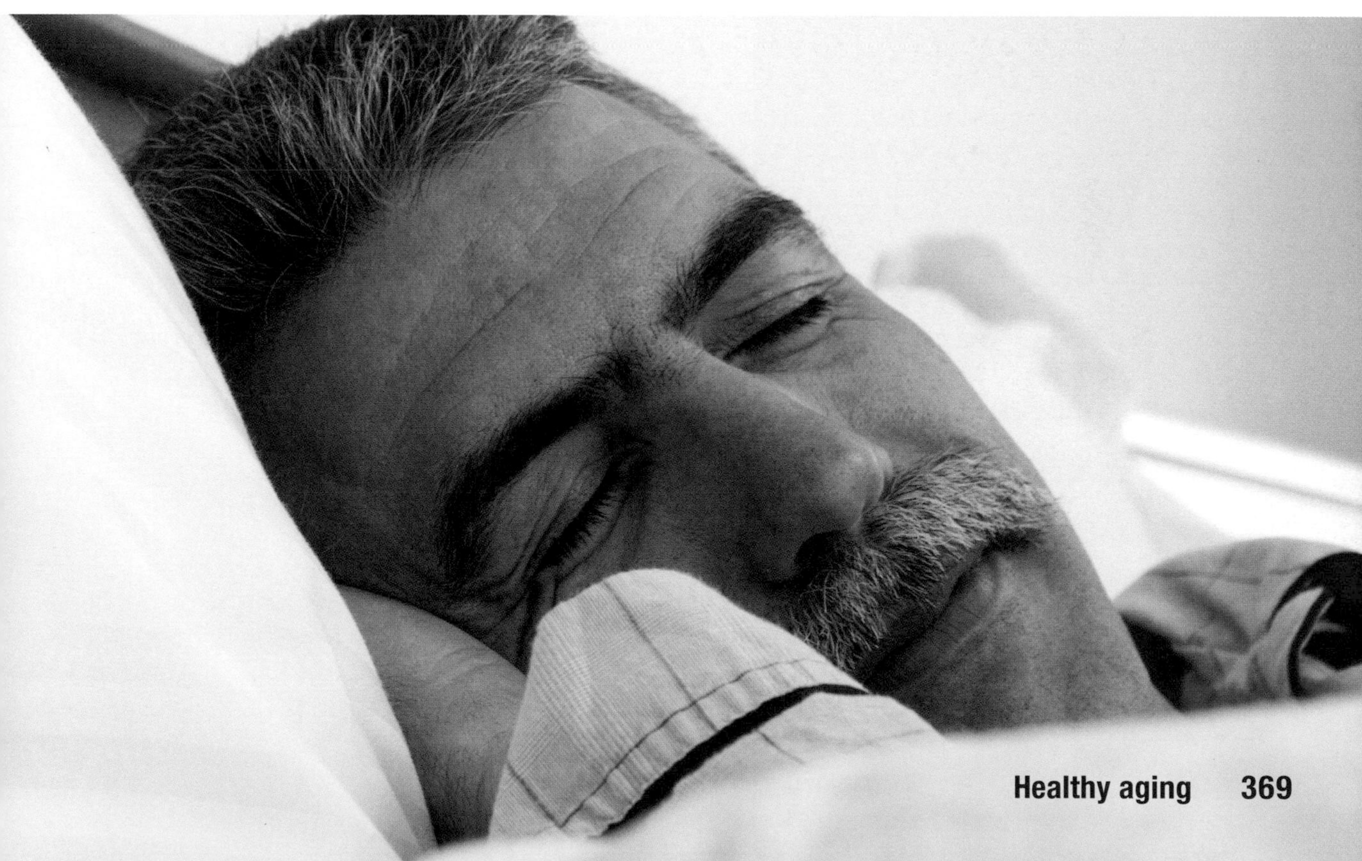

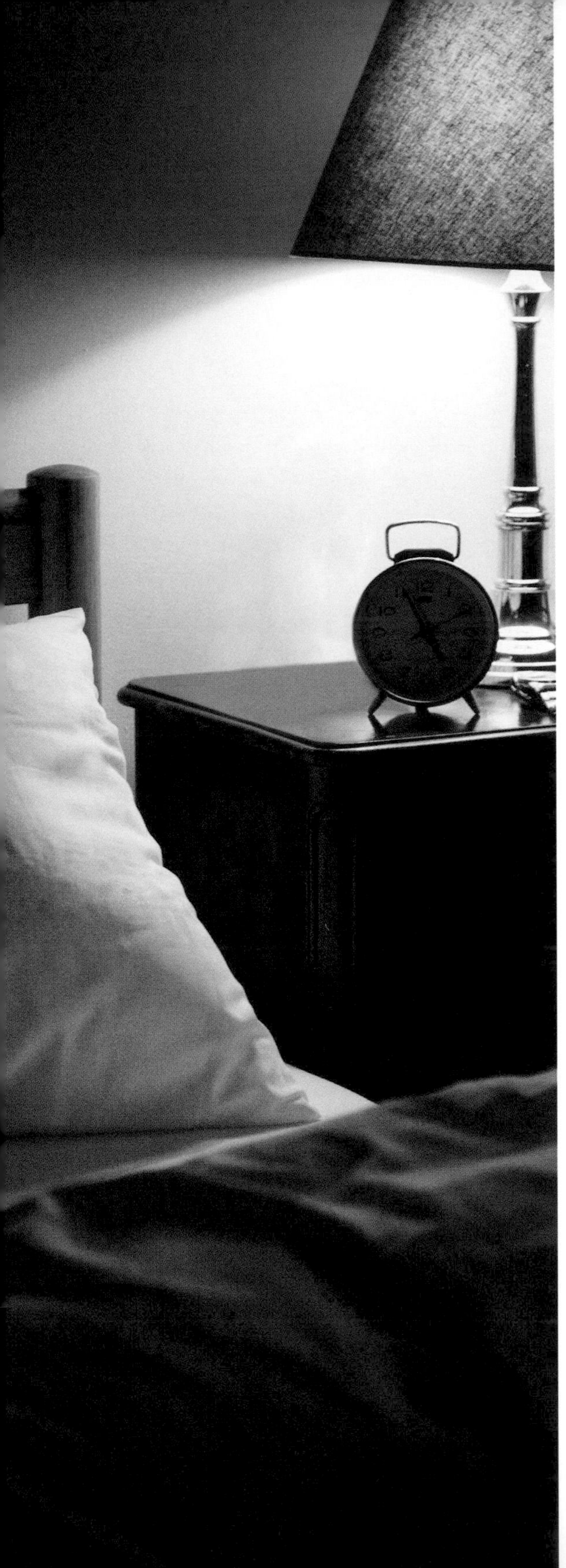

Set a schedule

Set a regular bedtime and wake time every day. It should be the same during the week as it is on the weekend.

Create the right sleep setting

A cool, dark, quiet room is best for sleeping. Not using electronic devices or watching TV for at least a half-hour before bed can also help improve sleep quality.

Watch what you eat and drink

Going to bed hungry or stuffed can make it harder to get a good night's sleep. Drinking alcohol or caffeine close to bedtime can have the same effect.

Lean on healthy daytime habits

Getting regular physical activity, spending time outdoors, limiting daytime naps and managing stress are all important for good overall health. Plus, these habits will help make it easier to get good sleep when bedtime arrives.

PREVENTION

Although damage to the brain can't be reversed, taking care of your brain and the blood vessels that nourish it can help. Taking care of your blood vessels is one way

“ADOPTING THESE HABITS CAN BENEFIT YOUR HEALTH AT ANY AGE — IT’S NEVER TOO LATE.”

you can reduce the risk of dementia. In a study of people who had Alzheimer's disease, researchers found that treating high blood pressure, high cholesterol, diabetes, smoking, and a buildup of fats and other substances in and on the artery walls (atherosclerosis) — conditions that make vascular disease more likely — helped slow the decline in thinking skills associated with Alzheimer's disease dementia.

Reduce the risk of stroke

Dementia is caused by brain disease, with Alzheimer's disease being the most common and most well-known. Diseases that affect the blood vessels — the same diseases that cause heart attacks and strokes — are the second most common cause of dementia after Alzheimer's.

Avoiding conditions that increase the risk of heart attacks and strokes may reduce your risk of dementia. Maintaining healthy levels of cholesterol and blood pressure, avoiding diabetes, not smoking, reaching and maintaining a healthy weight, and exercising regularly are all examples of ways to stay healthy.

Preventing stroke is so important that it may help keep symptoms of dementia from developing, even in people who show signs of dementia-related disease in the brain. For example, researchers following nearly 700 Catholic nuns for many years found that the nuns who had strokes were much more likely to develop symptoms of dementia. Nuns who didn't have any strokes were less likely to have symptoms of dementia — even if they had signs of dementia in their brains.

It's best to adopt habits that protect blood vessels early on and sustain them as you get older. If the health of your blood vessels deteriorates when you're younger, it's hard to mend that damage later on. In turn, damage to the brain's blood vessels can increase your risk of dementia. If your blood vessels are in good shape in young adulthood and midlife, they're more likely to stay in good shape as you age.

This is not to say that incorporating healthy choices won't make a difference later in life. Adopting these habits can benefit your health at any age — it's never too late. But the sooner you adopt these habits, the more benefit you'll likely gain.

Manage high blood pressure As you've already learned, controlling high blood pressure helps prevent a stroke, which helps lower the risk of dementia.

Don't smoke Smoking may increase the risk of stroke because it's linked to problems with the heart. In addition, neurotoxins found in cigarette smoke may harm the brain and make a stroke more likely. Either way, not smoking reduces your risk of stroke. Several years after stopping, a former smoker's risk of stroke is about the same as that of a nonsmoker.

While quitting smoking is never easy, a variety of tools, including medication and medication-free options, can help. The most successful quit-smoking plans tend to use both. Options range from medications like nicotine replacement therapy and bupropion to cognitive behavioral therapy and mindfulness-based approaches.

Control diabetes If you have diabetes, you're more likely to have a stroke, in part because diabetes can damage blood vessels. This alone makes managing diabetes an important way to reduce the risk of stroke — and, in turn, dementia. Diet, exercise, reaching and maintaining a healthy weight, and medication can all help. If you do have a stroke, you may have less damage to your brain if your diabetes is well controlled.

Diabetes also has other links to dementia. Excess blood sugar may cause more inflammation in the brain, which can cause problems with how well the brain functions. Plus, developing diabetes late in life also seems to be linked to a higher risk of dementia. This is an active area of research.

Maintain a healthy weight Being overweight contributes to many risk factors for stroke, including high blood pressure, heart disease and diabetes. Losing just 10 pounds can lower blood pressure and reduce the risk of dementia.

Reaching a healthy weight also reduces the risk of dementia in other ways. Research has linked obesity to metabolic syndrome, which is thought to contribute to a process that makes it hard for the brain to clear itself of beta-amyloid. Losing weight can help keep this process from taking place. Shedding excess pounds may also improve a number of factors linked to cognitive issues, like inflammation.

Also of note, obesity — a body mass index of 30 or higher — has been linked to a higher risk of cognitive impairment all on its own, especially in midlife.

Follow a healthy diet Getting regular physical activity and following a healthy diet are the keys to losing weight and keeping it off. You'll read more about physical activity next; as for diet, researchers think that the Mediterranean diet may help with weight *and* prevent dementia.

Earlier, you learned that following the Mediterranean diet — rich in fruits, vegetables, olive oil, legumes, whole grains and fish — is good for overall brain health. But it may do even more: Researchers think it may also play a role in the risk of dementia.

People who follow a Mediterranean diet seem to be less likely to have Alzheimer's disease dementia than those who don't follow it. Studies also suggest that following a Mediterranean diet may slow decline in older adults, keep mild cognitive impairment from progressing to Alzheimer's disease, and reduce the risk of mild cognitive impairment.

The food choices featured in the Mediterranean diet may be one reason why. Healthy food choices may lower cholesterol and blood sugar, which helps protect blood vessels and, in turn, reduces the risk of stroke, mild cognitive impairment and Alzheimer's disease. The Mediterranean diet may also help prevent the loss of brain tissue linked to Alzheimer's.

In particular, dementia researchers have been studying fish, one of the main components of the Mediterranean diet. Some studies suggest that people who carry the apolipoprotein E (APOE) gene — which is linked to a higher Alzheimer's risk — may have fewer Alzheimer's-related changes in their brains if they eat seafood on a regular basis.

But one area of concern with seafood is its mercury content. Mercury is a toxin, and in high amounts, it can harm the brain. With this in mind, research has focused on seafood intake and its link to the risk of Alzheimer's. Studies suggest that when eaten in moderate amounts, seafood helps prevent disease-related changes in the brain linked to Alzheimer's disease, even with its higher levels of mercury.

Exercise regularly While strong research has yet to emerge that definitively proves exercise prevents cognitive decline or dementia, some studies have found that exercise can significantly protect the brain against cognitive decline. The more exercise you get, the more benefits it seems to offer.

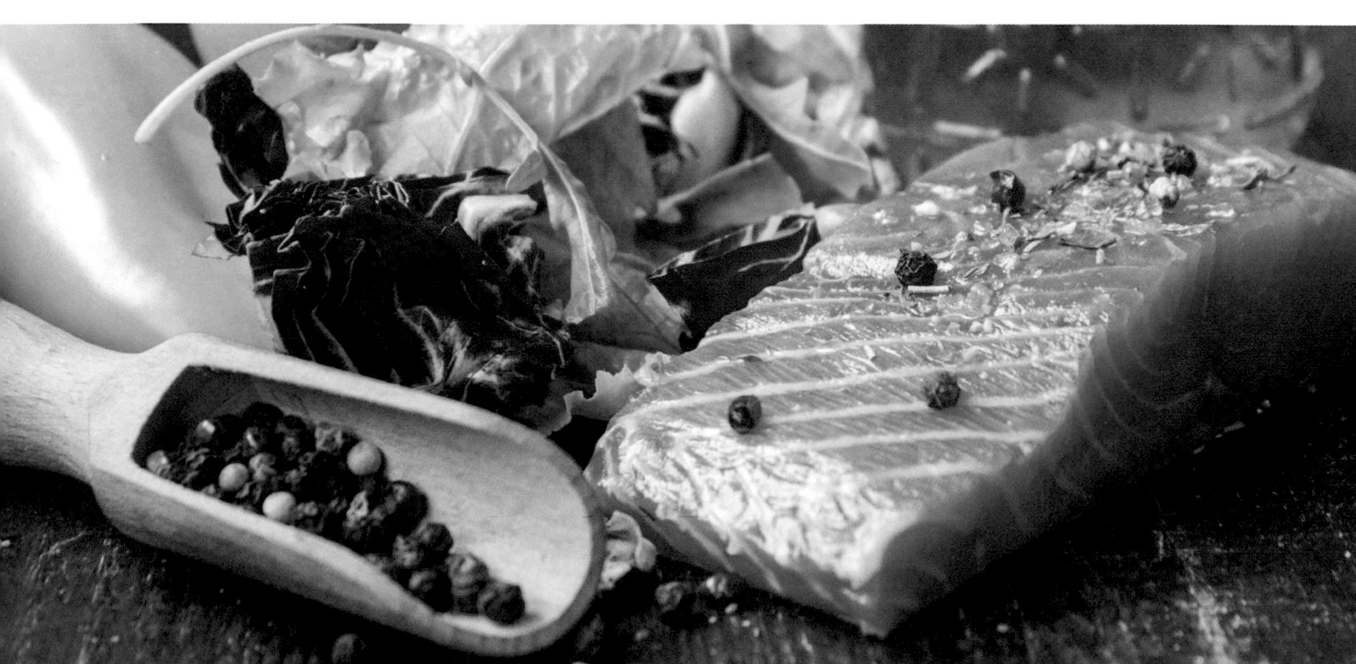

In general, older adults who exercise are more likely to maintain their thinking skills than those who don't exercise regularly.

A study of adults age 60 and older who either didn't have Alzheimer's disease or had early-stage Alzheimer's disease dementia suggests that those with better cardiorespiratory fitness had less brain shrinkage, a key marker of dementia.

Cardiorespiratory fitness is a way to measure a person's health by showing how well oxygen circulates throughout the body during physical activity. Another word for cardiorespiratory fitness is endurance.

Aerobic exercise is commonly used to improve endurance. It also improves the health of your blood vessels and heart and can reduce your risk of stroke. Aerobic activity can also lower blood pressure and help you lose weight, control diabetes, reduce stress, improve balance and reduce the risk of falls.

Any aerobic activity counts as long as it's something you enjoy enough to continue on a regular basis. Walking is a common choice, but any activity that makes you breathe a little harder and makes your heart beat a little faster is a good choice.

Exercise has also been shown to increase the size of the hippocampus, the part of the brain linked to memory. The hippocampus tends to shrink with age, which increases the risk of dementia. Aerobic activity seems to reverse this loss and improve memory even in older age.

Keep stress in check When you're faced with a stressful situation, a surge of hormones temporarily increases your blood pressure and causes your blood vessels to narrow. While there's no proof that stress can cause long-term high blood pressure on its own, it's linked to factors that can increase your risk of having high blood pressure. In times of stress, for example, some people turn to unhealthy habits like smoking, drinking too much alcohol and eating unhealthy foods. These unhealthy coping skills can all lead to high blood pressure.

Instead, strategies like deep breathing, exercising, meditation, yoga and simplifying your schedule are all examples of healthy ways to keep stress in check — and keep it from leading to high blood pressure.

Drink alcohol only in moderation While drinking small to moderate amounts of alcohol may protect you from a stroke, drinking too much can make a stroke more likely. It can also increase your risk of blood pressure, which can make a stroke more likely. Drinking too much alcohol also increases the risk of dementia and cognitive decline.

Take B vitamins B vitamins — B-6, B-12 and folic acid (folate) — can work together to reduce blood levels reduce blood levels of the protein homocysteine. Too much of this protein in your blood may increase your risk of blood vessel damage. However, there's no direct evidence that B vitamins can prevent stroke or vascular cognitive impairment, so taking this step may have little effect other than improved heart health.

"IN GENERAL, OLDER ADULTS WHO EXERCISE ARE MORE LIKELY TO MAINTAIN THEIR THINKING SKILLS."

If you take B vitamins, avoid taking more than 100 milligrams of B-6 a day. Currently, the World Health Organization doesn't recommend B vitamins and many other forms of nutritional supplements to reduce the risk of cognitive decline or dementia.

Don't use illicit drugs Many street drugs, like cocaine, can make a stroke more likely.

Can dementia medications help?

While medications like cholinesterase inhibitors and memantine can benefit those who've been diagnosed with dementia, they're not recommended for other cognitive issues or for preventing them. Clinical trials testing whether Alzheimer's drugs might prevent certain problems, like the progression of mild cognitive impairment to dementia, have generally shown no lasting benefit.

PUTTING IT ALL TOGETHER

It takes time to fully embrace lifestyle changes and new behaviors that can improve and protect your memory, but every little bit helps.

Start by reviewing what you've learned in this chapter and comparing it with your current habits and lifestyle. Are you already practicing the habits described here that can improve brain health? Identify all of the things you're already doing and give yourself credit for all the ways you're already nurturing your brain health.

Then focus on areas where you can improve. Start by listing behaviors that could use improvement. Then, identify new habits you want to try to incorporate on a regular basis.

Are there small steps you can take as you move toward making bigger, more healthful changes? For example, maybe joining a book club would help you socialize more. Or maybe you've set your sights on increasing your walking routine a little at a time. Or perhaps it's time to talk to your doctor about quitting smoking for good. All of these are examples of steps that can help your brain age well.

One more note: If you're interested in making several different improvements, start with just one first to keep from feeling overwhelmed and getting discouraged. Be patient with yourself, and take it one step at a time.

“WORLDWIDE RESEARCH INTO ALZHEIMER’S DISEASE AND OTHER CAUSES OF DEMENTIA IS ONGOING AND EXPANDING.”

CHAPTER 20

Research and trends

In the last chapter, you learned about the many factors involved in brain health, including the things you can do now to keep your brain healthy as you age. Researchers continue to pinpoint the best everyday choices for nurturing the brain. They've learned that while ideally it's best to take steps early on in life to keep the brain in good shape, it's never too late to adopt habits that are good for the brain. That's because brain health is a lifelong process.

Researchers are also unraveling the mystery of how and why dementia develops. While they're focused on ways to treat the diseases that cause dementia, they're also working on ways to prevent the diseases from taking shape in the first place.

This research is so critical that a national effort is underway to improve dementia prevention and treatment by 2025. This plan, called the National Plan to Address Alzheimer's Disease, has four overarching goals. First, establish effective ways to prevent and treat Alzheimer's disease and related dementias. Second, improve dementia care. Third, expand support for people with dementia and their families. And finally, educate the public more about dementia and its many causes.

All of these efforts to address dementia are critical. Around 50 million people worldwide are living with dementia now, and that number could triple by 2050.

This chapter highlights key trends in dementia research, including current developments and potential future directions. Each new effort brings more hope for finding ways to treat and prevent dementia.

DETECTING ALZHEIMER'S DISEASE BEFORE SYMPTOMS APPEAR

A lot of research is focused on detecting Alzheimer's and other forms of neurodegenerative disease in their earliest stages, before symptoms appear. Some researchers believe that medications may be most effective if they're given early in the disease process, before irreparable harm has been done to the brain. Early detection also would allow people to benefit from preventive therapies or treatments that may keep symptoms from becoming more severe.

You learned earlier that Alzheimer's disease begins long before any symptoms become apparent. This stage is known as preclinical Alzheimer's disease.

Typically, preclinical Alzheimer's is identified only in research settings. But imaging tests can now identify Alzheimer's trademark deposits of tau and beta-amyloid in this preclinical stage. As new treatments are developed for Alzheimer's disease, finding these early deposits becomes more critical.

Here are some of the newest factors linked to cognitive decline and how researchers may use these findings to detect the causes of cognitive impairment earlier.

A new risk factor for cognitive decline?

Researchers think that people who say they feel that their cognitive ability has changed may have a higher risk of developing mild cognitive impairment and Alzheimer's disease dementia in the future — even if their cognitive tests come back as normal. In medical literature, this is called subjective cognitive impairment.

A review of 10 years' worth of data suggests that a subjective decline in thinking and memory that doesn't show up in a cognitive test may actually indicate an early stage of Alzheimer's disease when it's paired with tests that show certain biomarkers in the brain.

At this point, telling the difference between subjective cognitive decline and typical everyday mistakes doesn't have any practical value. However, those who feel that their cognitive ability has changed may serve as a subset of individuals who should be screened for clinical trials because they're at higher risk of decline in the future.

The link between sleep and dementia

In the last chapter, you learned that getting enough regular, uninterrupted sleep may help prevent dementia. For example, some research suggests that people who don't get enough sleep are twice as likely to develop dementia. Researchers are continuing to uncover what makes the connection between sleep and dementia so important.

One answer may lie in how sleep affects levels of tau and beta-amyloid in the brain. Both, as you'll recall, are involved in the development of Alzheimer's disease. It's thought that sleep helps clear beta-amyloid from the brain before it hardens into plaques and eventually leads to Alzheimer's disease.

With this in mind, researchers are increasingly seeing sleep as a possible target for dementia prevention. Although more study is needed, it's possible that improving sleep quality may help delay and may even prevent some dementia-related changes.

Researchers studied a small group of adults with cognitive levels in the normal range to look for a link between sleep quality, measured in brain waves during sleep, and levels of tau and beta-amyloid in the brain. The researchers found that adults in their 50s who said they didn't sleep well had more beta-amyloid in their brains later in life. Those who said they slept less in their 60s had more tau in their brains later in life.

Although not everyone with beta-amyloid and tau goes on to develop dementia, impaired sleep may lead to changes in the brain associated with dementia.

In addition to not sleeping well at night, feeling sleepy during the day may be another risk factor for Alzheimer's disease.

Researchers have found that some people who appear to be healthy but have more beta-amyloid in the brain may be more tired during the day. Treating excessive daytime sleepiness may help with cognitive performance, but whether it will delay or prevent changes in the brain that lead to Alzheimer's disease is not yet known.

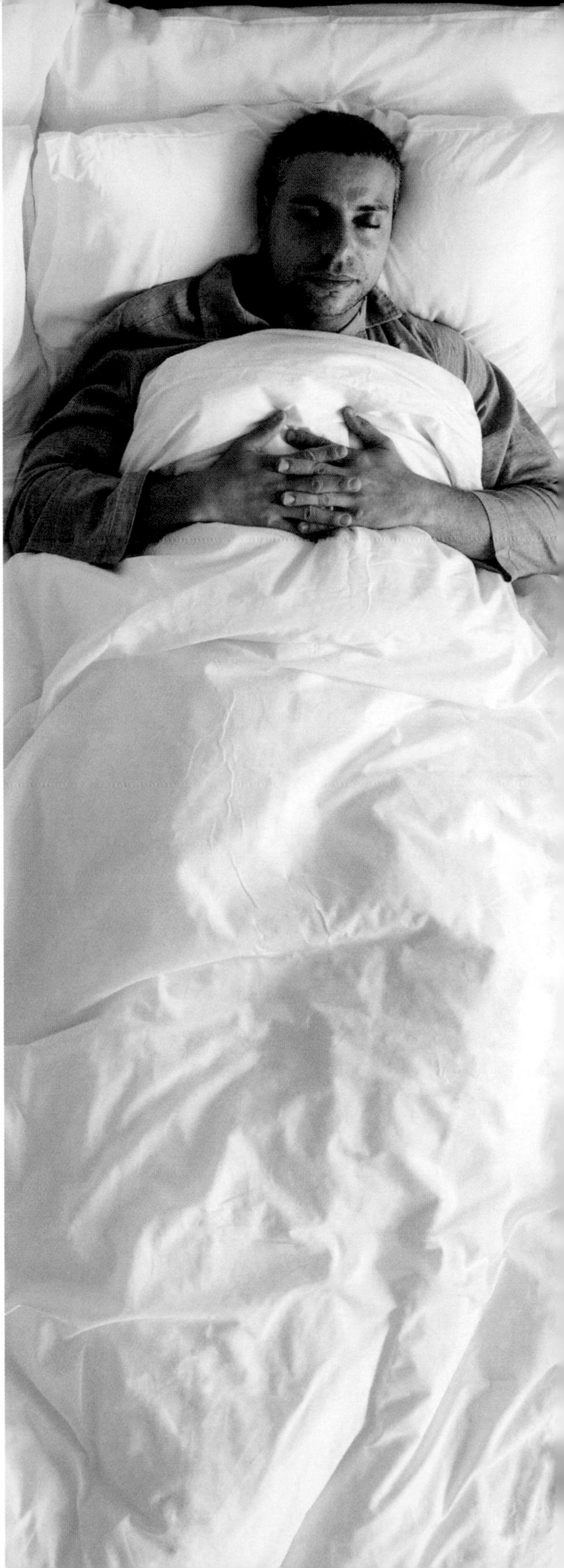

PROMISING BLOOD TESTS FOR ALZHEIMER'S DISEASE

Earlier, you learned about the tests that researchers are developing to diagnose Alzheimer's disease before it causes symptoms. Much of the research that's been done has focused on biomarkers and genetic changes that can be found long before someone has clinical symptoms of dementia.

While signs of Alzheimer's can be found in the fluid that surrounds the brain and spinal cord, the test required to find these signs involves placing a small needle in your lower back (spinal tap). PET scans are another option; they can show plaques in the brain that may lead to Alzheimer's disease. But a PET scan is expensive and uses radiation, and it's not available everywhere.

For these reasons, blood tests are a promising area of research. Blood tests may offer easier and more cost-effective ways to detect Alzheimer's disease or other causes of dementia. Researchers are studying several different substances in the blood that may be connected to Alzheimer's disease in an effort to develop blood tests.

Metabolites are one example. Metabolites are substances that are important for processes the body needs to maintain life (metabolism). Metabolism helps cells in the body grow, reproduce and stay healthy. It also helps rid the body of toxins. Researchers have identified 26 metabolites found in the blood and brain of someone with Alzheimer's disease. This information may lead to a new way of testing for — and treating — Alzheimer's.

The ability to spot beta-amyloid with a blood test is also under study. Researchers think a blood test that can detect beta-amyloid could one day be used as a screening tool to show if someone has amyloid in the brain and may have a higher risk of developing Alzheimer's disease dementia.

This type of blood test could be a simpler, more cost-effective way for doctors to gauge a person's risk of Alzheimer's disease or possibly diagnose Alzheimer's disease. It could also help identify people who should take part in research focused on developing new treatments. And it could offer a way to screen a large number of people and limit the need for more-invasive or costly tests.

A blood test that can measure the tau protein is also under study. As with beta-amyloid, a blood test that can track the amount of tau in someone's blood may help show tau deposits in the brain, a key sign of Alzheimer's disease.

Researchers think that a blood test that measures tau could serve as a screening test for Alzheimer's disease, similar to blood tests for beta-amyloid. It could also be a less invasive, lower cost way to identify people who should have other screening tests done.

Blood tests may help doctors screen for and diagnose the cause of someone's dementia. In turn, this could make treatment more accessible for those who need it.

“BLOOD TESTS MAY HELP DOCTORS SCREEN FOR AND DIAGNOSE THE CAUSE OF SOMEONE’S DEMENTIA.”

ADVANCES IN LEWY BODY DEMENTIA

The second most common cause of neurodegenerative dementia, Lewy body disease is often misdiagnosed. It doesn't start the same way for everyone, and it doesn't always take the same path. The symptoms — and when they appear — vary and can be similar to other causes of dementia.

Researchers studying the symptoms of Lewy body dementia are tackling these challenges. The hope is to find ways to diagnose it earlier, when treatment can be most helpful.

Researchers have learned that some symptoms of Lewy body dementia can appear long before it's diagnosed, during what's described as a prodromal stage. For example, color vision problems may affect an individual up to 12 years before a Lewy body dementia diagnosis. And rapid eye movement (REM) sleep behavior disorder may develop as many as 50 years before cognitive symptoms appear. REM sleep behavior disorder causes a person to physically act out vivid, often unpleasant dreams with vocal sounds and sudden, often violent arm and leg movements while sleeping.

Researchers are currently following people who have REM sleep behavior disorder and looking for clues with biomarkers to determine who might develop Lewy body disease and when it might develop.

Researchers are also working on new ways to help doctors navigate the symptoms of Lewy body dementia and diagnose it earlier, when treatment can be most effective. Doctors, like researchers, struggle with the challenges of Lewy body dementia. They often don't know much about the disease, and managing the array of symptoms is complex.

To address these challenges, a checklist available from the DIAMOND-Lewy research program may help.

DIAMOND stands for DIagnosis And Management Of Neurodegenerative Dementia. It's a research collaboration between Cambridge and Newcastle University funded by the National Institutes of Health Research.

The toolkit includes screening questions that help doctors tell if someone has any of the four core features of Lewy body dementia, which you learned about in Chapter 10: cognitive fluctuations, REM sleep behavior disorder, seeing things that aren't real (visual hallucinations) and parkinsonism.

Researchers are also looking into tests that can detect Lewy body disease earlier. For example, scientists are currently looking into whether they can detect and measure alpha-synuclein in cerebral spinal fluid samples to diagnose Lewy body disorders. In addition, researchers are looking into whether a skin biopsy can find changes to alpha-synuclein. This may help show if someone has Lewy body disease.

Heart rate variability is another area of interest; this is a measure of variations in heartbeat. Research suggests that a heart rate variability test may predict if someone with mild cognitive impairment will have Lewy body dementia or Alzheimer's disease.

PRIONS AND NEURODEGENERATIVE DISEASE

Prions (PRE-ons) are proteins that occur naturally in the brains of animals and people. Prions are usually harmless, but when they're misshapen, they can cause devastating illnesses. Prion disease has long been linked to rare, fatal brain disorders like Creutzfeldt-Jakob disease, which you learned about in Chapter 3. Researchers now think that the same processes may play a role in more common disorders that involve proteins in the brain, like Alzheimer's disease.

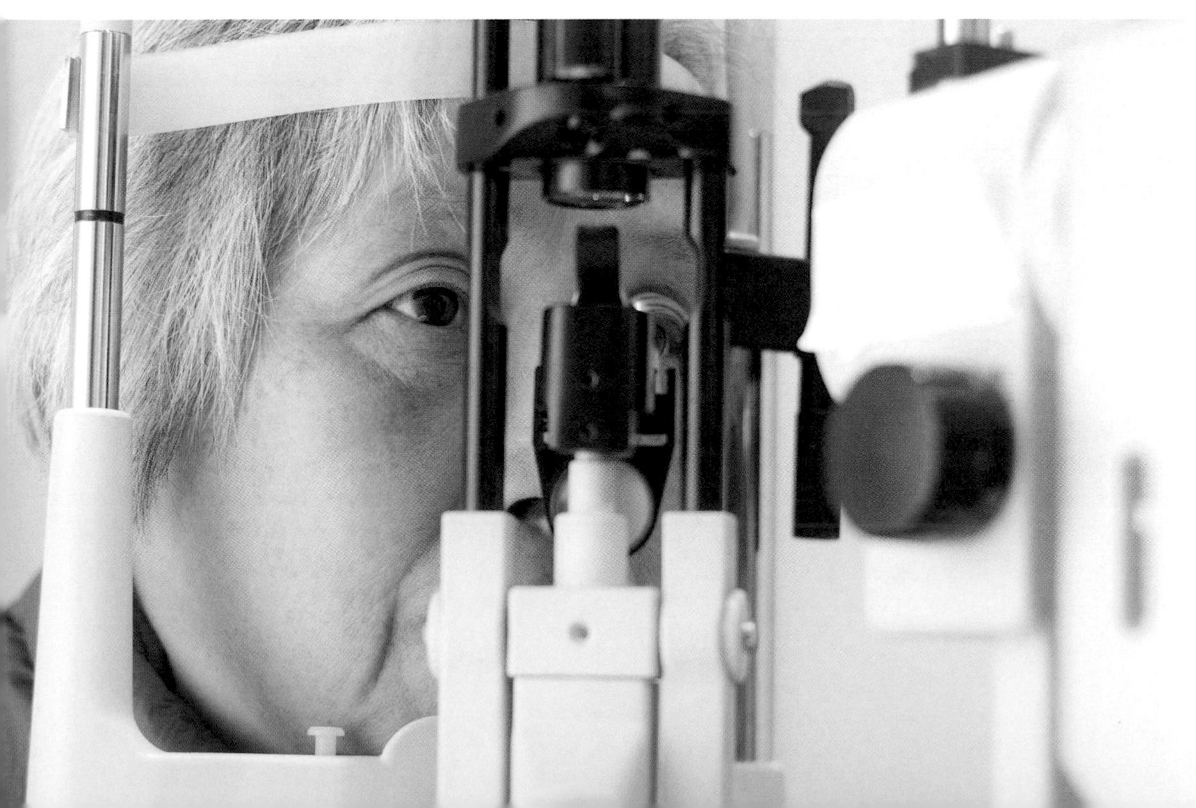

As you'll recall, the diseases that cause dementia generally start with proteins that are not processed properly. These proteins build up and damage healthy cells, causing them to stop working and die. Different proteins are linked to different causes of dementia. For example, beta-amyloid is a protein that's linked to Alzheimer's disease.

The relationship between beta-amyloid, tau, and alpha-synuclein and prions is one of the most active areas of current neurodegenerative research. Like prions, alpha-synuclein and tau misfold and may cause other cells in the brain to misfold, as well. This leads to changes in thinking and reasoning — changes that happen more slowly in Alzheimer's and Lewy body disease than they do in Creutzfeldt-Jakob disease.

Researchers think this may be a key part of the disease process in Alzheimer's and Lewy body disease. If prions and beta-amyloid, tau, and alpha-synuclein act in a similar way, they may have other characteristics in common, too. Researchers continue to study similarities between prions and the proteins linked to diseases that cause dementia. What they learn may offer more information about what happens early in the disease process and lead to earlier diagnosis and treatment for the causes of dementia.

INFECTIONS AND NEURODEGENERATIVE DISEASE

Researchers have long wondered if certain infections may be involved in causing Alzheimer's disease to take shape in the brain. As many as 30 years ago, researchers found herpes virus in the brains of people with Alzheimer's disease. Examples of herpes virus include chickenpox and shingles. While small studies suggest that herpes virus may increase the risk of dementia, research also shows that this risk is nearly eliminated when the infection is treated.

Larger studies are needed before researchers can be sure that these viruses play a role in the development of Alzheimer's disease.

GUM (PERIODONTAL) DISEASE

Several studies show that older people with gum disease have a higher risk of Alzheimer's disease dementia and cognitive decline. While researchers are still learning why, it appears that certain bacteria involved in gum disease may be able to make their way to the brain, where they cause inflammation that triggers the start of Alzheimer's disease.

While this is an active area of research, much is unknown. More study is needed before researchers can confirm this possible link.

GUT HEALTH AND DEMENTIA

Of the 30 to 50 trillion bacteria in the body, your gut holds by far the most. Good gut bacteria break down nutrients and drugs, help the immune system fend off infections, and keep the digestive system running smoothly. However, the gut also holds harmful bacteria. Too much bad bacteria in the gut has been linked to many disorders, including arthritis, irritable bowel syndrome, obesity, cancer and depression.

The delicate balance of gut bacteria may be tied to brain health. A proper balance may keep the blood-brain barrier strong. Some researchers think that this protective layer of cells keeps harmful substances, like those that cause Alzheimer's to form, from reaching the brain in the first place. Research also suggests that the right balance of gut bacteria reduces the amount of beta-amyloid in the brain, which may be helpful for people already living with Alzheimer's.

At this point, however, there's little agreement among researchers on the link between gut health and diseases of the brain. Not much is known about the connection between the two.

Diet is an important way to nurture gut health and reduce the risk of dementia at the same time. Studies show that a diet that's high in saturated fat and cholesterol, for example, increases the risk of Alzheimer's disease. Researchers think this may be due, in part, to the changes that this kind of diet makes to the balance of bacteria in the gut. Some researchers think that a diet high in these fats may also affect learning, memory and thinking ability. These findings offer opportunities to not only improve health but also keep changes from taking place in the brain that can lead to dementia.

Much more study on gut health and dementia is needed before possible therapies can be considered for clinical trials.

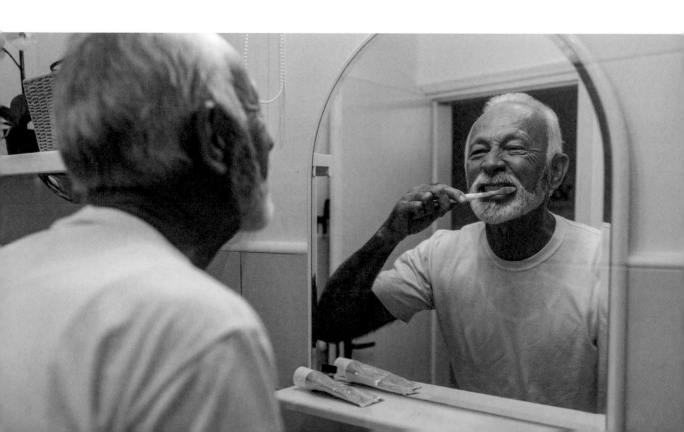

GENE THERAPY

You're already likely familiar with gene therapy. It involves changing the genes in your body's cells to treat or stop disease. Gene therapy holds promise for treating a range of diseases, including cancer, heart disease and diabetes. Researchers think gene therapy may one day be used to treat dementia-causing diseases and may even keep them from forming.

There are several ways gene therapy is used to cure a disease or help the body fight it. One way is by turning off certain genes before they have a chance to create disease in the body. In this way, gene therapy essentially blocks disease, preventing it from being made and helping to keep cells healthy.

Antisense therapy is an example of this approach. It uses small pieces of DNA or RNA called antisense oligonucleotides or antisense agents to change specific genetic products within a cell that are responsible for creating disease. The agent intervenes before a genetic product has a chance to cause damage, stopping the disease process before it starts.

Researchers have found early success in clinical trials for using antisense therapy with neurodegenerative disorders like Huntington's disease and amyotrophic lateral sclerosis (ALS). With this in mind, researchers are looking into ways that antisense therapy can be used to treat and prevent other neurodegenerative diseases, like those that cause dementia. Researchers are studying antisense treatments to target genetic forms of Alzheimer's and frontotemporal degeneration.

Specific targets of antisense therapy include the following:

- The amyloid precursor protein, which causes beta-amyloid to be produced.
- The gene variant of the apolipoprotein E, a gene linked to a higher risk of the late-onset form of Alzheimer's disease.
- Genes that cause frontotemporal degeneration, like the MAPT gene, which causes tangles to form in the brain.

This type of gene therapy does have some drawbacks. The agent that's injected may break down before it reaches its target. And it may not be able to completely change the genetic product in charge of causing disease. Even with these challenges, researchers feel that this therapy holds promise in treating and preventing diseases that cause dementia.

FRONTOTEMPORAL DEGENERATION AND RELATED DISORDERS

Frontotemporal degeneration, the overarching term for a group of neurodegenerative disorders that mostly affect areas of the brain linked to personality, behavior, memory and language, accounts for up to a fifth of dementia cases in the U.S.

As you learned earlier, frontotemporal dementia, progressive supranuclear palsy, primary progressive aphasia and corticobasal syndrome are disorders that are grouped under this umbrella. These disorders often affect adults in the prime of their lives — between their 40s and 60s — and no treatment has been shown to slow down, stop or prevent these diseases.

You also read earlier about the many genes linked to frontotemporal degeneration that runs in families. Researchers are using what they discover about these genes to develop biomarkers for early diagnosis and therapies that may delay this type of dementia.

For example, researchers have learned that in some people, cognitive decline starts as many as eight years before the first symptom of frontotemporal degeneration is noticed. These changes seem to be linked to genetic changes happening around the same time. Researchers are looking into cognitive tests that can be given to people who have frontotemporal degeneration in their families as a way to spot these changes — and the disease — earlier.

Researchers are also studying other changes that happen early on, before the first symptom of frontotemporal degeneration is noticed. Executive function is one example.

Trouble with executive function — organizing tasks, thinking abstractly, managing time and solving problems — seems to be affected early on in frontotemporal degeneration. With this in mind, testing executive function may be one way to find changes that may signal the beginning of frontotemporal degeneration. Research suggests that one test in particular, is known as Executive Abilities: Measures and Instruments for Neurobehavioral Evaluation and Research (EXAMINER). Sponsored by the National Institutes of Health (NIH), The EXAMINER may detect problems with executive function that are linked to frontotemporal degeneration better than other tests do.

As with other types of dementia, biomarkers are a focus of study for frontotemporal degeneration. Researchers are developing imaging, blood and cerebral spinal fluid biomarkers that can be used to detect frontotemporal degeneration early and track its progression.

Because research on frontotemporal disorders has been described as challenging, the NIH is funding a collaboration between two ongoing research efforts. The idea behind this collaboration, known as ALLFTD, is to integrate North American research on these diseases. This collaboration will help improve understanding of how the disorders take shape in the brain and ideally lead to treatments and preventive therapies.

Researchers in this collaboration are studying all forms of these disorders — those that run in families and those that don't. The hope is that researchers will uncover early signs that happen long before symptoms occur. This may enable effective treatment and preventive strategies to be created, tested and ultimately used by doctors.

As part of this effort, researchers want to test biomarkers — early signs of these disor-

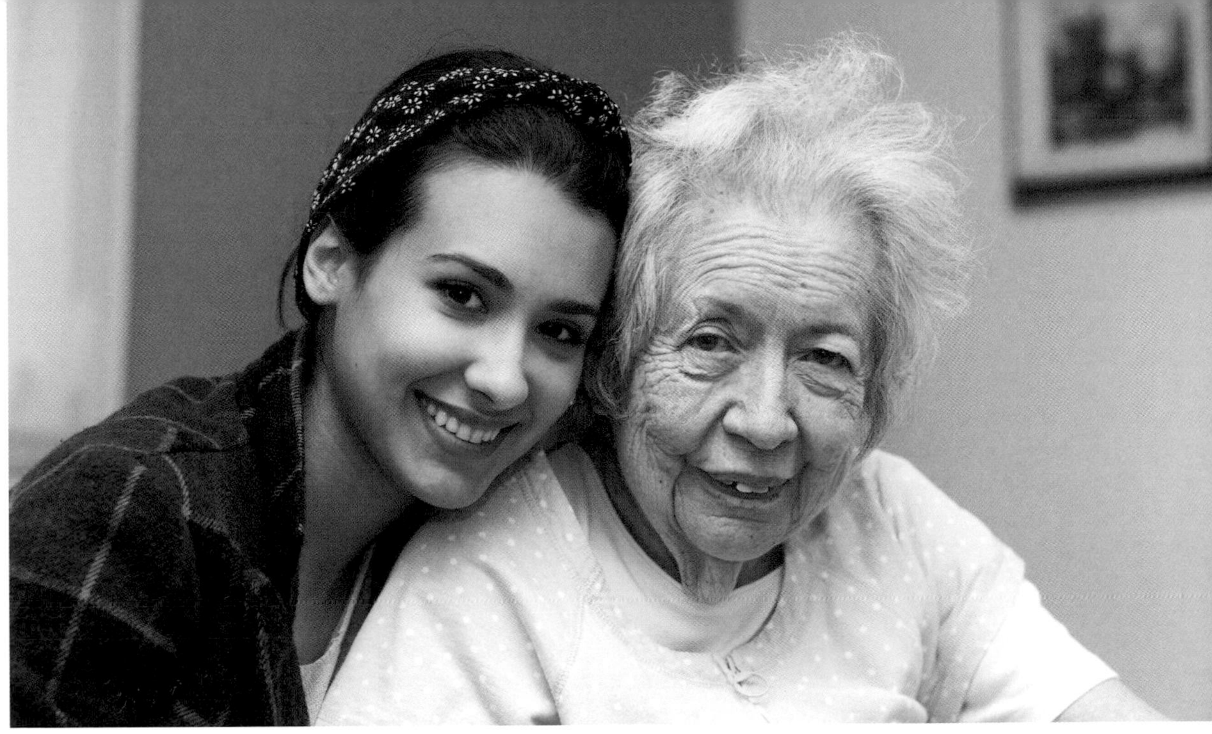

ders — and find ways to test for them and track them over time. This would offer more information about who's most at risk of developing these disorders and how symptoms of these diseases worsen over time.

THE ROLE OF BRAIN NETWORKS

Neurodegenerative diseases of the brain, like Alzheimer's disease, are defined by the symptoms they cause. As you've learned, symptoms include problems with memory.

But what's happening in the brain to cause symptoms like this? Researchers studying this aspect of Alzheimer's disease are starting to unravel this mystery, working toward a complete understanding of what goes into forming memories, specifically, and what happens in Alzheimer's disease to cause memory problems.

In earlier chapters, you learned about how memories are formed. As you'll recall, researchers have learned that several networks in the brain are involved in forming memories. No one network is responsible for memory; instead, several large-scale networks throughout the brain depend on each other to create memories.

Take, for example, memories of your grandmother. You can't pinpoint which cells in your brain hold all of the memories of your grandmother.

Instead, several different networks within your brain hold different types of information that provides context for the memories

PARTICIPATION IN CLINICAL TRIALS

It's impossible to conduct research without volunteers willing to participate in clinical trials. This is how the public plays a meaningful part in the fight against Alzheimer's disease and related dementias. Still, enrolling in a clinical trial requires careful consideration. In the case of Alzheimer's disease, the decision often rests with an entire family rather than one person.

To help families with this important decision, the Alzheimer's Association has prepared the following list of considerations:

- With your doctor, explore the pros and cons of participating in a particular study.
- Be prepared to answer questions about your loved one's condition.
- Expect further screening to determine eligibility. Only some people may qualify.
- Be aware of the time commitment and other responsibilities, such as making trips to the study site, administering the drug and reporting health-related changes to the study coordinators. Also ask about expenses.
- Understand that clinical studies may involve some risk, as they determine the effectiveness and safety of a drug.
- Be aware that not all participants are given the treatment being tested. In almost every study, one group receives an inactive substance (placebo), while another group receives the experimental medication. This allows researchers to compare the two groups. People receiving the placebo are just as important as those receiving the treatment. If the drug yields positive results, the participants who received a placebo may be given the option of receiving the experimental drug.
- Ask questions. Researchers should answer satisfactorily. If you feel uncomfortable at any point, you always have the option of not continuing with the study.

Find out more about clinical trials for Alzheimer's disease:

Alzheimer's Association
www.alz.org/research/clinical_trials/find_clinical_trials_trialmatch.asp
U.S. National Library of Medicine
www.clinicaltrials.gov

you have of your grandmother. Working together, the networks in your brain paint a picture of who your grandmother is, what you know about her, how you feel about her, and so on.

This simple illustration shows how several different networks — systems of cells spread across the brain — are needed to form memories. These networks in your brain work together and depend on one another.

The networks in your brain aren't that different from an electric power grid. If a hub of power goes down, then other nearby areas pick up the slack. If the power grid is robust enough, the lights in your house stay on. But if the burden is too high, other circuits get blown and the power goes out in your house.

Researchers think the same thing may happen with Alzheimer's disease — that a failure in one brain network increases the load on other brain networks. If the entire network system is robust enough, this doesn't necessarily cause problems — but any weak link in the brain's networks can cause Alzheimer's disease to take hold, spread and cause symptoms like memory loss.

Researchers hope that understanding brain networks and how they're affected in Alzheimer's disease may make it possible to help people make lifestyle choices that keep the brain's networks robust enough to prevent the spread of Alzheimer's in the brain.

NEXT STEPS FOR RESEARCH

Research into Alzheimer's disease and other causes of dementia is ongoing and expanding. New strategies for diagnosis and treatment take time to reach the people who need them most. After an initial discovery, many studies are needed to support findings and test the safety and effectiveness of a medication or procedure before it can be used.

To help accelerate research, the Coalition Against Major Diseases (CAMD) — an alliance of nonprofit foundations, pharmaceutical companies and government advisers — has formed a first-of-its-kind partnership to share data from Alzheimer's clinical trials. The CAMD has also collaborated with Clinical Data Interchange Standards Consortium (CDISC) to create data standards.

Researchers anticipate that these data standards and the sharing of data from more than 6,500 study participants will speed up development of therapies that can be used to effectively treat and prevent dementia-related diseases.

Additional resources

AARP

601 E St. NW
Washington, DC 20049
888-687-2277
www.aarp.org

ADMINISTRATION FOR COMMUNITY LIVING

330 C St. SW
Washington, DC 20201
202-401-4634
https://acl.gov

ADVANCE DIRECTIVE FORMS

From AARP
www.aarp.org/caregiving/financial-legal/free-printable-advance-directives
From the American Bar Association
www.americanbar.org/groups/law_aging/resources/health_care_decision_making/Stateforms

ADVANCING STATES

(formerly the National Association of States United for Aging and Disabilities)
241 18th St. S, Suite 403
Arlington, VA 22202
202-898-2578
www.advancingstates.org

AGENCY FOR HEALTHCARE RESEARCH AND QUALITY

Office of Communications
5600 Fishers Lane, Seventh Floor
Rockville, MD 20857
301-427-1104
www.ahrq.gov

ALZCONNECTED

225 N. Michigan Ave., Floor 17
Chicago, IL 60601
800-272-3900
www.alzconnected.org

ALZHEIMER'S AND RELATED DEMENTIAS EDUCATION AND REFERRAL CENTER

800-438-4380
www.alzheimers.gov

ALZHEIMER'S ASSOCIATION

225 N. Michigan Ave., Floor 17
Chicago, IL 60601
800-272-3900
www.alz.org

ALZHEIMER'S DISEASE INTERNATIONAL

64 Great Suffolk St.
London SE1 0BB
United Kingdom
011-44-20-7981-0880
www.alz.co.uk

ALZHEIMER'S FOUNDATION OF AMERICA

322 Eighth Ave., 16th Floor
New York, NY 10001
866-232-8484
https://alzfdn.org

THE ASSOCIATION FOR FRONTOTEMPORAL DEGENERATION

2700 Horizon Drive, Suite 120
King of Prussia, PA 19406
267-514-7221 or 866-507-7222
www.theaftd.org

BRIGHTFOCUS FOUNDATION

22512 Gateway Center Drive
Clarksburg, MD 20871
800-437-2423
www.brightfocus.org

CENTER FOR DRUG EVALUATION AND RESEARCH (CDER)

Division of Drug Information
Food and Drug Administration
Office of Communications
10001 New Hampshire Ave.
Hillandale Building, Fourth Floor
Silver Spring, MD 20993
855-543-3784 or 301-796-3400
www.fda.gov/Drugs

CENTERS FOR MEDICARE AND MEDICAID SERVICES

7500 Security Blvd.
Baltimore, MD 21244
www.cms.gov

COMMUNITY RESOURCE FINDER

www.communityresourcefinder.org

CREUTZFELDT-JAKOB DISEASE FOUNDATION INC.

3634 W. Market St., Suite 110
Akron, OH 44333
800-659-1991
https://cjdfoundation.org

CUREPSP

1216 Broadway, Second Floor
New York, NY 10001
347-294-2873 or 800-457-4777
https://www.psp.org

DEMENTIA ACTION ALLIANCE

732-212-9036
https://daanow.org

DEMENTIA FRIENDLY AMERICA

1100 New Jersey Ave. SE, Suite 350
Washington, DC 20003
202-872-0888
www.dfamerica.org/

DEPARTMENT OF VETERANS AFFAIRS

844-698-2311
www.va.gov/find-locations

ELDERCARE LOCATOR

Administered by the Administration on Aging
800-677-1116
https://eldercare.acl.gov

FAMILY CAREGIVER ALLIANCE

101 Montgomery St., Suite 2150
San Francisco, CA 94104
415-434–3388 or 800-445-8106
www.caregiver.org

FINANCIAL AND LEGAL PLANNING FOR CAREGIVERS

From the Alzheimer's Association
www.alz.org/help-support/caregiving/financial-legal-planning

GIVING VOICE INITIATIVE

7801 E. Bush Lake Road, Suite 120
Bloomington, MN 55439
612-440-9660
https://givingvoicechorus.org

HOUSE OF MEMORIES

345 W. Kellogg Blvd.
St. Paul, MN 55102
800-657-3773
www.mnhs.org/houseofmemories

THE I'M STILL HERE FOUNDATION

10 Tower Office Park, Suite 317
Woburn, MA 01801
781-674-2884
www.imstillhere.org

LEWY BODY DEMENTIA ASSOCIATION

912 Killian Hill Road SW
Lilburn, GA 30047
404-935-6444 or 800-539-9767
www.lbda.org

MAYO CLINIC

www.MayoClinic.org

MAYO CLINIC'S YOUTUBE CHANNEL

www.youtube.com/user/mayoclinic
Keyword search: dementia

MEALS ON WHEELS AMERICA

1550 Crystal Drive, Suite 1004
Arlington, VA 22202
888-998-6325
www.mealsonwheelsamerica.org

MEDICAID AND MEDICARE

7500 Security Blvd.
Baltimore, Maryland 21244-1850
877-267-2323 or 410-786-3000
www.medicaid.gov

MEDICALERT FOUNDATION

101 Lander Ave.
Turlock, CA 95380
800-432-5378
www.medicalert.org

NATIONAL ADULT DAY SERVICES ASSOCIATION

11350 Random Hills Road, Suite 800
Fairfax, VA 22030
877-745-1440
www.nadsa.org

NATIONAL APHASIA ASSOCIATION

P.O. Box 87
Scarsdale, NY 10583
www.aphasia.org/aphasia-resources/primary-progressive-aphasia

NATIONAL ASSOCIATION OF AREA AGENCIES ON AGING

1100 New Jersey Ave. SE, Suite 350
Washington, DC 20003
202-872-0888
www.n4a.org

NATIONAL COUNCIL ON AGING

251 18th St. S, Suite 500
Arlington, VA 22202
571-527-3900
www.ncoa.org

NATIONAL HOSPICE AND PALLIATIVE CARE ORGANIZATION

1731 King Street
Alexandria, VA 22314
703-837-1500
www.nhpco.org

NATIONAL INSTITUTE OF MENTAL HEALTH

Office of Science Policy, Planning, and Communications
6001 Executive Blvd.
Room 6200, MSC 9663
Bethesda, MD 20892-9663
866-615-6464
www.nimh.nih.gov

NATIONAL INSTITUTE OF NEUROLOGICAL DISORDERS AND STROKE

NIH Neurological Institute
P.O. Box 5801
Bethesda, MD 20824
800-352-9424
www.ninds.nih.gov

NATIONAL INSTITUTE ON AGING

31 Center Drive, MSC 2292
Building 31, Room 5C27
Bethesda, MD 20892
800-222-2225
www.nia.nih.gov

NATIONAL INSTITUTES OF HEALTH CLINICAL CENTER

10 Center Drive
Bethesda, MD 20892
301-496-4000
https://clinicalcenter.nih.gov

NATIONAL LIBRARY OF MEDICINE

8600 Rockville Pike
Bethesda, MD 20894
www.nlm.nih.gov

NATIONAL RESPITE NETWORK AND RESPITE LOCATOR

https://archrespite.org/respitelocator

PARKINSON'S FOUNDATION

800-473-4636
www.parkinson.org

THE PRESENCE CARE PROJECT

www.presencecareproject.com

SOCIAL SECURITY ADMINISTRATION

1100 W. High Rise
6401 Security Blvd.
Baltimore, MD 21235
800-772-1213
www.ssa.gov

SOCIETY FOR NEUROSCIENCE

1121 14th St. NW, Suite 1010
Washington, DC 20005
202-962-4000
www.sfn.org

SPARK!

800 W. Wells St.
Milwaukee, WI 53233
414-278-6943
www.sparkprograms.org

TIMESLIPS

www.timeslips.org

TRIALMATCH

From the Alzheimer's Association
www.alz.org/alzheimers-dementia/research_progress/clinical-trials/about-clinical-trials

WCG CENTERWATCH

Clinical Research and Drug Information
300 N. Washington St., Suite 200
Falls Church, VA 22046
617-948-5100 or 866-219-3440
www.centerwatch.com

WORLD HEALTH ORGANIZATION

525 Twenty-Third St. NW
Washington, DC 20037
www.who.int/mental_health/neurology/en

SELECTED RECOMMENDED READING

Ahlskog J Eric. *Dementia With Lewy Bodies and Parkinson's Disease Dementia: Patient, Family, and Clinician Working Together for Better Outcomes*. Oxford University Press; 2014.

Allen Power G. *Dementia Beyond Disease: Enhancing Well-Being*. Health Professions Press; 2014.

Ames Hoblitzelle O. *Ten Thousand Joys & Ten Thousand Sorrows: A Couple's Journey Through Alzheimer's*. TarcherPerigree; 2008.

Basting A. *Creative Care: A Revolutionary Approach to Dementia and Elder Care*. HarperOne; 2020.

Boss P. *Loving Someone Who Has Dementia: How To Find Hope While Coping With Stress and Grief*. Jossey-Bass; 2011.

Brackey J. *Creating Moments of Joy Along the Alzheimer's Journey.* 5th ed. Purdue University Press; 2016.

Bryden C. *Dancing With Dementia: My Story of Living Positively With Dementia*. Kingsley Publishers; 2005.

Buell Whitworth H, et al. *A Caregiver's Guide to Lewy Body Dementia.* Demos Medical Publishing; 2011.

Chang E, et al. *Living With Dementia: A Practical Guide for Families and Personal Carers*. ACER Press; 2013.

Cornish J. *The Dementia Handbook: How To Provide Dementia Care at Home*. CreateSpace Independent Publishing Platform; 2017.

Kuhn D, et al. *The Art of Dementia Care.* Delmar; 2008.

Manteau-Rao M. *Caring for a Loved One With Dementia: A Mindfulness-Based Guide for Reducing Stress and Making the Best of Your Journey Together*. New Harbinger Publications; 2016.

Neff K, et al. *The Mindful Self-Compassion Workbook: A Proven Way To Accept Yourself, Build Inner Strength, and Thrive*. The Guilford Press, 2018.

Pearce N. *Inside Alzheimer's: How to Hear and Honor Connections With a Person Who Has Dementia*. Forrason Press; 2010.

Powell T. *Dementia Reimagined: Building a Life of Joy and Dignity From Beginning to End.* Avery; 2019.

Snyder L. *Living Your Best With Early-Stage Alzheimer's: An Essential Guide*. Sunrise River Press; 2010.

Towne Jennings J. *Living With Lewy Body Dementia: One Caregiver's Personal, In-Depth Experience*. WestBow Press; 2012.

Zeisel J. *I'm Still Here: A New Philosophy of Alzheimer's Care*. Avery; 2009.

Index

A

B

C

D

E

F

G

H

M

N

Q

R

S

T

IMAGE CREDITS

The individuals pictured are models, and the photos are used for illustrative purposes only. There is no correlation between the individuals portrayed and the subjects being discussed.

All photographs and illustrations are copyright of MFMER, except for the following:

NAME: 761206651/PAGE: 14-15/CREDIT: © SHUTTERSTOCK — NAME: 220154653/PAGE: 16-17, 36-37, 48-49, 66-67, 96-97, 118-119, 136-137, 156-157, 176-177, 206-207, 238-239, 254-255, 262-263, 278-279, 292-293, 308-309, 318-319, 338-339, 360-361, 376-377, 390-391 /CREDIT: © SHUTTERSTOCK — NAME: 6892276/PAGE: 22/CREDIT: © SHUTTERSTOCK — NAME: 552942685/PAGE: 24/CREDIT: © SHUTTERSTOCK — NAME: 1092881093/PAGE: 26/CREDIT: © SHUTTERSTOCK — NAME: 535784338/PAGE: 28/CREDIT: © SHUTTERSTOCK — NAME: 794115388/PAGE: 31/CREDIT: © SHUTTERSTOCK — NAME: 261302252/PAGE: 32/CREDIT: © SHUTTERSTOCK — NAME: 649995802/PAGE: 39/CREDIT: © SHUTTERSTOCK — NAME: 204416887/PAGE: 40/CREDIT: © SHUTTERSTOCK — NAME: 545951080/PAGE: 44/CREDIT: © SHUTTERSTOCK — NAME: 115229260/PAGE: 46-47/CREDIT: © SHUTTERSTOCK — NAME: 535283767/PAGE: 51/CREDIT: © SHUTTERSTOCK — NAME: 381900463/PAGE: 57/CREDIT: © SHUTTERSTOCK — NAME: 81568180/PAGE: 59/CREDIT: © SHUTTERSTOCK — NAME: 599811197/PAGE: 62/CREDIT: © SHUTTERSTOCK — NAME: 1054761779/PAGE: 64/CREDIT: © SHUTTERSTOCK — NAME: 1443658877/PAGE: 68/CREDIT: © SHUTTERSTOCK — NAME: 1606120336/PAGE: 70/CREDIT: © SHUTTERSTOCK — NAME: 39882433/PAGE: 74/CREDIT: © SHUTTERSTOCK — NAME: 1530211733/PAGE: 79/CREDIT: © SHUTTERSTOCK — NAME: 222228898/PAGE: 88/CREDIT: © SHUTTERSTOCK — NAME: 130170572/PAGE: 92/CREDIT: © SHUTTERSTOCK — NAME: 1382449433/PAGE: 94-95/CREDIT: © SHUTTERSTOCK — NAME: 493516783/PAGE: 104/CREDIT: © SHUTTERSTOCK — NAME: 599810918/PAGE: 108-109/CREDIT: © SHUTTERSTOCK — NAME: 1010232652/PAGE: 110/CREDIT: © SHUTTERSTOCK — NAME: 681049993/PAGE: 112/CREDIT: © SHUTTERSTOCK — NAME: 52420438/PAGE: 115/CREDIT: © SHUTTERSTOCK — NAME: 1436329454/PAGE: 117/CREDIT: © SHUTTERSTOCK — NAME: 1080411422/PAGE: 121/CREDIT: © SHUTTERSTOCK — NAME: 1147381970/PAGE: 123/CREDIT: © SHUTTERSTOCK — NAME: 611163263/PAGE: 125/CREDIT: © SHUTTERSTOCK — NAME: 1200390274/PAGE: 127/CREDIT: © SHUTTERSTOCK — NAME: 132295121/PAGE: 130/CREDIT: © SHUTTERSTOCK — NAME: 387245194/PAGE: 133/CREDIT: © SHUTTERSTOCK — NAME: 754752016/PAGE: 134/CREDIT: © SHUTTERSTOCK — NAME: 1354555811/PAGE: 138/CREDIT: © SHUTTERSTOCK — NAME: 1454751020/PAGE: 140/CREDIT: © SHUTTERSTOCK — NAME: 1506117983/PAGE: 142/CREDIT: © SHUTTERSTOCK — NAME: 792204943/PAGE: 147/CREDIT: © SHUTTERSTOCK — NAME: 507817354/PAGE: 148/CREDIT: © SHUTTERSTOCK — NAME: 1243951663/PAGE: 150/CREDIT: © SHUTTERSTOCK — NAME: 402621055/PAGE: 154/CREDIT: © SHUTTERSTOCK — NAME: 120091201/PAGE: 158/CREDIT: © SHUTTERSTOCK — NAME: 62078386/PAGE: 160/CREDIT: © SHUTTERSTOCK — NAME: 140194663/PAGE: 163/CREDIT: © SHUTTERSTOCK — NAME: 1044110854/PAGE: 164/CREDIT: © SHUTTERSTOCK — NAME: 1067089391/PAGE: 166/CREDIT: © SHUTTERSTOCK — NAME: 1085344457/PAGE: 169/CREDIT: © SHUTTERSTOCK — NAME: 680555875/PAGE: 170/CREDIT: © SHUTTERSTOCK — NAME: 173814815/PAGE: 172/CREDIT: © SHUTTERSTOCK — NAME: 71197978/PAGE: 174-175/CREDIT: © SHUTTERSTOCK — NAME: 438753733/PAGE: 180/CREDIT: © SHUTTERSTOCK — NAME: 1560859382/PAGE: 183/CREDIT: © SHUTTERSTOCK — NAME: 726155047/PAGE: 188/CREDIT: © SHUTTERSTOCK — NAME: 430949605/PAGE: 196-197/CREDIT: © SHUTTERSTOCK — NAME: 624305585/PAGE: 199/CREDIT: © SHUTTERSTOCK — NAME: 1454750087/PAGE: 202/CREDIT: © SHUTTERSTOCK — NAME: 520348207/PAGE: 210/CREDIT: © SHUTTERSTOCK — NAME: 777145744/PAGE: 213/CREDIT: © SHUTTERSTOCK — NAME: 606857867/PAGE: 214/CREDIT: © SHUTTERSTOCK — NAME: 573890437/PAGE: 217/CREDIT: © SHUTTERSTOCK — NAME: 483706777/PAGE: 220/CREDIT: © SHUTTERSTOCK — NAME: 704578852/PAGE: 225/CREDIT: © SHUTTERSTOCK — NAME: 701444587/PAGE: 227/CREDIT: © SHUTTERSTOCK — NAME: 143404885/PAGE: 229/CREDIT: © SHUTTERSTOCK — NAME: 341357261/PAGE: 230/CREDIT: © SHUTTERSTOCK — NAME: 334800716/PAGE: 232/CREDIT: © SHUTTERSTOCK — NAME: 261353090/PAGE: 234/CREDIT: © SHUTTERSTOCK — NAME: 166336454/PAGE: 236/CREDIT: © SHUTTERSTOCK — NAME: 137226314/PAGE: 240/CREDIT: © SHUTTERSTOCK — NAME: 1243951690/PAGE: 247/CREDIT: © SHUTTERSTOCK — NAME: 1070726507/PAGE: 250/CREDIT: © SHUTTERSTOCK — NAME: 180833294/PAGE: 252-253/CREDIT: © SHUTTERSTOCK — NAME: 1364110391/PAGE: 257/CREDIT: © SHUTTERSTOCK — NAME: 500115082/PAGE: 261/CREDIT: © SHUTTERSTOCK — NAME: 1024749082/PAGE: 265/CREDIT: © SHUTTERSTOCK — NAME: 371777050/PAGE: 266/CREDIT: © SHUTTERSTOCK — NAME: 1562124094/PAGE: 267/CREDIT: © SHUTTERSTOCK — NAME: 1179377293/PAGE: 270-271/CREDIT: © SHUTTERSTOCK — NAME: 1448581820/PAGE: 273/CREDIT: © SHUTTERSTOCK — NAME: 181675625/PAGE: 274-275/CREDIT: © SHUTTERSTOCK — NAME: 1450164884/PAGE: 276/CREDIT: © SHUTTERSTOCK — NAME: 1054764995/PAGE: 281/CREDIT: © SHUTTERSTOCK — NAME: 1367530361/PAGE: 284/CREDIT: © SHUTTERSTOCK — NAME: 39882433/PAGE: 294/CREDIT: © SHUTTERSTOCK — NAME: 188300012/PAGE: 296/CREDIT: © SHUTTERSTOCK — NAME: 194862401/PAGE: 301/CREDIT: © SHUTTERSTOCK — NAME: 1258018522/PAGE: 303/CREDIT: © SHUTTERSTOCK — NAME: 683169130/PAGE: 305/CREDIT: © SHUTTERSTOCK — NAME: 1070212811/PAGE: 306-307/CREDIT: © SHUTTERSTOCK — NAME: 1016721946/PAGE: 310/CREDIT: © SHUTTERSTOCK — NAME: 1372581620/PAGE: 311/CREDIT: © SHUTTERSTOCK — NAME: 1092927950/PAGE: 313/CREDIT: © SHUTTERSTOCK — NAME: 225478723/PAGE: 315/CREDIT: © SHUTTERSTOCK — NAME: 210431020/PAGE: 316-317/CREDIT: © SHUTTERSTOCK — NAME: 245391928/PAGE: 323/CREDIT: © SHUTTERSTOCK — NAME: 238898230/PAGE: 325, 326, 330, 336/CREDIT: © SHUTTERSTOCK — NAME: 499896445/PAGE: 327/CREDIT: © SHUTTERSTOCK — NAME: 226310848/PAGE: 333/CREDIT: © SHUTTERSTOCK — NAME: 209352988/PAGE: 340/CREDIT: © SHUTTERSTOCK — NAME: 734789518/PAGE: 344/CREDIT: © SHUTTERSTOCK — NAME: 686367931/PAGE: 350/CREDIT: © SHUTTERSTOCK — NAME: 1623196279/PAGE: 354/CREDIT: © SHUTTERSTOCK — NAME: 113221057/PAGE: 356/CREDIT: © SHUTTERSTOCK — NAME: 1379588399/PAGE: 357/CREDIT: © SHUTTERSTOCK — NAME: 1185179275/PAGE: 358-359/CREDIT: © SHUTTERSTOCK — NAME: 520251157/PAGE: 362/CREDIT: © SHUTTERSTOCK — NAME: 175926254/PAGE: 363/CREDIT: © SHUTTERSTOCK — NAME: 1012270567/PAGE: 365/CREDIT: © SHUTTERSTOCK — NAME: 1304502961/PAGE: 366/CREDIT: © SHUTTERSTOCK — NAME: 146332514/PAGE: 368-369/CREDIT: © SHUTTERSTOCK — NAME: 1071960113/PAGE: 370/CREDIT: © SHUTTERSTOCK — NAME: 324500189/PAGE: 373/CREDIT: © SHUTTERSTOCK — NAME: 1060490900/PAGE: 379/CREDIT: © SHUTTERSTOCK — NAME: 573422434/PAGE: 381/CREDIT: © SHUTTERSTOCK — NAME: 1019252857/PAGE: 382/CREDIT: © SHUTTERSTOCK — NAME: 1198840801/PAGE: 384/CREDIT: © SHUTTERSTOCK — NAME: 283061759/PAGE: 387/CREDIT: © SHUTTERSTOCK